APPENDICITIS – A COLLECTION OF ESSAYS FROM AROUND THE WORLD

Edited by **Anthony Lander**

Appendicitis – A Collection of Essays from Around the World
Edited by Anthony Lander

Published by InTech
Janeza Trdine 9, 51000 Rijeka, Croatia

Publishing Process Manager Ivana Zec

Technical Editor Teodora Smiljanic

Cover Designer InTech Design Team

Additional hard copies can be obtained from orders@intechopen.com

Appendicitis – A Collection of Essays from Around the World, Edited by Anthony Lander
p. cm.
ISBN 978-953-307-814-4

For EU product safety concerns:
IN TECH d.o.o., Prolaz Marije Krucifikse Kozulić 3, 51000 Rijeka, Croatia,
info@intechopen.com or visit our website at intechopen.com.

Meet the editor

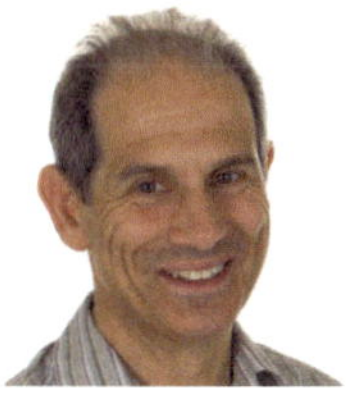

Dr Lander was appointed as a consultant pediatric surgeon in July of 1997 at Birmingham Children's Hospital in the UK after completing his training and PhD in Teratology. His department has a busy clinical practice with the hospital covering a local population of over five million. He has held the following educational titles: Training Program Director, Chair of the Specialist Training Committee for the West Midlands, Raven Tutor at the Royal College of Surgeons of England, Clinical Lead for e-Learning in Pediatric Surgery at the Department of Health, and Chair of the Education and Training Committee for the British Association of Pediatric Surgeons. He has been Clinical Lead for Pediatric Surgery and Urology and is currently the Clinical Director for Surgical Services.

Contents

Preface

This book is a collection of essays and papers from around the world, written by surgeons who look after patients of all ages with abdominal pain, many of whom have appendicitis. Some of these authors are previously unpublished and this route has given them a voice. In these pages, there are some novel thoughts and something for all surgical readers. I have enjoyed working with the authors to help shape their thoughts into publishable papers. Much of the correspondence has been stimulating and a privilege for me. I have learned new things.

All general surgeons maintain a fascination with this important condition because it is so common and yet so easy to miss. All surgeons have a view on the literature and any gathering of surgeons embraces a spectrum of opinion on management options. Many aspects of the disease and its presentation and management remain controversial. This book does not answer those controversies, but should prove food for thought. The reflections of these surgeons are presented in many cases with novel data. The chapters encourage us to consider new epidemiological views and explore clinical scoring systems and the literature on imaging. Appendicitis is discussed in patients of all ages and in all manner of presentations.

I remain a Luddite who believes that a good history and clinical examination, including a temperature properly taken, followed by repeated clinical examination by the same surgeon over the subsequent 24 hours, will lead to few negative appendicectomies. However, with shorter training, and the European working directive, there may be a real role for scoring systems. Persistent guarding in the right illiac fossa on repeated examination is the key to the diagnosis, but imaging is getting better and is more widely used. Laparoscopic appendicectomy is now the treatment of choice if equipment and skills are available, but the arguments for conservative management are by no means weak. These are all explored in this book.

I do hope you enjoy this collection of papers.

Dr. Anthony Lander
Birmingham Children's Hospital,
UK

1

Epidemiologic Features of Appendicitis

Robert B. Sanda
Department of Surgery, Institute of Health,
Ahmadu Bello University Teaching Hospital, Zaria,
Nigeria

1. Introduction

Though appendicitis is common many important questions remain unanswered. When is the appendix normal and when is it the cause of abdominal pain? Why does appendicitis primarily affect older children and young adults? Why is appendicitis uncommon in those under five years of age and in those over sixty years of age? Why are boys affected more often than girls? Why does appendicitis appear to run in some families? Why is appendicitis more common in affluent parts of the world and rare in parts where poverty and poor hygiene are prevalent? The epidemiology of appendicitis is complex and its cause is not explained by any single factor. The peak incidence of appendicitis coincides with the age when the immune system is most efficient and the lymphoid follicles are at their maximum development. Could this implicate immunological factors in the pathogenesis and, therefore, the epidemiology of appendicitis?

Obstruction of the lumen of the appendix is believed to be the trigger initiating the processes that culminate in inflammation of the appendix. Fecaliths are a specific cause of appendicitis in about one-third of specimens (Mitros & Rubin, 2009) and are composed of fats (coprosterols), inorganic salts (calcium phosphate) and organic residue (vegetable fibres) in a proportion of 50%, 25% and 20%, respectively (Berg, RM., & Berg, HM., 1957). Their physical consistency varies from soft to hard concretions. The reported incidence of fecaliths depends on whether the data was obtained from intraoperative palpation of the organ, from histological analysis of operative specimens or from autopsy reports. It is suggested that vegetable matter entering the lumen of the appendix forms the nucleus around which glandular secretions in the lumen desicate to form the calculi (Lowenberg, 1949). In the other two-thirds of instances where fecaliths are absent, the obstruction is thought to be caused by hypertrophy of mural lymphoid follicles in response to a host of causes that are discussed elsewhere in this book.

This chapter aims to understand the environmental, demographic, cultural and genetic factors that make the appendix susceptible to obstruction and inflammation. To understand the epidemiology of appendicitis is to look at the possibility of moving beyond treating it operatively to entertaining non-operative treatments and to foresee a future when some cases of appendicitis can be prevented.

2. What is a normal appendix ?

The histological features of pathological inflammation in most tissues are well defined. The inflammatory cell types encountered and the tissue architecture enable a precise diagnosis of acute or chronic inflammation. For organs at the frontline of the fight against invasion by pathogens, however, a distinction has to be made between what is pathological and what is physiological. All would agree that transmural inflammation with edema, congestion and infiltration of polymorphs, intramural abscesses, mucosal ulceration, fibrinopurulent peritonitis and vascular thrombosis are pathological. When present these findings establish the diagnosis of appendicitis beyond doubt. However, when inflammation is confined to the mucosa, a finding that is reported in up to 35% of specimens (Day, et al., 2003), the question has to be asked whether this is early appendicitis or something entirely different. Likewise, reports of 'appendicitis' in specimens taken from well patients undergoing incidental appendectomies suggests that some histological 'appendicitis' might represent a normal physiological inflammatory response. The term 'sub-acute appendicitis' is used by some pathologists to circumvent this dilemma. Describing the appendix as either 'normal' or 'inflamed' may not sufficiently reflect the heterogeneity of the physio-pathological features of the appendix.

Wide differences in negative appendicectomy rates are reported in the literature. Low rates are variously attributed to good clinical skills (repeated clinical examination by an experienced surgeon) (Lander 2007) or attributed to the higher specificity of diagnostic tests (Seetahal, et al., 2011). This section argues that some of this difference may be due to variation in the histological reporting of mild inflammation. For example, negative appendicectomy rates vary from Spain (4.3%) to Nigeria (52.3%) and it has been hypothesised that these differences are unlikely to be due to difference in training, clinical skills or the availability of diagnostic technological accessories (Andreu-Ballester, et al., 2009; Uba, et al., 2006). This argument is supported by the observation that the diagnostic accuracy of appendicitis has largely been unaffected by technological innovations (Hale, et al., 1997; Gnanalingham, et al., 1997). Even in recent literature the negative appendicectomy rate varies from as low as 3% (6/190) (Cleeve et al 2011) through 4% (Whisker, et al., 2009) to as high as 44 % (76/172) (Gopal and Jaffrey2011). A large part of this variation in diagnostic rate may come from differences in clinical practice but some may come from variations in histological reporting. In departments where pathologists report superficial inflammation as "early appendicitis" there will be a lower negative appendectomy rates while others who regard it as a normal variant will report higher values.

In a 1961-study of 1000 consecutive appendectomy specimens in Ottawa, Canada, this problem was encountered and the authors concluded that appendicitis is an imprecise diagnosis (Campbell JS et al., 1961). The authors observed that 6.2% of specimens of primary appendectomies and 6.6% of specimens from incidental appendectomies showed evidence of superficial inflammation. In the same series during the year 1960, the authors encountered 40% (27/65) cases of superficial appendicitis from a total of 141 specimens after exclusion of 76 cases with diffuse inflammation of the appendix from primary appendectomy meeting the criteria for appendicitis. The same lesion was found in 35% (24/68) cases of incidental appendectomy. The findings in both periods of study suggested an almost equal incidence of superficial inflammation of the appendix in specimens from primary appendectomy as from incidental appendectomy. The authors wondered, "When is a superficial appendicitis responsible for symptoms and when is it not?" They were reproached by their clinical colleagues for "adding to the iatrogenic diseases produced in the laboratory". This same observation would be made in subsequent publications on incidental appendectomy by other workers.

In a study involving 90 pregnant women who were randomly assigned to undergo caesarean section alone or with prophylactic appendectomy three cases of "appendicitis" were encountered that were not accompanied by symptoms, clinical signs or positive laboratory tests (Pearce, et al., 2008). In a more remarkable study comprising of 772 women in the state of Illinois undergoing laparoscopic examination for primary infertility who also underwent incidental appendectomy, 585 (75%) had histologic evidence of superficial appendicitis even though none of them presented with features that would suggest appendicitis preoperatively (Song, et al., 2009).

There are suggestions that this superficial inflammation of the appendix may be an extension of colitis caused by bacteria such as salmonella and campylobacter into the lumen of the appendix (Campbell LK et al., 2006; Chan, et al., 1983; Lau, et al., 2005).

Without agreement on the categorization of superficial appendicitis the basis for comparative epidemiological studies of appendicitis is shaky. The reported findings of inflamed appendices in specimens taken during incidental appendectomies will continue to be a nagging problem.

3. Etiologic hypotheses on appendicitis

Numerous hypotheses have been proposed to explain the etiology of appendicitis. Three of these have a measure of credibility and deserve discussion.

3.1 Mechanical hypothesis

The association between low-fibre diet and appendicitis was first proposed by Rendle Short in 1920 which was spurred by the observation of an upsurge of appendicitis in Britain at the beginning of the twentieth century (Short, 1920). He hypothesized a causal relationship with low cellulose content of imported food. About half a century later another British surgeon working in East and Southern Africa in the early 1970's, Denis Burkitt, built on this hypothesis by observing a low prevalence of diseases like appendicitis, diverticular disease, colon cancer and varicose veins among native Africans in comparison to the population he was used to back in Europe. He attributed this to the high fibre-content of the diet of Africans making for low transit time for gastrointestinal contents and softer consistency of stool which assuaged the need for straining at defecation (Burkitt, 1977a; 1977b; Burkitt, et al., 1979).

The mechanical hypothesis implicates two factors in the etiology of appendicitis: fecaliths and high intra-colonic pressure. In the first instance, Burkitt and his team demonstrated a significant difference in the incidence of fecaliths in appendicitis and in non-pathological specimens of the vermiform appendix in a comparative study of patients in Toronto and Johannesburg (Jones, et al., 1985). This study has been cited almost exclusively by many authors to defend the unproved claim that fecaliths in the appendix have a particular geographic distribution. On closer scrutiny, however, the publication is beset by a number of inadequacies that include; the small sample size, insensitive measurement (intraoperative palpation of the appendix to determine the presence of fecaliths) and inter-observer bias (one surgeon in Toronto and another in Johannesburg worked independently). Moreover, neither Toronto nor Johannesburg are representative of a North American and an African population, respectively.

The percentage of minorities (non-Aboriginal and non-Caucasian Canadians) in Toronto has been steadily rising and was estimated at 46.9% of the City's 2.5 million people in 2006 (Wikipedia Foundation Inc., 2011). In addition it is questioned whether the epidemiology of appendicitis and appendicular fecaliths in Aboriginal Canadians based on dietary habits resembled Caucasian Canadians at all. Similarly, Johannesburg during the period of study had a population that was not representative of the native African continent. The US Bureau of

Census estimated that as at 1992, 48% of all black South Africans lived in the ten nominally independent homelands under the segregation of the Apartheid system which limited their access to healthcare within urban Johannesburg (Byrnes, 1996). Thus, the conclusion drawn from this study is not from a representative sample reflecting racial or geographical characteristics. Another point of note is that, descriptively, the study showed a discordant mean age of the samples of the two populations. The African population were younger than their Canadian counterparts (with mean ages of 31 years versus 55 years, respectively) which may have skewed the observation to show a higher proportion of incidental fecaliths in Canadians since the prevalence of fecaliths in normal appendix specimens increases with age (vide infra).
High intra-colonic pressure as the main cause of diverticulosis has an inverse relationship with diets high in fibre, typical for native Africans. Acquired diverticulosis is an age-dependent disease that is most noticeable after the third decade of life unlike appendicitis. While this explains the rarity of diverticulosis in rural Africans the role of high intra-colonic pressure in the pathogenesis cannot be deduced because of the differences in the peak age of incidence.
A recent retrospective study claimed to have found an epidemiological similarity between appendicitis and diverticulitis in terms of low-fibre diets and better hygiene suggesting a common causal factor (Livingston, et al., 2011). The authors acknowledge that the peak incidence of the two diseases differ considerably. Fecaliths occupy the lumens of diverticuli as well as about a third of appendicitis specimens and that is where their etiologic similarities end. Even if a powerful cohort study or a case-control study finds a strong association, a causal relationship will be hard to sell simply because the diseases occupy opposite ends of the age spectrum. Why would the same causal factor produce appendicitis in the young and not in old and vice versa with diverticulosis?

3.2 Infection hypothesis

Specific infections with viruses, bacteria and parasites have been linked to appendicitis prompting the suggestion that local invasion could trigger appendicitis. Dengue, Influenza, Epstein-Barr, Rota and Cytomegaloviruses has been linked to appendicitis (Alder, et al., 2010; Boon-Siang, et al., 2006; Livingston, et al., 2007; Thalayasingam, 1985). Similarly, bacteria such as Campylobacter, Brucella and Salmonella (Campbell LK et al., 2006; Chan, et al., 1983; Lau, et al., 2005; Pourbagher, et al., 2006) as well as parasites like Entameba histolytica, Schistosoma mansonii/japonicum, and Enterobius vermicularis (Andrade, et al., 2007; Elazary, et al. 2005; Gali, et al., 2008; Gotohda, et al., 2000; Isik, et al., 2007; McCarthy, et al., 2002; Sah & Bhadani, 2006; Terada, 2009) have been isolated in specimens or indirectly implicated in the pathogenesis of appendicitis. These pathogens are thought to cause appendicitis by invading the lamina propria and inciting edema to cause obstruction of the narrow lumen of the appendix to result in appendicitis.
If infectious agents have a causal relationship with appendicitis, then infections by airborne viruses with known seasonal variations might show a temporal pattern coincident with that of appendicitis. This issue was studied in two recent publications that showed a decreasing incidence of non-perforated appendicitis (but not perforated appendicitis) in the 10-19 years age-group from 1970 to 1995 coincident with a decreasing incidence of influenza infections in the United States (Livingston, et al., 2007; Alder, et al., 2010). These studies also observed a falling rate of negative appendectomy after 1995 which they attributed to CT scanning and laparoscopy. Consequently the authors made a distinction between perforated and non-perforated appendicitis by suggesting that they may be etiologically distinct implying that viruses like influenza may be causally related to the latter but not the former (Livingston, et

al. 2007, 2011). A critique of one of these papers (Alder, et al., 2010) observed that hospital discharge records fail to take note of the fact that patients with appendicitis will require admission but most people with influenza will not and that while appendicitis is predominantly a disease of the young, influenza is a disease of the old (Britt, 2010). Similarly, enteric viruses (rotavirus) and outbreaks of entero-invasive bacteria like some strains of Escherichia and Shigella should show similarity to outbreaks of appendicitis.

Lymphotropic viruses like Epstein-Barr and Cytomegaloviruses should show an epidemiological pattern that mimics the seasonal variation of appendicitis. Evidence for an association with these pathogens is scant. It is suggested that because of the latency period from infection with these viruses to induction of appendicitis the link between the two is missed because we do not routinely perform studies to determine recent infections with these viruses (Thalayasingam, 1985; Dzabic, et al., 2008).

The infection hypothesis may explain why some patients with a good history and signs of appendicitis recover spontaneously without operation and may be the explanation for the finding of fibrosis in the submucosa of the appendix showing that previous inflammation had occurred. To this end, florid mesenteric lymphadenitis with an unimpressive appearance of the appendix on the one hand and gangrene or perforation of the appendix on the other may represent extremes of the pathological spectrum of appendicitis. The difference between what is appendicitis and what is not maybe dependent in part on the temporal stage of the illness and the pathological diagnostic criteria used.

The relationship between childhood appendicitis/appendectomy and subsequent low incidence of ulcerative colitis is intriguing and is the subject of a recent large population-based study in Sweden and Denmark (Frisch, et al., 2009). The study confirmed the reported observation that people who underwent appendectomy in childhood had a lower incidence of ulcerative colitis as adults than those who did not. The authors concluded that appendicitis and mesenteric lymphadenitis in childhood, and not appendectomy, accounts for the lower incidence of ulcerative colitis in later adulthood.

The infection hypothesis outlined above is closely related to the hygiene hypothesis below.

3.3 Hygiene hypothesis

At the beginning of the 1980s another British physician with past clinical experience in East Africa, David Barker, sought to elucidate the link between diet and certain diseases. He published a cross-sectional study with team members at the Medical Research Council's Environmental Epidemiology Unit of the University of Southampton on the incidence of appendicitis in England and Wales. They found that despite similar dietary habits the distribution of appendicitis did not follow other diseases associated with low-fibre consumption (Barker & Liggins, 1981). In a subsequent case-control study they concluded that infection and familial predisposition, rather than the fibre-content of the diet, may enhance susceptibility to appendicitis (Nelson, et al., 1984, 1986). Barker followed this by proposing an alternative hypothesis commonly referred to as the hygiene hypothesis in which he looked at historical data that showed a steep increase in appendicitis in Britain from 1895 through 1930 before declining. He declared that "*...dietary changes do not explain the time trends in appendicitis and that the epidemiology of the disease is more readily explained by a primary infectious aetiology*" (Barker, 1985). In subsequent publications, Barker and his team suggested that the observed increase in the incidence of appendicitis at the end of the 19th century was a consequence of the adoption of a housing policy in Britain and Ireland which enforced the provision of safe-drinking water and sanitary measures like sewage and waste disposal (Barker, et al. 1982, 1988a; Morris, et al.,

1987). In another paper they proclaimed "*We conclude that our findings support the hypothesis that appendicitis is primarily caused by Western housing rather than by Western diet. This would explain the international distribution of the disease which is one of industrialized communities. It explains the rarity of the disease in blacks in South Africa despite their adoption of aspects of Western lifestyle, including low consumption of fiber. It predicts that communities in which children still grow up in conditions of Third World hygiene will experience outbreaks of appendicitis when housing improves*" (Barker, et al. 1988b). With this, Barker and his team offered an attractive hypothesis by hinting that the immune system may be induced by prevailing circumstances to reach a compromise with gut pathogens and commensals through adaptation.

If appendicitis is simply a disease that results from the obstruction its lumen, akin to obstruction of the common bile duct or the ureters by calculi, we should expect that the mere presence of a calculus in its lumen is sufficient to trigger appendicitis. However it does not always cause it. The appendix, with a lumen estimated at 1-2 mm in diameter when compared to the supra-duodenal portion of the common bile duct (6mm) and the middle third of the ureters (3-4mm), is small. Unlike the calcular diseases of the common bile duct and the ureter, appendicitis shows a population distribution not easily explained by the prevalence of luminal calculi alone. While the lumens of the ureters and the CBD tend to dilate proximally in response to obstruction by stones the only time they narrow is during peristaltic movements to aid the downward movement of their contents. The lumen of the appendix, on the other hand, will become narrow when the lymphoid follicles become hypertrophic in response to remote or local infection.

Autopsy studies show that the prevalence of asymptomatic fecaliths in the elderly exceeds what should be expected in surgically resected specimens in younger populations on the basis of the prevalence of appendicitis in the general population (Andreou, et al., 1990). Unlike the appendix where calculi can remain silent, silent calcular diseases of the ureters and the common bile duct are a rarity. This would suggest that the presence of calculi does not trigger appendicitis per se. A recent follow up study of the finding of incidental appendicoliths on pelvic CT scans in patients younger than 18 years at the Children's Medical Center of the University of Utah, found that of 75 patients who met the inclusion criteria, only 16 patients (21%) subsequently developed clinical symptoms and signs suggestive of appendicitis and of these only 6 patients (8%) had histological evidence of appendicitis (Rollins, et al., 2010).

This perspective may offer an explanation as to why the incidence of appendicitis is low not only in Africa but also in other developing countries in Latin America, the Middle East and Southeast Asia. The prediction of an increase in the incidence of appendicitis in emerging economies with rapid industrialization, urbanization and higher standards of living maybe the explanation for the recent observation of a high incidence of appendicitis in South Korea with 227 cases per 100,000 people (Lee JH, et al. 2010). This figure is more than 12 times the rate in Ghana (Ohene-Yeboah & Abantanga, 2009). Saudi Arabia, another country that is attaining rapid improvement in health indices, maybe showing this trend as a post-hoc analysis of the data in our study shows that in the city of Hail with a population of around 356,000 an estimated average of 526 cases of appendicitis were recorded annually from 2000 to 2006 giving an incidence rate of 147/100,000 people; a figure that is similar to figures obtainable from European countries and higher than figures from sub-Saharan Africa by as much as a factor of 10 (Sanda, et al., 2008). This observation fits in with the hypothesis offering an explanation for the propensity of appendicitis in the age group with the most developed immune system and, conversely, explains its rarity at the extremes of age.

4. Comparative incidence and temporal trends of appendicitis

The epidemiology of appendicitis is best studied by comparing national incident rates from different regions of the world with low and high incidences of appendicitis. Fidelity of medical databases and accurate population counts at multiple points in time are necessary to calculate incidence rates and trend. Ideally this should be based on age-specific annual rates but since the peak incidence of appendicitis appears to vary slightly from one region of the world to another, a crude rate using all cases is an acceptable alternative. Because of the variable negative appendectomy rates it is ideal to compare rates of histologically confirmed cases. These data are unfortunately not frequently reported in various publications. A search of the literature from around the world using the standardized annual incidence rates shows a wide range of estimates of the incidence of appendicitis.

Importantly, most publications reporting incidence rates do not differentiate between calcular appendicitis and the non-calcular variety. Table 1 shows a comparison of annual incidence rates from around the world in the last 25 years. What can possibly account for the huge difference in the annual incidence rates of appendicitis between European and African countries as represented by Ireland (174/100,000) and Ghana (18/100,000) ? (Morris, et al., 1987; Ohene-Yeboah & Abantanga, 2009). Why is the incidence rate higher for white South African children (215-395 per 100,000) in comparison to black children (5-19 per 100,000) in the same country (Walker, et al. 1989)? Why does appendicitis run in families? (Basta, et al., 1990; Brender, et al., 1985) Why is the rate lower in girls compared to age-matched boys? (Hale, et al., 1997; Humes & Simpson, 2006)

5. Innate immunity insights

5.1 Toll-like receptors

For over a century after the discovery of phagocytes and endotoxin by Ilya Mechnikov and Richard Pfeifer, respectively, research in immunology focused on adaptive immunity to the neglect of innate immunity. Perceived as an archaic, passive, non-discriminatory pathway, the importance of innate immunity was under-appreciated until recently. The insight derived contributed to our understanding of the hygiene hypothesis as proposed by Barker and his team.

Charles Janeway led the way in this renewed interest in innate immunity just over two decades ago (Janeway Jr., 1989). He postulated that the cells of the first line of defence such as those of the gastrointestinal tract possessed molecules he termed "pattern recognition receptors" (PRRs) and the ligands on the surfaces of those pathogens that they are capable of reading as "pathogen associated molecular patterns" (PAMPs). Inspired by earlier work on the Drosophila Toll antigen in regards to the dorsal-ventral polarity in the embryo of that species (Anderson, et al, 1985), Janeway's team identified the product of the human homologue of this gene calling it "the Toll-like receptor" (TLR) and characterized it as a trans-membrane protein that replicates the functions of the PRRs in adaptive immunity (Medzhitov, et al., 1997). Through these molecules the innate and the adaptive arms of the immune system are able to share information and collaborate in defence. They ensure that when pathogens breach the first line of defence they are eliminated or contained to minimize further invasion and harm. This collaboration ensures that the inflammatory response mounted against invading pathogens is appropriate and proportionate so as to minimize collateral damage from immunological over reaction.

It is possible that inflammatory bowel disease (ulcerative colitis and Crohn's disease) is a consequence of an inappropriate and excessive immune response to pathogens that are mildly harmful or harmless to the host.

Country	Incidence per 100,000	Year or Period	Data Scope	Author(s)	Observation/Remarks
Italy	570 370	1955 1987	National	Basoli, et al., 1993	Decline in incidence from two-point incidence rates.
Finland	340	1987-2007	National	Ilves, et al., 2011	32% decline over 21 years.
Ethiopia	307 (M) 327 (F)	1971-1988	Provincial	Horntrich & Schneider, 1990	46% decline between 1971 and 1988.
South Korea	227	2005-2007	National	Lee JH, et al., 2010	No change in rate
United States	97	1979-1981	Provincial (South Carolina)	Sugimoto & Edwards, 1987.	Noted a high incidental appendectomy with 75 NNT at a cost of $20 million.
	233	1979-1984	National	Addiss, et al., 1990.	14.6% decline in rate.
Australia	180	1986-1990	Provincial (NSW)	Close, et al., 1995.	Decline from 1986 to 1990.
Germany	130		West Germany	Haussler, et al., 1989.	
	165		National	Sahm, et al., 2011	
Greece	652 (70) 164 (99)	1970-1999	National	Papadopoulos, et al., 2008	75% decline in incidence rate over 30 years.
Turkey	149.8	2004-2007	National	Sulu, et al., 2010.	
Norway	140	1977-1978	National	Soreide, 1984	Decline attributed to better quality of data.
	84	1989-1993	Provincial (Rogaland)	Korner, et al., 1997.	
	117	1990-2001	National	Bakken, et al., 2003.	Covered period of introduction of laparoscopic appendectomy
Spain	79.6			Osta et al., 1991	
	117.5	2000	Provincial		
	132.1	2003		Andreu-Ballester, et al., 2009.	Difference not significant.
Sweden	116	1984-1989	Meta-analysis	Andersson, et al., 1994.	Data from meta-analysis of six studies.
Canada	75	1991-1998	Provincial (Ontario)	Al-Omran, et al., 2003	Noted decreasing incidence rate with increasing perforation rate.
	93.2	1993-2000	Provincial (Ontario)	To & Langer, 2010.	Data calculated exclusively for appendicitis in children younger than 19 years.
Poland	61.6	1989-1998	Provincial (Cracow)	Anielski, et al., 2001.	Authors noted a decreasing incidence rate.
Israel	37.5	1973-1983	Provincial (Negev)	Freud, et al., 1988.	Higher incidence in Jewish versus Israeli Arabs. Noted seasonal variation related to humidity as well as viral/bacterial infections.
Papua New Guinea	39		Provincial (North Solomons)	Foster & Webb, 1989.	
Thailand	32 & 37		Meta-analysis	Chatbanchai, et al., 1989	The figures were derived from rural population.
South Africa	5-19 (Black) 215-395 (White)	1985-1987	Provincial (Free State, North West)	Walker, et al., 1989a	Authors also noted a decline in dietary fibre in blacks without a rising incidence.
Central African Republic	36.5	1991	Provincial (Bangui)	Zoquereh, et al., 2001	
Ghana	18	2000-2005	Provincial (Ashanti)	Ohene-Yeboah & Abantanga, 2009	Rising incidence was claimed
Madagascar	77		Hospital	Langenscheidt, et al., 1999.	Negative appendectomy rate of 85%by histological assessment.

NNT = Number Needed to Treat; NSW = New South Wales.

Table 1. Comparison of annual incidence rates of appendicitis from around the world.

Ten subtypes of TLRs have been identified in man with TLRs1, 2, 4, 5, and 6 known to be present on the cell membrane surface and recognize microbial components such as lipids, lipoproteins and proteins. They function to identify bacterial lipopolysaccharide (LPS) in Gram-negative bacteria, peptidoglycans, lipoprotein and lipoteichoic acid in Gram-positive bacteria. TLRs 4, 5 and 6 identify HSP60, flagellin and diacyllipopeptides in chlamydia, bacteria and mycoplasma, respectively. In addition TLR4 recognizes respiratory syncytial virus fusion proteins. On the other hand, TLRs 3, 7, 8, and 9 appear to be confined to the intracellular compartment where they recognize microbial nucleic acid. TLRs 3, 7 and 8, identify single-stranded RNA viruses. The function of TLR10 is still unclear (Yoon, 2010).

5.2 Nucleotide-binding oligomerization domain-containing proteins

Another group of molecules thought to work intimately with the TLRs are the intracellular Nucleotide-binding Oligomerization Domain-containing proteins 1/2 (NOD1/NOD2). NOD1 mediates innate immunity by recognizing bacterial molecules containing the D-glutamyl-meso-diaminopimelic acid (iE-DAP) moiety while NOD2 recognizing muramyl dipeptide (MDP) found on the surfaces of certain bacteria. Signals transduced by these two groups of molecules trigger a response from the cells of the innate immune system such as macrophages, monocytes and dendritic cells (DCs). This response produces cytokines which initiate inflammation, phagocytosis of bacteria and subsequent presentation of the antigens to CD4+T cells or, in the case of viruses, switching off the mechanism of induction of protein synthesis or apoptosis of the infected cell (Damgaard & Gyrd-Hansen, 2011; Le Bourhis, et al., 2007; Kawai & Akira, 2009).

5.3 Role of dendritic cells and other immune effectors in the induction of tolerance

TLR signals and the immune effector responses to them contribute to the well-being of the gut ecosystem and the integrity of the intestinal epithelial barrier which confers tolerance to commensals. NOD2 signalling contributes to this by exerting antimicrobial activity and prevents pathogenic invasion (Cario, 2005). The pathogenesis of both Crohn's disease and Blau syndrome have been linked to mutations in the genes coding for NOD2 and the resulting imbalance of these groups of molecules produces the chronic mucosal inflammation that characterize these two diseases. (Blau syndrome is a rare autosomal dominant granulomatous polyarthritis with panuveitis, cranial neuropathies, and exanthema with Crohn's disease seen in 30%.) TLRs are thought to be constitutively expressed and inducible throughout the gastrointestinal tract by absorptive enterocytes, Paneth cells, goblet cells, neuroendocrine cells, myofibrobalsts, as well as in immune cells such as monocytes, macrophages, DCs, and CD4+ T cells in response to the load of commensal and pathogenic cell wall antigens (Cario, 2010). It has been observed that the pattern of TLR expression by some of these cells is variable in different anatomic sites. While DCs may develop from a number of distinct precursors, most of them go through distinct maturation stages that are shaped by the local conditions of the tissues in which they reside or migrate through. The two subsets of DCs are plasmacytoid (pDCs) and conventional myeloid DCs (cDCs). The key features of pDCs are their expression of TLR7 which binds ssRNA in endosomes and TLR9 which binds unmethylated Cytosine-phosphate-Guanine (CpG) regions of the DNA as well as their production of interferon-1 (INF-1). Both pDCs and cDCs localize to intestine immune inductive and effector sites. The microbiota in combination with CD8+ T cells cooperate to regulate systemic numbers of pDCs (Garrett et al., 2010) When differentiating into immature dendritic cells, monocytes progressively lose the expression of some TLRs, but gain the expression of others (Visintin, et al., 2001). Bone-marrow derived CD11c+ DCs express TLR4 to pathogens but, in contrast, CD11c+ DCs in the lamina propria do not express TLR4 to LPS. Thus, the gut responds to the presence of different commensal and pathogenic ligands by modulating its immune response against real threats and ignoring low level ones by mounting mild attack responses. Host innate and adaptive immunity thus cooperate to limit bacterial overgrowth and to prevent mucosal penetration by pathogens. They do this by the elaboration of α-defensins from Paneth cells and the induction of IgA secretion coordinated by regulatory T lymphocytes. In this way both arms of the immune system collaborate to maintain the luminal ecosystem for the mutual benefit of the host and the commensals (Cerovic, et al., 2009; Uematsu, et al., 2006; Yanagawa, et al., 2007)

5.4 Response to endemicity of gut commensals and pathogens

It can be hypothesised that in communities with poor levels of hygiene through poor waste disposal and perpetual exposure to gut pathogens from contaminated water that the maturing immune system of growing children and young adults has the capability to adapt and avoid further damage to the gut by limiting the severity of the immune response. This is the postulated role of T-reg cells in adaptive immunity. In genetically susceptible individuals it is thought that this process is compromised and may be the underlying mechanism by which pathogens cause IBD (Matricon et al, 2010; Fava & Danese, 2011). The immune response to the ubiquitous enteric pathogens such as viruses (rota, hepatitis and polio), bacteria (Salmonella, Shigella, and Escherichia) and protozoans (Entamoeba and Giardia) have to be kept in check to limit the inflammatory reaction to the minimum necessary to prevent invasion. The immune response of long-term residents in these parts of the world may be controlled to attain balance between letting these organisms invade the individual and the individual succumbing to excess immune response. It is increasingly recognized that during early childhood and early adulthood gut bacteria shape the tissues, cells and the molecular profile of the gastrointestinal immune system. This partnership was forged over thousands of years of coevolution based on molecular exchange involving bacterial signals that are recognised by host receptors to mediate beneficial outcomes to both commensals and humans and are tolerated (Lee YK & Mazmanian, 2010; Round & Mazmanian, 2010; Round et al., 2011).

This is the premise by which it is being suggested that the gut of people living in areas with low standards of hygiene eventually attain a level of tolerance to gut commensals that results in a controlled reaction to the presence of pathogens and commensals. In the case of the appendix this means that its lumen is not at the risk of occlusion by lymphoid hyperplasia in response to common local or remote infections in people living under conditions of low hygiene and may explain the low incidence of appendicitis in the Third World.

5.5 Gene polymorphism and severity of appendicitis

It is tantalizing to attempt to detect differences in the susceptibility of individuals to infections by studying the differences in the levels of gene products that are elaborated in response to localized inflammation like appendicitis. In a study involving 56 patients with pathologically-confirmed appendicitis of whom 85% of the patients met the criteria for systemic inflammatory response syndrome, the authors compared the levels of soluble pro- and anti-inflammatory cytokines in the serum and peritoneal fluids of the patients. The pattern of the soluble cytokines and the effect of the plasma on monocyte activation by LPS led the authors to conclude that a difference exists in the elaboration of these cytokines between mild localized infections in comparison to the severe form of the disease (Rivera-Chavez, et al., 2003). In a subsequent publication, the authors studied the relationship of the severity of local inflammation in appendicitis with the occurrence of single nucleotide polymorphism that account for microbial recognition and local inflammation in the innate response. They demonstrated polymorphism in the IL-6 gene was associated with the severity of acute appendicitis even after adjustment for duration of symptoms (Rivera-Charvez, et al., 2004). The suggestion that the human response to a local infection, such as appendicitis, is influenced by inherited differences in innate immunity genes such as IL-6 supports the hypothesis that that children growing up in environments that predispose them to rampant and sustained exposure to gastrointestinal pathogens as is common in developing countries, may have their innate immune effectors subject to regulation to modify their responses to gut pathogens to a point that makes for less likelihood of their lymphoid follicles to hypertrophy and occlude the lumen of the organ and cause appendicitis. This would both explain the rarity of appendicitis in developing countries and the higher incidence rates in developed nations with higher standards of public health.

6. Distribution and variation of appendicitis in populations

6.1 Age distribution

Appendicitis is overwhelmingly a disease of childhood and early adulthood. This is a consistent finding in almost all publications on the subject regardless of the population studied (Hale, et al., 1997; Lee JH, et al., 2010; Smink, et al., 2005; Uba, et al., 2006). As discussed earlier, the lymphoid follicles are most developed in this age group. The presence of local infections probably stimulates the lymphoid follicles to hypertrophy and occlude the lumen of the appendix more commonly in this age group. The efficiency of the immune system in this age group is also a plausible explanation for the tendency for remote agents like air-pollution and sandstorms to be associated with significant variations in the incidence of appendicitis (Kaplan, et al., 2009; Sanda, et al., 2008). On the other hand the immaturity of the immune system before the age of five years and immunosenescence as well as the atrophy of the wall and obliteration of the lumen of the appendix as seen intra-operatively or at autopsy in aged individuals may explain why appendicitis is less common in these age groups.

6.2 Sex distribution

The consistent observation of a slight preponderance of appendicitis in boys is not explained by a difference in fecalith formation. Since the peak incidence of appendicitis coincides with sexual maturity with the sex hormones being most active, it maybe that they play a role in the pathogenesis of appendicitis. Whether this has any relationship to the high incidence of autoimmune diseases like systemic lupus erythematosus, Grave's disease, multiple sclerosis and myasthenia gravis being predominant in women in this age group is not clear. Since the 17-ketosteroids estrogen and progesterone have been implicated in the modulation of the immunosuppressive state of pregnancy, it maybe that different levels of estrogens and androgens between boys and girls may be responsible for this observed difference in incidence (Ben-Hur, et al., 1995; Jara, et al., 2006; Zen, et al., 2010). Furthermore, antigen-presenting cells which play key roles in innate and adaptive immunity as well as tolerance have been found to express estrogen receptors on their surface implying that their functions may be modulated by sex hormones and would explain the purported immunological dimorphism between genders (Bouman, et al., 2005; Kovats & Carreras, 2008). One study suggests that the better prognosis in females following infectious challenge may be due to gender-specific differences in LPS-induced TNF-α and IL-1β but not IL-6 and suggests that the underlying mechanism may be due to alterations in mitogen-activated protein kinase phosphorylation (Imahara, et al., 2005).

6.3 Familial appendicitis

Appendicitis runs in some families (Andersson et al., 1979; Basta et al., 1990; Ergul, 2007). A very neat prospective study noted a significant familial relationship when comparing three groups of children aged 2-19 years admitted to a single large center whose family histories were taken at admission over a 52-month period (Gauderer, et al., 2001). Group A (n=166) comprised of children who underwent appendectomy, group B (n=117) comprised of children who presented with an acute abdomen and with a tentative diagnosis of appendicitis but did not undergo appendectomy due to resolution of symptoms, and group C (n=141) was made of children who were seen in the same hospital over the same period for unrelated complaints. A positive parental history was obtained from 59 patients (36%) in group A, 24 patients (21%) in group B, and 20 patients (14%) in group C. The odds ratios (OR) were 2.0 (p=0.035), and 2.9 (p<0.001) for groups A versus B and A versus C, respectively. Of the 13 patients whose sibling had had acute appendicitis, 9 were in group A while 2 each were in groups B and C. The OR for any family history (siblings, parents) in groups A versus B was 1.9 (p=0.028) and for groups A versus C was 2.9 (p<0.001). The authors concluded that children with appendicitis are three times more likely to have a positive family history of appendicitis in first degree relatives than controls. Similar observations had been made in smaller studies earlier (Andersson, et al., 1979; Brender, et al., 1985; Basta, et al., 1990). These familial associations, however, do not prove a genetic component since members of families often share similar environments.

6.4 Twin studies

Twin studies have attributed both genetic and environmental factors in the predisposition to appendicitis. The evidence suggests that environmental and genetic factors may account for about 70% and 30% of the predisposition to appendicitis, respectively. The ratio attributable to genetic factors appears to be consistent (Basta, et al., 1990; Duffy, et al., 1990; Oldmeadow, et al., 2009; Sadr-Azodi, et al., 2009). An interesting observation linked the incidence of appendicitis to cigarette smoking in 3808 pairs of Australian twins after controlling for sex, age and year of birth. This was not affected by socioeconomic status or the father's occupation and the effect was stronger in females (Oldmeadow, et al., 2008).

6.5 Racial variation

Racial variation in the incidence of appendicitis is difficult to investigate. Poverty and low levels of public hygiene are difficult to separate for many peoples of African, Hispanic or Asian ancestry. One study from the USA comparing the incidence of appendicitis in various ethnic groups concluded that the rate was lower in Negroes and Asians in comparison to Caucasians and Hispanics (Luckmann & Davis, 1991). A case-control study from Brazil comparing the people of that country on the basis of skin colour claimed that race was a factor in the incidence of appendicitis. After excluding native Indians the study found a significantly lower incidence of appendicitis in Negroes in comparison to Caucasians (Petroianu, et al., 2004). This finding has to be interpreted in the context of social differences and genetic variables between black and white Brazilians. Figures showing comparative economic indices of Brazilians among its races are hard to find. A study on phenotypes as an indicator of genotypes in the same country concluded: "Our data suggest that in Brazil, at an individual level, color, as determined by physical evaluation, is a poor predictor of genomic African ancestry, estimated by molecular markers" (Parra, et al., 2003). From the Republic of South Africa, another multiracial society, some publications suggest that appendicitis has racial associations. The incidence of appendicitis in Black children was estimated at 8.2 per 100,000 which is 10-20 times less than the incidence in their White compatriots (Walker, et al. 1989a, 1989b, Walker & Segal, 1995). It should be remembered that the Apartheid political system in the country at the time left the native Africans economically and social disenfranchised with a standard of living that was not comparable to their White counterparts. What these studies share is the inability to separate race from poverty.

6.6 Geographic distribution

The different incidences found across geographic regions are possibly explained by economic and public health factors rather than by environmental factors. As table 1 shows the incidence of appendicitis increases with the level of sophistication of the health system across nations (Barker, et al., 1988a & 1988b). That appendicitis is less common in sub-Saharan Africa and Asia may have more to do with shared poverty and underdevelopment and less to do with geography.

6.7 Seasonal variation

Seasonal variations in appendicitis are reported in several studies across many regions. Most studies report a summer peak with a winter nadir; USA (Luckmann & Davis, 1991), Canada (Al-Omran, et al., 2003), Italy (Gallerani, et al., 2006), Israel (Freud, et al., 1988) and Russia (Khaavel & Birkenfeldt, 1978). Our own study in northern Saudi Arabia showed a winter low but a spring peak which coincides with the sandstorm season characterized by rise in infections and allergic conditions of the upper respiratory tract which concur with earlier studies on the spread of allergens during this season in Saudi Arabia (Kwaasi, et al., 1992a, 1992b, 1993, 1998; Sanda, et al., 2008). A similar seasonal variation to ours was reported four decades earlier in Britain (Ashley, 1967). Our observation of an association between appendicitis and air pollution was corroborated by a study from Western Canada (Kaplan, et al., 2009). The significance of these observations is underscored by pathological studies linking appendicitis to eosinophilic degranulation (Santosh & Aravindan, 2008; Aravindan, et al., 2010). Seasonal variation of appendicitis with its peak associated with a season characterized by high ambient pollen and other phyto-allergens or sandstorm is an observation that can neither be explained by diet nor fecaliths but may have a bearing on immune modulation playing a role.

7. Conclusion

The epidemiology of appendicitis is important but ill understood. We can study the incidence of appendicectomies but this is not to say we are studying appendicitis. To measure the incidence of appendicitis a definition of the disease is required and a confidence that all cases are ascertained. These criteria are not well met. Finding mucosal inflammation in the appendix in a significant portion of incidental appendectomies challenges the definition of a "normal appendix". Furthermore variation in histopathological reporting may account for some of the variation in negative appendicectomy rates. Finding fibrous adhesions around the appendix in unrelated operations and at autopsy proves that appendicitis does not always run an inevitable course to perforation and surgery.

It is difficult to deduce the causes of appendicitis from the associations but we can make hypotheses. Fecaliths accompany appendicitis in only a third of cases suggesting that they are only one risk factor. It is also important to note that not all obstructed appendices develop appendicitis that ends in an appendicectomy.

A temporal relationship between some viral infections and non-perforated appendicitis gives credence to the belief that some infections can cause a luminal appendiceal obstruction leading to appendicitis. However, an inverse relationship between the incidence of appendicitis and the prevalence of some enteric infections exists and may be explained by an adaptive immunological response. A mechanism for this may involve the TLRs and T-reg Lymphocytes. A better understanding of these two phenomena may lead to novel non-operative treatments for a subset of cases of appendicitis.

8. References

Abantanga, FA., Nimako, B., & Amoah, M. 2009. The range of abdominal emergencies in children older than 1 year at the Komfo Anokye teaching hospital, Kumasi, Ghana. *Ann Afr Med*. Vol. 8, issue 4 (2009):236-42.

Addiss, DG., Shaffer, N., Fowler, BS., et al. 1990. The epidemiology of appendicitis and appendectomy in the United States. *Am J Epidemiol*. Vol. 132:910-25.

Alder, AC., Fomby, TB., Woodward, WA., et al. (2010). Association of viral infection and appendicitis. *Arch Surg*. 2010;145(1):63-71.

Al-Omran, M., Mamdani, M., & McLeod, RS. (2003). Epidemiologic features of acute appendicitis in Ontario, Canada. *Can J Surg*. 2003;46(4):263-8.

Anderson, KV., Jurgens, G., & Nusslein-Volhard, C. (1985). Establishment of dorsal-ventral polarity in the Drosophila embryo:genetic studies on the role of the Toll gene product. *Cell*. 1985 Oct;42(3):779-89.

Andersson, N., Griffiths, H., Murphy, J., et al. 1979. Is appendicitis familial? *British Medical Journal*, 1979, 2 (22 sep), 697-8.

Andrade, JE., Mederos, R., Rivero, H., et al. (2007). Amebiasis presenting as acute appendicitis. *South Med J*. 2007;100(11):1140-2.

Andren-Sandberg, A. & Korner, H. 2004. Quantitative and qualitative aspects of diagnosing acute appendicitis. *Scand J Surg*.2004;93:4-9.

Andreou, P., Blain, S., & du Boulay, CE. (1990). A histopathological study of the appendix at autopsy and after surgical resention. *Histopathology*. 1990 Nov;17(5):427-31.

Andreu-Ballester, JC., Gonzales-Sanchez, A., Ballester, F., et al. 2009. [Epidemiology of appendectomy and appendicitis in the Valencian community (Spain), 1998-2007]. *Dig Surg*. 2009;26(5):406-12.

Anielski, R., Barczynski, M., Cichon, S., et al. (2001). [Acute appendicitis in Crakow population]. Przeql Lek. 2001;58(12):1034-7.

Aravindan, KP., Vijayaraghavan, D., & Manipadam, MT. Acute eosinophilic appendiciticis and the significance of eosinophil-edema lesion. *Indian J Pathol Microbiol.* 2010;53:258-61.
Ashley, DJB. (1967). Observations on the epidemiology of appendicitis. *Gut.* 1967;8:533-8.
Azodi Sadr, O., Andren-Sandberg, A., & Larsson, H. (2009). Genetic and environmental influences on the risk of acute appendicitis in twins. *Br J Surg.*2009;96:1336-40.
Bakken, IJ., Skjeldestad, FE., Mjaland, O., et al. (2003). [Appendicitis and appendectomy in Norway 1990-2001]. Tidsskr Nor Laegeforen. 2003;123(22):3185-8.
Barker, DJP., & Liggins, A. (1981). Acute appendicitis in nine British towns. *Br Med J;* 1981;283:1083-5.
Barker, DJP., & Morris, J. (1982). Acute appendicitis, bathrooms, and diet in Britain and Ireland. *Br Med J* 1982;296:953-5.
Barker, DPJ. (1985). Acute appendicitis and dietary fibre: an alternative hypothesis. *Br Med J* 1985;290:1125-7.
Barker, DJP., Morris, JA., Simmonds SJ., et al. (1988a). Appendicitis epidemic following introduction of water in Anglesey. *J Epidemiol Comminity Health.* 1988;42():144-8.
Barker, DJP., Osmond, C., Golding, J., et al. (1988b). Acute appendicitis and bathrooms in three samples of British children. *Br Med J* 1988; 296:956-8.
Basoli, A., Zarba-Meli, E., Slavio, A., et al. (1993). [Trends in the incidence of appendicitis in Italy during the past 30 years]. *Minerva Chir.* 1993;48(3-4):127-32.
Basta, M., Morton, NE., Mulvihill, JJ., et al., 1990. Inheritance of acute appendicitis: familial aggregation and evidence of polygenic transmission. *Am J Hum Genet.* 1990. 46:377-82.
Ben-Hur, K., Mor, G., Insler, V., et al. (1995). Menopause is associated with a significant increase in blood monocyte number and a relative decrease in the expression of estrogen receptors in human peripheral monocytes. *Am J Reprod Immunol.* 1995 Dec;34(6):363-9.
Berg, RM., & Berg, HM. (1957). Coproliths. *Radiology.*1957;68:839-44.
Boon-Siang, K., Jien-Wei, L., Ing-Kit, L., et al. (2006). Dengue hemorrhagic fever patients with acute abdomen: clinical experience of 14 cases. *Am J Trop Med Hyg.* 2006;74(5):901-4.
Bouman, A., Heineman, MJ., & Faas, MM. (2005). Sex hormones and the immune response in humans. *Hum Reprod Update.* 2005;11(4):411-23.
Brender, JD., Marcuse, EK., Weiss, NS., et al. 1985. Is Childhood appendicitis familial? *Am J Dis Child.* 1985 Apr. 139(4):338-40.
Britt RC. (2010). Still looking for reasons in appendicitis. *Arch Surg.* 2010; 145(1):71.
Burkitt, DP. (1977a). Relationships between diseases and their etiological significance. *Am J Clin Nutr.*1977 Feb;30:262-7.
Burkitt, DP. (1977b). Appendicitis and diabetes. *Br. Med J.* 1977;28:1413-4.
Burkitt, DP, Moolgaokar, AS., & Tovey, FI. (1979). Aetiology of Appendicitis. *Br Med J.* 1979;3:620.
Byrnes, RM. (1996). South Africa: a country study. Washington: GPO for the Library of Congress. http://countrystudies.us/south-africa/ (accessed May 30, 2011).
Campbell, JS., Fournier, P., & da Silva, T. 1961. When is the appendix normal? *Canad M A J.* 1961;85:1155-7.
Campbell, LK., Havens, JM., Scott, MA., et al. (2006). Molecular detection of Campylobacter jejuni in archival cases of acute appendicitis. *Modern Pathology.* 2006;19:1042-6.
Cario, E. (2005). Bacterial interactions with cells of the intestinal mucosa: Toll-like receptors and NOD2. *Gut* 2005;54:1182-93.

Cario, E. (2010). Toll-like Receptors in Inflammatory Bowel Disease: a decade later. *Inflamm Bowel Dis* 2010;16:1583-97.

Cerovic, V., Jenkins, CD., Barnes, AG., et al. (2009). Hyporesponsiveness of intestinal dendritic cells to TLR stimulation is limited to TLR4. *J Immunol.* 2009;182:2405-15.

Chatbanchai, W., Hedley, AJ., Ebrahim, SB., et al. (1989). Acute abdominal pain and appendicitis in north east Thailand. Paediatr Perinat Epidemiol. 1989;3(4):448-59.

Chan, FTH., Stringel, G., & Mackenzie, AMR. (1983). Isolation of Campylobacter jejuni from an appendix. *J Clin Microbiol.* 1983 Aug;18(2):422-4.

Cleeve, S., Jones, N., Joshi, A., Misra, D., Phelps, S., and Ward H. Trends in Childhood appendicitis. Abstract 108 British Association of Paediatric Surgeons 58th International Conference Belfast 2011.

Close, GR., Rushworth, RL,. Rob, MI. (1995). Paediatric appendicectomy in NSW: changes in practice over time and between groups. *J Qual Clin Pract.* 1995;15(1):29-36.

Damgaard, RB., & Gyrd-Hansen, M. (2011). Inhibitor of apoptosis (IAP) proteins in regulation of inflammation and innate immunity. *Discov Med.* 2011;11(58):221-31.

Day, DW., Jass, JR., Price, AB., et al. Eds. (2003). *Morson and Dawson's Gastrointestinal Pathology, 4th Edition,* Blackwell Science, ISBN 0-632-04204-4 Massachusetts USA, Oxford UK, Victoria Australia & Berlin Germany.

Duffy, DL., Martin, NG., & Mathews, JD. (1990). Appendectomy in Australian Twins. *Am J Hum Genet.*1990;47:590-2.

Dzabic, M., Bostrom, L., & Rahbar, A. (2008). High prevalence of an active cytomegalovirus infection in the appendix of immunocompetent patients with acute appendicitis. Inflamm Bowel Dis. 2008;14:236-41.

Elazary, R., Maly, A., Khalaileh, A., et al. (2005). Schistosomiasis and acute appendicitis. *IMAJ* 2005;7:533-4.

Ergul E. (2007). Heredity and familial tendency of acute appendicitis. Scand J Surg. 2007; 96:290-2.

Fava F, Danese S. Intestinal microbiota in inflammatory bowel disease: friend of foe? World J Gastroenterol. 2011; 17(5):557-66.

Foster, HM., & Webb, SJ. (1989). Appendicitis and appendicectomy in a Melanesian population. Br J Surg. 1989;76(4):368-9.

Freud, E., Pilpel, D., & Mares, AJ. Acute appendicitis in childhood in the Negev region: some epidemiological observations over an 11-year period (1973-1983). *J Pediatr Gastroenterol Nutr.* 1988;7(5):680-4.

Frisch, M., Pedersen, BV., & Andersson, RE. (2009). Appendicitis, mesenteric lymphadenitis, and subsequent risk of ulcerative colitis: cohort studies in Sweden and Denmark. BMJ. 2009;338:b716.

Gallerani, M., Boari, B., Anania, G., et al. (2006). [Seasonal variation in onset of acute appendicitis]. *Clin Ter.* 2006;157(2):123-7.

Gali, BM., Nggada, HA., & Eni EU. Schistosomiasis of the appendix in Maiduguri. *Trop Doct.* 2006 Jul;36 (3):162-3.

Garrett WS, Gordon JI & Glimcher LH. (2010). Homeostasis and inflammation in the intestine. Cell. 2010; 140(6):859-70.

Gauderer, MW., Crane, MM., Green, JA., et al. 2001. Acute appendicitis in children: the importance of family history. *J. Pediatr Surg,* 36, 8(Aug 2001),1214-7, PMID: 11479859.

Gnanalingham, KK., Biddlecombe, G., & Hancock, BD. 1997. Are we overinvestigating appendicitis. *Lancet.* 1997;349:1918.

Gotohda, N., Itano, S., Okada, Y., et al. (2000). Appendicitis caused by amebiasis. *J Gastroenterol.* 2000; 35(11):861-3.

Gopal, M., & Jaffrey, B. (2011). The consequences of ignoring evidence base in management of acute appendicitis in children. Abstract 100 British Association of Paediatric Surgeons 58th International Conference Belfast 2011.

Hale, DA., Molloy, M., Pearl, RH., et al. (1997). Appendectomy: a contemporary appraisal. *Ann Surg.* 225,3(1997):252-61.

Haussler, B., Schrader, WF., & Witt, K. (1989). [Incidence of appendectomy and length of hospital stay in a region of West Germany]. *Soz Praventivmed.* 1989;34(3):131-5.

Horntrich, J., & Scheneider, W. (1990). [Appendicitis from an epidemiologic viewpoint]. *Zentralbl Chir.* 1990;115(23):1521-9.

Horton, LWL. (1977). Pathogenesis of appendicitis. *BMJ.* 1977 Dec 24-31;1672-3.

Humes, DJ., & Simpson, J. (2006). Acute appendicitis. *BMJ.* 333 (2006):530-4.

Ilves, I., Paajanen, HE., Herziq, KH., et al. (2011). Changing incidence of acute appendicitis and nonspecific abdominal pain between 1987 and 2007 in Finland. *World J Surg.* 2011;35(4):731-8.

Imahara, SD., Jelacic, S., Junker, CE., et al. (2005). The influence of gender on human innate immunity. Surgery. 2005;138(2):275-82.

Isik, B., Yilmaz, M., Karadaq, N., et al. (2007). Appendiceal Enterobius vermicularis infestations in adults. *Int Surg.* 2007 Jul/Aug;92(4):221-5.

Janeway Jr., CA. (1989). Approaching the asymptote? Evolution and revolution in immunology. *Cold Springs Harb Symp Quant Biol.* 1989;54 Pt 1:1-13.

Jara, LJ., Navarro, C., Medina, G., et al. (2006). Immune-neuroendocrine interactions and autoimmune diseases. *Clin Dev Immunol.* 2006;13(2-4):109-23.

Jones, BA., Demetriades, D., Segal, I., et al. (1985). The Prevalence of Appendiceal Fecaliths with and without Appendicitis. *Ann Surg,* 202, 1(Jul 1985):80-2.

Kaplan, GG., Dixon, E., Panaccione, R., et al. (2009). Effect of ambient air pollution on the incidence of appendicitis. *CMAJ* 2009;181:591-7.

Kawai, T., & Akira, S. (2009). The roles of TLRs, RLRs and NLRs in pathogen recognition. *Int Immunol.* 2009;21(4):317-37.

Khaavel, AA., & Birkenfeldt, RR. [Nature of the relation of acute appendicitis morbidity to meteorological and heliogeographical factors]. *Vestn Khir Im I I Grek.* 1978;120(4):67-70.

Korner, H., Sondenaa, K., Soreide, JA., et al. (1993). Incidence of acute nonperforated and perforated appendicitis: age-specifi and sex-specific analysis. *World J Surg.* 1997;21(3):313-7.

Kovats, S., & Carreras, E. (2008). Regulation of dendritic cell differentiation and function by estrogen receptor ligands. *Cell Immunol.* 2008;252(1-2):81-90.

Kwaasi, AAA., Tipirneni, P., Harfi, H., et al. (1992a). Date palm (*Phoenix dactylifera L*) is a potent allergen. *Ann Allergy.* 1992;68:78.

Kwaasi, AAA., Parhar, RS., Tipirneni, P., et al. (1992b). Characterization of antigens and allergens of date palm (*Phoenix dactylifera L*) pollen: immunological assessment of atopic patients using whole extracts or its fractions. *Allergy.* 1992;47:535-44.

Kwaasi, AAA., Tipirneni, P., Harfi, H., et al. (1993). Major allergens of the date palm (*Phoenix dactylifera L*) pollen: identification of IgE binding components by ELISA and immunoblot analysis. *Allergy.* 1993;48:511-8.

Kwaasi, AAA., Parhar, RS., Al-Mohanna, FAA., et al. (1998). Aeroallergens and viable microbes in sandstorm dust. *Allergy.* 1998;53:255-65.

Lambertucci, JR., dos Santos Silva, LC., & Miranda, D. (2008). [Schistosomiasis mansoni of the appendix in a patient with acute appendicitis]. *Rev Soc Bras Med Trop.* 2008;41(2):217-8.

Lander A. (2007). The role of imaging in children with suspected appendicitis: the UK perspective. Pediatr Radiol. 2007 Jan;37(1):5-9.

Langenscheidt, P., Lang, C., Puschel, W., et al. (1999). High rates of appendicetomy in a developing country: an attempt to a more rational use of surgical resources. *Eur J Surg.* 1999;165(3):248-52.

Lau, SKP., Woo, PCY., Chan, CYF., et al. (2005). Typhoid fever associated with acute appendicitis caused by an H1-j strain of Salmonella enterica serotype typhi. *J Clin Microbiol.* 2005 Mar;43(3):1470-2.

Le Bourhis, L., Benko, S., & Girardin, SE. (2007). Nod1 and Nod2 in innate immunity and human inflammatory disorders. *Biochem Soc Trans.* 2007;35:1479-84.

Lee YK & Mazmanian SK. (2010). Has the microbiota played a critical role in the evolution of the immune system? Science. 2010;330:1768-73.

Lee, JH., Park, YS., & Choi, JS. (2010). The epidemiology of appendicitis and appendectomy in South Korea: National registry data. *J Epidemiol.* 2010;20:97-105.

Livingston, EH., Woodward, WA., Sarosi, GA., et al. (2007). Disconnect between incidence of nonperforated and perforated appendicitis - implications for pathophysiology and management. *Ann Surg.* 2007 Jun;245(6):886-92.

Livingston, EH., Fomby, TB., Woodward, WA., et al.. (2011). Epidemiological similarities between appendicitis and diverticulitis suggesting a common underlying pathogenesis. Arch Surg. 2011;146(3):308-14.

Lowenberg, RI. (1949). Appendicular Calculi; their pathologic and clinical significance. *Ann Surg.* 1949 Nov;975-9.

Luckmann, R., & Davis, P. The epidemiology of acute appendicitis in California: racial, gender, and seasonal variation. *Epidemiology.* 1991;2(5):323-30.

Matricon J, Barnich N, Ardid D. (2010). Immunopathogenesis of inflammatory bowel disease. Self Nonself. 2010; 1(4):299-309.

McCarthy, JS., Peacock, D., Trown, KP., et al. (2002). Endemic invasive amoebiasis in northern Australia. *MJA.* 2002;177(10):570.

Medzhitov, R., Preston-Hurlburt, P., & Janeway Jr., CA. (1997). A human homologue of the Drosophila Toll Protein signals activation of adaptive immunity. *Nature.*1997; 388:394-7.

Mitros, FA., & Rubin, E. (2009). The Gastrointestinal Tract, In: *Essentials of Rubin's Pathology, 5th Edition,* Emanuel Rubin & Howard M. Reisner, ISBN-13: 978-0781773249. pp 275-308,

Moertel, CG., Dockerty, MB., & Judd, ES. (1968). Carcinoid tumours of the vermiform appendix. *Cancer.* 1968;21:270.

Morris, J., Barker, DJ., & Nelson, M. (1987). Diet, infection, and acute appendicitis in Britain and Ireland. *J Epidemiol.* 1987; 41:44-9.

Nelson, M., Barker, DJ., & Winter, PD. (1984). Dietary fibre and acute appendicitis: a case-control study. *Hum Nutr Appl Nutr.* 1984; 38(2):126-31.

Nelson, M., Morris, J., Barker, DJ., et al. (1986). A case-control study of acute appendicitis and diet in children. *J Epidemiol Community Health.* 1986;40(4):316-8.

Ohene-Yeboah, M., & Abantanga, FA. (2009). Incidence of acute appendicitis in Kumasi, Ghana. *West Afr J Med.* 2009;28:122-5.

Oldmeadow, C., Wood, I., Mengersen, K., et al. (2008). Investigation of the relationship between smoking and appendicitis in Australian twins. *Ann Epidemiol.* 2008;18(8):631-6.

Oldmeadow, C., Mengersen, K., Martin, N., et al. (2009). Heritability and linkage analysis of appendicitis utilizing age at onset. *Twin Res Hum Genet.* 2009; 12(2):150-7.
Osta, PA., Redondo, MJ., Ladron, E., et al. (1991). [A retrospective study of 469 cases of acute appendicitis. Importance of primary care]. *Aten Primaria.* 1991;8(2):123-7.
Papadopoulos, AA., Polymeros, D., Kateri, M., et al. (2008). Dramatic decline of acute appendicitis in Greece over 30 years: index of improvement of socioeconomic conditions or diagnostic aids? *Dig Dis.* 2008;26(1):80-4.
Parra, FC., Amado, RC., Lambertucci, JR., et al. (2003). Color and genomic ancestry in Brazilians. *Proc Natl Acad Sci.* 2003;100(1):177-82.
Pearce, C., Torres, C., Stallings, S., et al. (2008). Elective appendectomy at the time of caesarean delivery: a randomized controlled trial. *Am J Obstet Gynecol.* 2008;199:491.e1-491.e5.
Petroianu, A., Oliveira-Neto, JE., & Alberti, LR. (2004). [Comparative incidence of acute appendicitis in a mixed population, according to skin color]. *Arch Gastroenterol.* 2004; 41(1):24-6.
Pisacane, A., de Luca, U., Impagliazzo, N., et al. (1995). Breast feeding and acute appendicitis. *BMJ* 1995;310:836-7.
Pourbagher, MA., Pourbagher, A., Savas, L., et al. (2006). Clinical pattern and abdominal sonographic findings in 251 cases of Brucellosis in Southern Turkey. *AJR.* 2006;187:W191-W194.
Rivera-Chavez, FA., Wheeler, H., Lindberg, G., et al. (2003). Regional and systemic cytokine responses to acute inflammation of the vermiform appendix. *Ann Surg.* 2003;237(3):408-416.
Rivera-Chavez, FA., Peters-Hybki, DL., Barber, RC., et al. (2004). Innate immunity genes influence the severity of acute appendicitis. *Ann Surg.* 2004;240(2):269-77.
Rollins, MD., Andolsek, W., Scaife, ER., et al. (2010). Prophylactive appendectomy: unnecessary in children with incidental appendicoliths detected by computed tomographic scan. *J Pediatr Surg.* 2010 Dec;45(12):2377-80.
Round JL, Lee SM, Li J, et al. (2011). The Toll-like receptor 2 pathway establishes colonization by a commensal of the human microbiota. Science. 2011;332:974-7.
Round JL & Mazmanian SK. (2010). Inducible Fox3+ regulatory T-cell development by a commensal bacterium of the intestinal microbiota. Proc Natl Acad Sci USA. 2010;107(27):12204-9.
Sah, SP., & Bhadani, PP. (2006). Enterobius vermicularis causing symptoms of appendicitis in Nepal. *Trop Doct.* 2006 Jul;36(3):160-2.
Sahm, M., Pross, M., & Lippert, H. (2011). [Acute appendicitis - changes in epidemiology, diagnosis and therapy]. *Zentralbl Chir.* 2011;136(1):18-24.
Sanda, RB., Zalloum, M., El-Hossary, M., et al. (2008). *Ann Saudi Med.* 28,3(Mar-Apr 2008):140-1.
Sanda, RB. (2010). Appendicitis as an Immunological Disease: why it is uncommon in Africans. *Ann Afr Med,* 9,4(Oct-Dec 2010):200-2.
Santosh, G., & Aravindan, KP. Evidence of eosinophil degranulation in acute appendicitis. *Indian J Pathol Microbiol.* 2008;51:172-4.
Seetahal, SA., Bolorunduro, OB., Sookdeo, TC., et al. (2011). Negative appendectomy: a 10-year review of nationally representative sample. Am J Surg. 2011;201(4):433-7.
Segal, I., & Walker, ARP. (1982). Diverticular disease in urban Africans in South Africa. *Digestion.* 1982;24(1):42-6.
Short, AR. (1920). The causation of appendicitis. *Br J Surg.* 1920; 8:171-88.

Smink, DS., Fishman, SJ., Kleinman, K., et al. 2005. Effect of race, insurance status, and hospital volume on perforated appendicitis in children. *Pediatrics;* 115,4(Apr 2005):920-5. ISSN 0031 4005.

Song, JY., Yordan, E., & Rotman, C. (2009). Incidental appendectomy during endoscopic surgery. *JSLS.* 2009;13:376-83.

Soreide, O. (1984). Appendicitis - a study of incidence, death rates and consumption of hospital resources. *Postgrad Med J.* 1984;60(703):341-5.

Sugimoto, T., & Edwards, D. (1987). Incidence and cost of incidental appendectomy as a preventive measure. *Am J Public Health.* 1987;77(4):471-5.

Sulu, B., Gunerhan, Y., Palanci, Y., et al. (2010). Epidemiological and demographic features of appendicitis and influences of several environmental factors. *Ulus Travma Acil Cerrahi Derg.* 2010;16(1):38-42.

Terada, T. (2009). Schistosomal appendicitis: incidence in Japan and a case report. *World J Gastroenterol.* 2009 Apr; 15(13):1648-9.

Thalayasingam, B. (1985). Acute appendicitis and infectious mononucleosis. *BMJ* 1985 Jul 13;291:140-1.

To, T., & Langer, JC. (2010). Does access to care affect outcomes of appendicitis in children? A population-based cohort study. *BMC Health Serv Res.* 2010; 10:250.

Uba, AF., Lohfa, LB., & Ayuba, MD. (2006). Childhood acute appendicitis: is routine appendicectomy advised? *J Indian Assoc Pediatr Surg.* 11, 1(Jan-Mar 2006):27-30.

Uematsu, S., Jang, MH., Chevrier, N., et al. (2006). Detection of pathogenic intestinal bacteria by Toll-like receptor 5 on intestinal CD11c+ lamina propria cells. *Nat Immunol.* 2006;7:868-74.

Visintin, A., Mazzoni, A., Spitzer, JH., et al. (2001). Regulation of Toll-like Receptors in Human Monocytes and Dendritic Cells. *J Immunol.* 2001;166:249-55.

Walker, AR., Shipton, E., Walker, BF., et al. 1989. Appendicectomy incidence in black and white children aged 0 to 14 years with a discussion on the disease's causation. *Trop Gastroenterol.* 1989;10:96-101.

Walker, ARP., Walker, BF., Manetsi, B., et al. (1989). Appendicitis in Soweto, South Africa. Traditional healers and hospitalization. *J R Soc Hlth.* 1989;109:190-2.

Walker, ARP., & Segal, I. Appendicitis: an African perspective. *J R Soc Med.* 1995;88:616-9.

Wikkipedia Foundation Inc.. http://en.wikipedia.org/wiki/Demographics_of_Toronto (Accessed on May 11, 2011)

Whisker L, Luke D, Hendrickse C, Bowley DM, Lander A. (2009). Appendicitis in children: a comparative study between a specialist paediatric centre and a district general hospital. *Journal of Pediatric Surgery.* 2009;44(2):362-7.

Yanagawa, Y., & Onoe, K. (2007). Enhanced IL-10 production by TLR4- and TLR2-primed dendritic cells upon TLR restimulation. *J Immunol.* 2007;178:6173-80.

Yoon, HS. (2010). Neonatal innate immunity and toll-like receptor. *Korean J Pediatr.* 2010;53(12):985-8.

Zen, M., Ghirardello, A., Iaccarino, L., et al. (2010). Hormones, immune response, and pregnancy in women and SLE patients. *Swiss Med Wkly.* 2010 Apr 3;140(13-14):187-201.

Zoquereh, DD., Lemaitre, X., Ikoli, JF., et al. (2001). [Acute appendicitis at the National University Hospital in Bangui, Central African Republic: epidemiologic, clinical, paraclinical and therapeutic aspects]. *Sante.* 2001;11(2):117-25.

2

Diagnostic Challenges in Acute Appendicitis

Sanjay Harrison[1] and Harrison Benziger[2]
[1]*Sunderland Royal Hospital*
[2]*Queen Elizabeth the Queen Mother Hospital*
United Kingdom

1. Introduction

Acute appendicitis is one of the commonest surgical problems (Humes et al, 2007) and though less common at the extremes of age, it can present classically or in an atypical manner in the very young and the elderly. Making a diagnosis of appendicitis is not always easy and it has led to the development of clinical scoring systems and a wider use of imaging techniques.

A raised white cell count and C-reactive protein level reflect inflammation and raise the probability that a patient with right iliac fossa pain has appendicitis. These markers have been joined by serum levels of novel markers such as interleukin-6 and procalcitonin (Erkasap, 2000; Paajanen, 2002). Importantly, it should be realised that no test has a 100% sensitivity or specificity.

The diagnosis of acute appendicitis can be missed leading to morbidity and mortality especially at the extremes of age sometimes with medico-legal consequences. It is estimated that a missed or delayed diagnosis of acute appendicitis is among the top five most frequent malpractice claims made against emergency department clinicians (Chung, 2000). This highlights the need for improving our ability to diagnose this condition.

Missed or delayed diagnoses sometimes follow classical presentations and reveal an education gap in training. Missed or delayed diagnoses following atypical presentations are well documented (Alloo, 2004; Paulson, 2003; Rusnak, 1994). All clinicians involved in the initial assessment of patients with abdominal pain need a good understanding of the pathophysiology of appendicitis, appropriate investigations and imaging.

2. Methods

A Pubmed and Medline search of papers utilising the keywords appendicitis, atypical appendicitis, appendicitis in pregnancy, appendicitis in the elderly, pathophysiology appendicitis, scoring systems appendicitis, imaging appendicitis, ultrasound appendicitis, computerised tomography appendicitis, causes of appendicitis were used for this review. The bibliographies of relevant articles were also searched.

3. The classical presentation

The typical history usually attributed to an underlying inflamed appendix is a central abdominal pain which gets progressively worse and localises to the right iliac fossa. This is usually associated with anorexia, nausea, vomiting and a low grade pyrexia. The initial central abdominal pain is described as dull and becomes sharp once localised to the right iliac fossa where it is exacerbated by movement, coughing or sneezing. There may be a history of one or two episodes of loose stools. The vomiting occurs once the abdominal pain has been noticed. Vomiting preceding the pain should raise suspicion of the symptoms being due to gastroenteritis. The frequencies with which these occur is illustrated in table 1.

On physical examination, the patient may appear slightly dehydrated and in pain. A low grade pyrexia with an accompanying tachycardia might be noted. Tenderness is elicited on palpation of the right lower abdomen. Signs of localised peritonism include guarding and rebound tenderness. Other signs that have been described are a characteristic oral fetor and facial expression (Terry, 1983). Occasionally, there might be an increased urinary frequency and urinalysis may demonstrate the presence of white blood cells in the urine (Puskar, 1995).

The signs and symptoms of the classical presentation of acute appendicitis are understood in terms of the underlying pathophysiology. The initial triggering factor is often the obstruction of the appendiceal lumen by a faecolith. This results in the accumulation of appendiceal secretions. Continued distension of the lumen stimulates the nerve endings of visceral afferent pain fibres which accounts for the initial central pain. As the distension progresses, the pressure within the appendix exceeds the venous pressure but not the arterial pressure. This results is a continued inflow of blood to the appendix but a very limited or no outflow. This leads to engorgement and vascular congestion and distension of this magnitude triggers a reflex nausea and vomiting. This distension exacerbates the diffuse visceral abdominal pain. Bacterial overgrowth occurs and an inflammatory reaction is triggered which spreads across the mucosa of the appendix through to the serosa and the overlying peritoneum. This is perceived by the patient as the initial central abdominal pain migrating to the right lower abdomen.

The clinical presentation can vary with the position of the appendix (Ahmed, 2007). An inflamed appendix lying in the pelvis can sometimes irritate the rectum causing loose stools. If the inflamed appendix comes in contact with the right ureter or bladder, it causes a localised inflammatory response which can result in a urinalysis positive for white cells and sometimes blood (Puskar, 1995). Irritation of the bladder by the inflamed appendix can result in an increased urinary frequency. Classically, the point of maximal tenderness is described as being at McBurney's point but this is very variable (Karim, 1990).

Sign or Symptom	**Frequency (%)**
Abdominal pain	99 - 100
Right lower quadrant pain/tenderness	96
Anorexia	24 - 99
Nausea	62 - 90
Low grade pyrexia	67 - 69
Vomiting	32 - 75
Migration of pain to right iliac fossa	50
Rebound tenderness	26
Right lower quadrant guarding	21

Table 1. The frequencies with which the 'classical signs' present in acute appendicitis (Old et al, 2005)

4. Anatomical variations of the vermiform appendix

Clinicians involved in the assessment of patients suspected of having acute appendicitis should be familiar with the variations that can occur in the anatomy of the appendix. The variable position of the appendix is attributed to developmental processes (Schumpelick, 2000; Devlin, 1971). The structure that develops into the caecum and appendix is called the caecal diverticulum or the 'bud of the caecum'. This structure lies in the distal segment of the umbilical loop. The appendix appears as a distinct structure and becomes visible only in the eighth week of gestation. The embryonic gut undergoes rotations that bring the duodenal curve to its classic "C" shape and a rotation that brings the early caecum to the right. The caecum descends into the right iliac fossa as described below.

As a result of these morphological movements, the caecal diverticulum comes to occupy a region in the right half of the abdominal cavity. This is in close apposition to the liver. The liver in the developing fetus takes up a large proportion of the abdominal cavity. During subsequent development, the liver migrates cranially and separates from the caecum and appendix. The intervening bowel elongates to form the ascending colon. The appendix along with the caecum is pushed downwards and occupies the right lower quadrant. At this stage, the position of the appendix is determined by chance (Kozar, 1999). During the post partum period, the caecum grows in the lateral direction which results in the vermiform appendix being displaced medially. This movement of the appendix in the medial direction and its acquisition of a position that borders the caecum is believed to play a major role in placing the appendix in a retrocolic position, especially in later life (Herrinton, 1991).

Results of studies in humans looking at the relative frequencies with which the appendix occupies various anatomical positions demonstrate considerable variability (Nayak, 2010). Given the complexity of the underlying embryological processes this finding should not be surprising. In a post mortem study of ten thousand cases, Wakeley (1933) found the retrocaecal position to be the most common. Given our current understanding of the embryological processes this is to be expected. However, several other studies indicate that there might be other factors involved and that the final position of the appendix is not the result of purely embryological development as suggested by Wakeley.

Most authors follow the variations described by Sir Frederich Treaves but alternative descriptions have been suggested (Sahana's Human Anatomy, 1994). In his paper, Treaves considers the caecum to be analogous to the dial of a clock and the appendix as the hour arm. Therefore, the positions of the appendix are described as in Figure 1.

- 11 O'clock position or para colic or para caecal. The appendix is directed upwards and lies to the right side of the caecum in close apposition. In this position, the appendix can even lie in front of the right kidney. In this position, a long appendix can irritate the ureter resulting in leucocytes detected on urinalysis or may even mimic the presentation of pyelonephritis (Jones, 1988).
- 12 O'clock position or retro caecal. The appendix lies behind the caecum or the ascending colon and may be intraperitoneal or lie behind the peritoneum.
- 2 O'clock position or splenic. The appendix lies directed towards the spleen or towards the left upper quadrant and may lie in front of the terminal ileum (pre-ileal) or behind the terminal ileum (post-ileal).
- 3 O'clock position or promonteric. The appendix is directed transversly in a medial direction towards the sacral promontory.

- 4 O'clock position or pelvic. The appendix hangs just at the brim of the pelvis and projects into the pelvic cavity. This position is of clinical importance as the tip of the appendix lies on the psoas muscle. Irritation of the psoas muscle by an inflamed appendix on flexion of the hip is the basis of the 'psoas test' (Sharma, 2005, Smith, 1965).
- 6 O'clock or midiguinal. The appendix passes inferiorly towards the midpoint of the inguinal ligament. This is also referred to as the sub-caecal position. In this position, the appendix lies in the iliac fossa, separated from the iliacus muscle only by the intervening peritoneum. This is of clinical importance as an inflamed appendix in this position can irritate the iliacus muscle which would be indicated by worsening pain when the right hip is flexed (Smith, 1965).

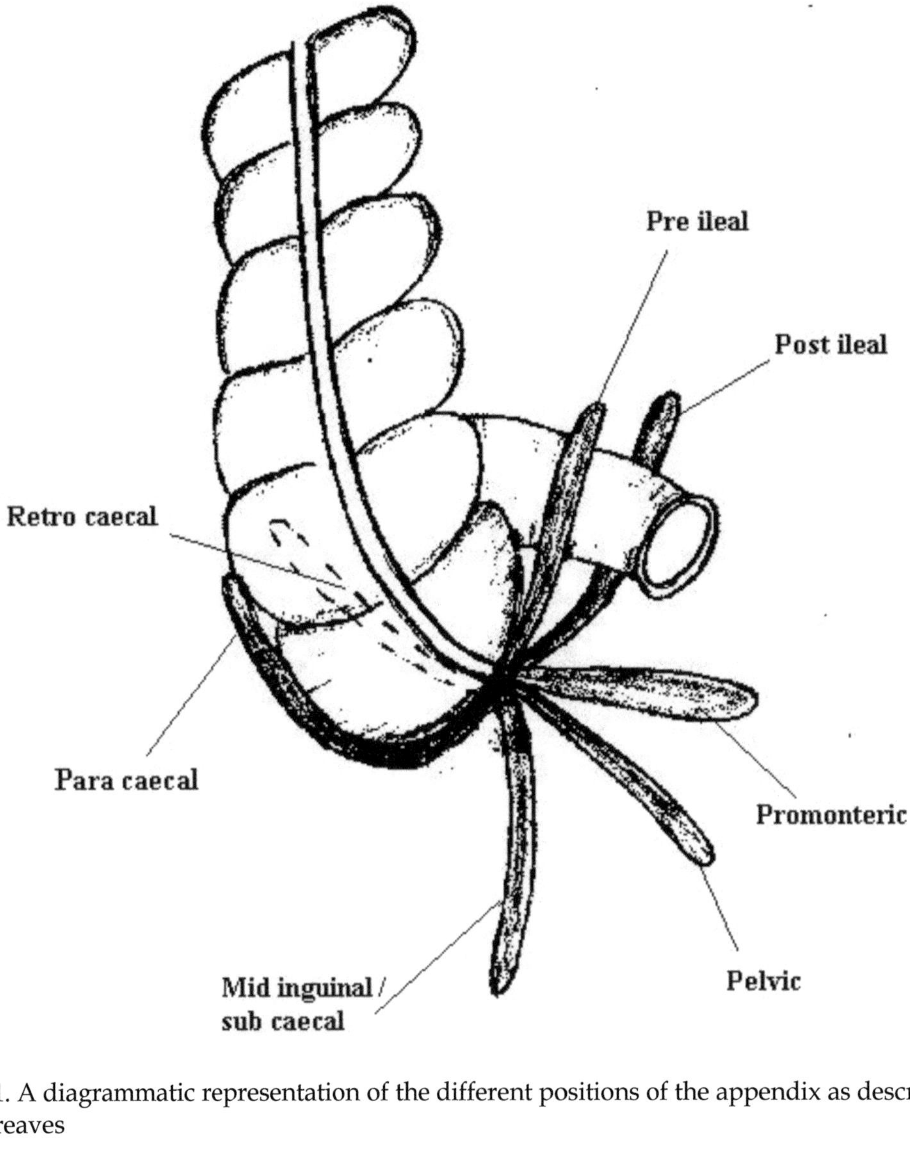

Fig. 1. A diagrammatic representation of the different positions of the appendix as described by Treaves

Based on his analysis of ten thousand cases, Wakeley (1933) also noted the presence of ectopic appendices. These are rare and accounted for only five cases out of the ten thousand. Of these five, two were found to be pre-hepatic in position. Another two were noted to be with the caecum in the umbilical region just below the stomach and transverse colon. The remaining one was in the left side of the abdomen and was the result of a complete transposition of the abdominal viscera.
The results from various studies summarising their results on the different positions of the vermiform appendix are given in table 2.
In addition to the considerable variability of the eventual position of the appendix, various authors have also noted that there is a corresponding heterogeneity in the length of the appendix as well (Alzaraa, 2009). In a classic study by Collins (1932) of 4680 specimens, the length was found to vary from 0.3 cm to 24.5 cm with around 61% of the specimens having a length between 6 cm and 9 cm. The length of the appendix is just as important as its position in influencing the clinical presentation of acute appendicitis. This is because, a long appendix in the paracolic position can abut the right kidney and sometimes even the duodenum giving the clinical impression of cholecystitis or a pathology related to the duodenum (Hsu, 2011). Likewise, an inflamed pelvic appendix which extends deep enough into the pelvis can irritate the rectum causing the loose stool which is sometimes observed in acute appendicitis (Codon & Telford, 1991). These kind of symptoms that appear to localise in areas far removed from the' traditional' or 'classical' position of the appendix can mislead the clinician who is not aware of the anatomical variations.

Authors	**Year**	**Country**	**Number**	**Retro caecal**	**Pelvic**	**Para caecal**	**Pre ileal**	**Post ileal**
Liertz	1909	Germany	2092	35.0	42.1	9.0	13.9	
Smith	1911	USA	882	24.2	19.4	2.9	50.9	
Ajmani & Ajmani	1983	India	100	58.0	23.0	7.0	2.0	10.0
Ojeifo	1989	Nigeria	548	44.5	25.0	8.7	1.8	1.6
Wakeley	1933	UK	10,000	65.3	31.0	12.3	1.4	
Peterson	1934	Finland	373	31.0	42.2	0.0	26.8	
Shah & Shah	1945	India	405	61.2	3.7	5.4	26.9	
Waas	1960	South Africa	103	26.7	58.0	5.0	28.0	
Solanke	1970	Nigeria	203	38.4	31.2	11.2	29.2	
Bakheit & Warille	1996	Sudan	60	58.3	21.7	11.7	11.7	
Delic	2002	Croatia	50	52.0	32.0	8.0	10.0	

Table 2. The above table shows the relative frequencies (%) of the different positions of the appendix (see Old et al, 2005)

The results of various studies that have reported on the length of the vermiform appendix are summarised below (table 3). Although most anatomical studies of the appendix were done several decades ago, their results are still relevant today as it is the knowledge gained from such studies that guides our diagnostic reasoning to a very large extent.

Author	Shortest	Longest	Average
Monks & Blake	1.0	24.0	7.9
Deaver	1.0	23.0	8.9
Lewis	2.0	20.0	8.3
Robinson	1.8	23.0	9.2
Royster	2.5	29.4	7.5
Hafferl	2.5	20.0	9.0
Solanke	4.0	20.0	9.6

Table 3. Lengths of the appendix (in cm) (Thyagaraj, 2005)

5. The pathophysiological mechanisms of acute appendicitis

It is widely believed that acute appendicitis is the result of an obstruction of the appendiceal lumen, usually by a faecolith (Larner, 1988) but some have found a faecolith only in a minority of cases of acute appendicitis (Chang, 1981). Furthermore, faecoliths need not always cause appendicitis since they have been demonstrated to be present in the appendix in the absence of any inflammation (Fraser, 2004). Obstruction can also be the result of lymphoid hyperplasia (Humes, 2007; Walker, 1990), or rarely caecal tumours can obstruct the lumen (Sieren, 2010). A number of authors find little convincing evidence that appendiceal obstruction is the principle cause of acute appendicitis (Carr, 2000; Andreou, 1990). In a small series by Horton (1997) the lumen was empty in 25% of 44 cases and faecoliths were only found in 9% and in the rest, only purulent material or soft faeces were found within the lumen of the appendix. Other important possible factors include: the role of infection, hygiene, genetics and diet.

Interestingly Chang found lymphoid hyperplasia to be more common in non inflamed appendices and he estimated it to occur in only 6% of cases of acute appendicitis (Chang, 1981).

Experimental work by Arnbjornsson and Bengmark (1983, 1984) provided evidence for an etiology other than just luminal obstruction. In their study, the pressure within the lumen of the appendix was measured with a U-tube manometer. Their results showed that there was no increase in intraluminal pressure in 19 out of the 21 cases of phlegmonous appendicitis. The other two cases of phlegmonous appendicitis along with all six cases of gangrenous appendicitis however, had intraluminal pressures of over 20 cm saline. No increase in intraluminal pressure was noted in the normal appendices. The results of this study are not consistent with luminal obstruction as a major cause of acute appendicitis. The finding of increased intraluminal pressure in the gangrenous appendices suggests that increases in pressures within the appendiceal lumen might be a late change and could result from an inflammatory process.

There has been much speculation about the cause of the early mucosal ulceration seen in acute appendicitis. A study by Sisson et al (1971) demonstrated that mucosal ulceration happens before any distension of the appendix. Moreover, it has been observed in several studies that cases of acute appendicitis tend to cluster in manner that is suggestive of a transmissible infective agent (Anderson, 1995). Such investigations led to the idea of the mucosal ulceration being the result of a viral infection which is then followed by a secondary bacterial infection which aides the perpetuation of the inflammatory response. Various infectious agents have been implicated in the etiology of acute appendicitis (Lamps, 2010). This theory would to a certain degree explain the seasonal variations of the incidence of acute appendicitis reported by some (Sulu, 2010). Periods of high incidence might be because certain associated gut infections are more common during these periods. While there is substantial evidence demonstrating the role played by different infectious agents in the pathogenesis of acute appendicitis, the effects of season, altitude and temperature are yet to be conclusively established.

Closely connected with the role of a possible infectious etiology of acute appendicitis is the 'hygiene hypothesis' which also proposes that enteric infections during childhood and early adulthood trigger acute appendicitis (Raynor, 2010). The appeal of this hypothesis is that it provides an explanation for certain epidemiological characteristics of appendicitis. The epidemiology of acute appendicitis shows a rising incidence accompanies increasing industrialisation (Barker et al, 1988). This is believed to be because as increasing industrialisation and improved socio-economic conditions arise there is a concomitant improvement in hygiene. This in turn leads to a reduced immunity in adult life as infections rates during childhood decrease. This decreased resistance predisposes to appendicitis. The theory remains controversial (Coggon et al, 1991).

The observation that the incidence of acute appendicitis is a lot less common in developing countries compared to the Western world led to the suggestion that diet may play an important role in the etiology (Burkitt 1971). The initial suggestion was that a diet relatively low in fibre and high in unrefined food predisposed to the development of acute appendicitis (Larner, 1988). This was inferred primarily from the observation that there was a decrease in the incidence of acute appendicitis during the second world war when there was an increase in the use of high fibre and unrefined food (Burkitt, 1971). There has however, been evidence to suggest the contrary as the decrease in incidence of acute appendicitis in the United States and Western Europe in the last few decades has not been associated with any significant alteration in diet (Larner, 1988). Moreover, studies in South Africa demonstrate a lower incidence of acute appendicitis among the urban black population despite their diet being relatively low in fibre (Walker & Segal, 1995). High fibre diets decrease the stool transit times and also have the effect of reducing faecal viscosity. This impairs the formation of faecoliths and could therefore provide a theoretical basis for the association with appendicitis (Burkitt et al, 1972). Epidemiological studies have suggested a protective role for green vegetables and tomatoes which might be partly due to alterations in the gut flora (Barker et al, 1986). It is possible that diet works in conjunction with other predisposing factors and exerts a modulatory role.

Vascular compromise is a factor that might play a role in triggering acute appendicitis. Histological examinations of certain appendicectomy specimens have noted an association between an obstructed blood supply and morphological changes resembling that of ischaemic colitis (Carr, 2000). The role of vascular compromise in the pathogenesis of acute appendicitis is also illustrated by the fact that appendicitis appears to progress more rapidly to perforation in patients with sickle cell anaemia (Al Salem et al 1998). It has been suggested that this is due to the ischaemia that results when the blood vessels get blocked by the sickled red blood cells. Abdominal trauma has also been seen to result in acute appendicitis (Toumi et al, 2010). This is believed to be mediated by processes that result in the obstruction of the appendiceal lumen. However, it must also be noted that bruising, edema and rupture of the mesoappendix are very often seen with these cases and can occur without any luminal obstruction. The result would be compromise to the vascular supply of the appendix which would then promote bacterial invasion of the appendiceal wall and subsequent inflammation.

Some authors have suggested a genetic component in the pathogenesis of acute appendicitis (Azodi et al, 2009). It has been suggested that certain individuals could be more susceptible to developing appendicitis. Some studies demonstrate differences in the incidence of acute appendicitis between different races and also on the observation of a familial tendency (Hiraiwa et al, 1995). Some studies report that for individuals with a close family member who has had appendicitis, their likelihood of developing the condition is higher than average (Ergul, 2007). While it is possible that genetic factors play a role in determining an individual's response to inflammation and other pathogenic factors such as bacteria, it is very difficult to isolate the effects of genetics from that of the environment.
Rare causes of obstruction include foreign bodies with the following reported: nails, pins, screws, shot gun pellets, condoms and teeth (Klinger et al, 1997). Barium has been implicated in appendicitis following its use for investigation for other bowel pathology (Fang et al, 2009). 'Barium appendicitis' is more common in children as they tend to retain the barium for longer periods than adults.

6. The role of imaging

Studies have demonstrated that history and examination alone has an accuracy for diagnosis of between 78 to 92 percent in males and between 58 to 85 percent in females (Birnbaum & Wilson, 2000). Imaging has improved diagnostic accuracy to over 95% (Old, 2005). Imaging should be interpreted in conjunction with the history, clinical examination and blood test results.

6.1 Plain radiography

The use of plain radiography is generally not indicated when appendicitis is suspected unless there is clinical evidence to suspect a co-existing pathology such as an obstruction or perforation. Plain radiography is not cost effective and can be misleading (Rao et al, 1999). An incidental finding of faecal loading in the right hemicolon might mistakenly be labelled as the cause of the right iliac fossa pain. Faecoliths are visible on plain radiography in less than 5% of cases of appendicitis (Rao et al, 1999). Therefore, the routine use of abdominal films is not indicated as part of the initial assessment.

6.2 Ultrasonography (USS)

Diagnostic accuracy with ultrasonography in identifying an inflamed appendix varies between 71% and 97% (Rao et al, 1998a, Wilson et al, 2001). This large variation is due in part to the operator dependency of this imaging modality. While the biggest advantage of ultrasonography is the absence of any ionising radiation, its use is limited by the requirement for well trained staff out of normal working hours. Importantly, ultrasound can identify other causes of right iliac fossa pain such as ovarian cysts, ectopic pregnancies and tubo-ovarian abscesses. USS is also ideal for assessment during pregnancy.
The features suggesting a diagnosis of acute appendicitis on ultrasonography are well established and when observed, are very reliable (Puylaert, 1986). One highly suggestive feature is the presence of a distended appendix with an outer diameter of 6 mm or greater when viewed in the cross sectional plane (Kessler et al, 2004). Other features include evidence of inflammatory changes in the vicinity of the appendix especially in the surrounding fat. Ultrasonography can also be used to identify a perforated appendicitis with evidence of a loculated fluid collection around the caecum, prominent pericaecal fat or

the presence of an abscess. Loss of the submucosal layer in a circumferential manner apparent on ultrasonography has also been associated with a perforated appendicitis. The presence of a phlegmon is identified as an ill defined structure very closely apposed to the appendiceal wall (Rumack et al, 1998).
The pressure exerted by the transducer can cause discomfort for the patient (Wise et al, 2001). Visualisation of the appendix can be limited by a variety of factors which include a co-existent ileus or in the obese (Fefferman et al, 2001). Bowel gas in the overlying dilated small bowel loops can cast an ultrasonographic shadow which can obscure the appendix. Also, if the appendix occupies a retrocaecal position, it can be difficult to identify. Inflammatory bowel disease, caecal diverticulitis, pelvic inflammatory disease and endometriosis can not only mimic the clinical presentation of acute appendicitis but also its ultrasonographical findings.

6.3 Computed Tomography (CT)

CT has an accuracy between 93% and 98% (Rao et al, 1998b) which is superior to that of ultrasonography in cases of suspected acute appendicitis (Terasawa et al, 2004). There has been a shift towards the use of CT in clinical practice with ultrasonography usually being reserved for cases where exposure to ionising radiation is contra indicated. The success of CT is due largely to its ability to visualise the appendix (Friedland & Siegel, 1997). An inflamed appendix usually appears to be larger than 6 mm in diameter and there will also tend to be evidence of inflammatory changes in the surrounding tissues (Choi et al, 2003; Haaga et al, 2003). These changes include the presence of a phlegmon, inflammatory fat stranding, free fluid, abscess formation and in the case of a perforated appendicitis even the presence of small amounts of free air (Haaga et al, 2003). CT also has the advantage of being able to detect other pathologies, for instance, luminal obstruction leading to acute appendicitis due to a caecal malignancy should be identifiable on computed tomography. Also, any associated adenopathy or metastasis could be detected as well. Figure 2 is a computed tomography scan that demonstrates acute appendicitis.
The main disadvantage of CT is that it involves ionising radiation and its use in children has to be weighed against the potential risks. Cost is also an issue however, at present the cost of a CT scan is less than the costs associated with performing a negative laparotomy or diagnostic laparoscopy. Another disadvantage of using computed tomography scans is the need for administering a contrast agent to which there may be a reaction. The administration of rectal contrast is also associated with patient discomfort The presence of intra abdominal fat can be used as a contrast agent and therefore even very subtle inflammatory changes can be detected.. One factor that might lead to a diagnosis of acute appendicitis being missed on a CT scan is the lack of intra abdominal fat. This is usually encountered in children and very slim patients (Levine et al, 2005). In such cases an ultrasonography scan would seem to be more beneficial.

6.4 Magnetic Resonance Imaging (MRI)

There are no large studies conclusively demonstrating a superiority for MRI over other imaging modalities (Rothrock & Pagane, 2000). A recent study by Pedrosa et al (2009) studied 148 pregnant patients with suspected acute appendicitis. Their results showed that the use of magnetic resonance imaging did lower the incidence of negative laparotomies and perforation rates and thereby suggested a potential benefit. MRI however, is time consuming and its cost effectiveness is yet to be evaluated.

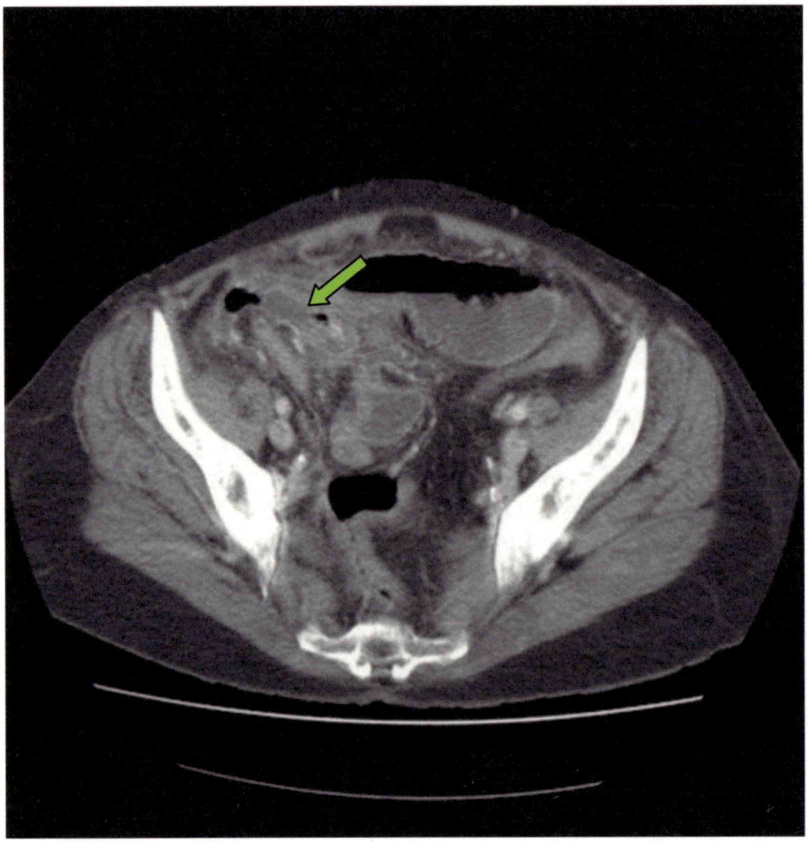

Fig. 2. A computed tomography scan of a patient with acute appendicitis. The arrow illustrates the position of the appendix.

7. The role of blood tests

Numerous studies have looked at the role of blood tests such as the serum levels of certain inflammatory markers like the white cell count and the C-reactive protein level (Andersson, 2004). From a pathophysiological point of view one would expect the serum levels of these inflammatory markers to rise in a patient with acute appendicitis. This indeed is the case in the majority of cases and has been confirmed in various studies (Sack et al, 2006; Beltran et al, 2007). A study by Dueholm et al (1989) which looked at patients between the ages of 15 and 45 reported that the patients with acute appendicitis had higher white cell counts than those who did not have appendicitis. It must be noted that taken on their own, the elevated values of these inflammatory markers have a poor predictive value for acute appendicitis (Beltran, 2007). There are also contradictory reports on the value of the white cell count as a marker of severity of the disease (Sasso et al, 1970; Vermeulen et al, 1995)). The value of these inflammatory markers is appreciated only when they are interpreted together and not in isolation. Studies have demonstrated that elevated levels of the white cell count and the C-reactive protein together improve the predictive value (Andersson, 2004; Peitola et al, 1986).

The converse however which is if the patient does not have elevated serum levels of the relevant inflammatory markers then they are unlikely to have acute appendicitis needs to be interpreted with caution. While there are studies that suggest the absence of raised inflammatory markers indicates a low likelihood of acute appendicitis (Sengupta, 2009), one must be wary when encountering a patient with a suggestive history but normal blood tests. There are reports in the literature suggesting that 21% to 65% of patients with acute appendicitis have a normal white cell count (Merlin et al, 2010).

Similar results have been demonstrated for the serum levels of the C-reactive protein (Old, 2011). Studies indicate that it is a poor predictor of acute appendicitis when looked at in isolation but in conjunction with the white cell count it increases the likelihood ratio considerably (Vissers & Lennarz, 2010). Other studies have also indicated that normal levels of the white cell count, C-reactive protein and the neutrophil count have a high negative predictive value (Dueholm et al, 1989). One reason for the varying results between studies could be the heterogeneity of the sample population. Factors known to influence the levels of these inflammatory markers include the patient's age and the duration of symptoms (Paajanen et al, 1997). The temporal relation that the serum levels of the inflammatory markers bear with the onset of symptoms is that the white cell count appears to rise early on in acute appendicitis with the C-reactive protein levels following later on. Persistently rising or high C-reactive levels could indicate the possibility of an appendiceal perforation (Chung et al, 1996, Sanjuan et al, 1999). This temporal relation does not seem to be so clear cut in children and therefore making a diagnosis in children poses additional problems (Kharbanda et al, 2011).

As always, it should be emphasised that blood tests alone cannot be used to diagnose acute appendicitis and therefore what should be employed is a holistic approach which takes into account the patients history and also the results of any other investigations.

8. Appendicitis scoring systems

The need to collate information obtained from the patients history, clinical examination and investigation results, which should then be interpreted as a coherent whole when assessing a patient with suspected appendicitis, has been recognised by many investigators (Zimmermann, 2008). Attempts to simplify the process and quantify the likelihood of a positive diagnosis for acute appendicitis led to the development of various scoring systems. All these systems allocate particular numerical values to a feature. These are then added to give a final number which should give the clinician an idea of the likelihood of the patient having acute appendicitis. The most commonly used in clinical practice is the Alvarado score or the MANTRELS (**M**igratory pain, **A**norexia, **N**ausea/vomiting, **T**enderness in right iliac fossa, **R**ebound tenderness, **E**levated temperature, **L**eucocytosis shift to the left) score (Alvarado, 1986). The scoring system is illustrated in table 4. Currently there are many variants of the Alvarado score, specifically modified to address certain groups of patients like children (Macklin et al, 1997). It must be noted that none of these modified scoring systems have demonstrated an increased accuracy in diagnosing acute appendicitis.

A multicentre prospective study conducted by Ohmann et al (1995) looked at 1254 patients with acute abdominal pain and assessed various appendicitis scoring systems such as the Alvarado score, the Lindberg score, the Fenyo score and the Christian score against certain pre-set criteria. The pre-set standardised criteria included a negative laparotomy rate of 15% or less, a potential perforation rate of 35% or less, an initial missed perforation rate of 15% or less and a missed appendicitis rate of 5% or less. The results of this study indicated that there were marked differences between the different scoring systems and that none of them satisfied the standardised criteria. However, when the published data was evaluated, many of the scoring systems demonstrated better agreement with the standardised criteria. The authors conclude that the original published data is 'optimistically biased' and that further large scale studies are required to validate these scoring systems.

Symptoms	**Score**
Migratory right iliac fossa pain	1
Nausea/vomiting	1
Anorexia	1
Signs	
Tenderness in right iliac fossa	2
Rebound tenderness in right iliac fossa	1
Pyrexia	1
Blood Test Results	
Elevated white cell count	2
Shift to the left of neutrophils	1
TOTAL	10

Table 4. The Alvarado score (Alvarado, 1986; Malik et al, 2000)

A more recent study by Horzic et al (2005) looked at the value of appendicitis scoring systems in diagnosing acute appendicitis in women. This study involved 126 female patients admitted with abdominal pain and looked at the Alvarado score, the Ohmann score and the Eskelinen score. This study too gave variable results in terms of accuracy but did report that the scoring systems, when used in conjunction with each other can be used to determine whether the patient would require surgery immediately or if observation would suffice initially. This potentially has the advantage of avoiding delays in operation and further investigations. It must be noted that the relatively small number of patients in this study does mean that further studies are required before such a strategy is adopted in clinical practice.

While clinical scoring systems appear to be useful adjuncts in diagnosing acute appendicitis, one should always bear in mind the variable diagnostic accuracy for each scoring system and therefore the limitations associated with them. As with all investigations, the different scoring systems should only play an ancillary role in the diagnosis. Clinical decisions should not be made solely on the basis of the value obtained on the application of a single scoring system.

9. Appendicitis at the extremes of age

While a diagnosis of acute appendicitis is considered rare in the elderly population, it is still common enough to be included in the differential diagnosis in an elderly patient presenting with an acute abdomen. It is estimated that 7% of elderly patients with acute abdominal pain have acute appendicitis (Doria et al 2006; Vissers & Lennarz, 2010). The diagnosis of acute appendicitis in the elderly population is particularly difficult as the clinical picture is often complicated by comorbidities. These include conditions which can mask or suppress the normal inflammatory reaction, such as diabetes or immunosuppression (Binderow & Shaked, 1991; Tsai et al, 2008). In such cases, the symptoms tend to be rather non specific. The damped inflammatory reaction demonstrated by certain elderly patients often complicates the clinical picture as palpation of the abdomen may not elicit marked tenderness or signs of peritonism.

The physical examination can be complicated, and for the unwary clinician even misleading at times , by the fact that many elderly patients have a weak abdominal musculature. This would mean that the expected signs of rigidity and guarding in a patient with peritonitis may not be present. It should also be noted that the rates of perforation are much higher in the elderly population and so many of the patients can also present with diffuse abdominal tenderness and peritonism (Korner et al, 1997; Hiu et al, 2002). The differential diagnosis for elderly patients presenting with abdominal pain is much broader and therefore when such a patient presents, especially with a non specific history, a computed tomography scan is the imaging modality of choice (Paranjape et al, 2007). In such circumstances, the presence of any other pathology can be assessed with a computed tomography scan and the appropriate management can be planned accordingly. Also, the benefits of the scan outweigh the risks associated with exposure to ionising radiation.

Appendicitis in the very young child can pose considerable challenges. The signs and symptoms of acute appendicitis are age dependent (Blab et al, 2004). From the age of around six and over the signs and symptoms are more reliable and tend to conform to the classical presentation. In younger children, nausea and vomiting seem to be constant features. Rothrock et al (1991) report that vomiting tends to precede the abdominal pain, and very often it is the vomiting that is noticed first by parents before a history of abdominal pain. In the 2 to 5 age group, the pain tends to be more localised which is in contrast to the children of ages 2 and younger where the abdominal pain tends to be more diffuse. Localised tenderness has been reported to be present in less that 50% in this age group (Barker & Davey, 1988; Horwitz et al, 1997). Patients in this age group or even younger tend to also exhibit lethargy, abdominal distension, diarrhoea and fever. Acute appendicitis has a higher rate of perforation with subsequent diffuse peritonism in the very young patient. This is partly due to the fact that in such young patients, the omentum has not reached sufficient maturity and therefore is unable to wall off any leakage that occurs during a perforation. This leads to the enteric contents being spread throughout the abdominal cavity. Other misleading signs in the very young patient include irritability and pain or stiffness in the right hip (Daehlin, 1982; Rothrock & Pagane, 2000).

Misdiagnosing acute appendicitis in young children can result in considerable morbidity and has been the subject of numerous medicolegal investigations. An understanding of the variations that occur in the very young should alert the astute clinician to the possibility of an underlying acute appendicitis when encountering a child with non specific symptoms.

10. Acute appendicitis in pregnancy

The pathophysiology and presentation of acute appendicitis in the pregnant patient can be very similar to that of the non pregnant patient (Mourad et al, 2000). The appendix can be displaced upwards as the uterus enlarges and therefore it may give rise to pain and tenderness in unexpected positions. There are however, studies that report the location of pain in pregnant patients with acute appendicitis to be predominantly in the right iliac fossa

(Hodjati et al, 2003; Oto et al 2006). White cell counts can be misleading as they are raised as a consequence of the pregnancy. A delay in the diagnosis of acute appendicitis can put the fetus at risk and a ruptured appendicitis is associated with a fetal loss rate of between 20% and 25% (Kilpatrick et al, 2007). It is therefore essential to confirm the diagnosis by ultrasonography. This avoids ionising radiation but can be difficult due to the displaced anatomy. Not visualising the appendix does not rule appendicitis out and therefore the diagnosis would still be in question. In such cases the use of computed tomography would need to be considered with due consideration given to the associated risks and benefits. Magnetic resonance imaging is another possibility however, large scale studies demonstrating its accuracy in pregnant patients are lacking and therefore no definitive conclusion can be made regarding its usefulness (Blumenfeld et al, 2011).

11. Atypical presentations of acute appendicitis

The literature detail numerous atypical presentations. Akbulut et al (2010) report a case of a 21 year old lady with congenital situs inversus presenting with acute appendicitis. She had a one day history of mid epigastric pain which migrated to the left iliac fossa. Her white cell count was normal on admission although clinical examination revealed tenderness and guarding in the left iliac fossa. The diagnosis was confirmed on ultrasonography and she subsequently underwent an open appendicectomy. What is notable about this case is that the patient's history was 'classical' apart from the migration of the pain to the left iliac fossa. Given her situs inversus, the reason for her left sided migratory pain is obvious. It is worthy of note that her chest radiograph demonstrated dextrocardia and a right sided gastric bubble. In patients presenting with such histories, dextrocardia can be deduced either from plain radiographs or from the clinical examination of the cardio-respiratory system. One should bear in mind that as the vermiform appendix can end up in the left side of the abdomen as a result of midgut malrotation, dextrocardia may not always be present.

Chae et al (2007) report a case of a 49 year old lady who underwent a colonoscopy as part of a bowel screening programme. The colonoscopy was uneventful and all caecal landmarks were identified. The lady was well post procedure and discharged home the same day. She developed progressively worsening right sided abdominal pain and was seen in the outpatient department four days later. Her blood tests were within normal limits but physical examination revealed tenderness in her right iliac fossa. Appendicitis was confirmed on ultrasonography and the patient subsequently underwent an appendicectomy and was discharged 3 days later. The potential mechanisms suggested for this rare complication of colonoscopy are increased intra-luminal pressure due to gas insufflation and possible displacement of faecoliths into the appendiceal lumen. The authors also suggest that ulceration of the appendiceal mucosa by the colonoscope was a possibility.

Another unusual presentation of acute appendicitis is as a small bowel obstruction with raised inflammatory markers. Harrison et al (2009) describe two elderly patients presenting with small bowel obstruction diagnosed on computed tomography scans to be due to an acute appendicitis (Figure 3). Often the inflammatory process that accompanies acute appendicitis can result in small bowel obstruction. A similar case has been reported by Assenza et al (2005) who suggested that adherence of the inflamed tip of the appendix to the posterior peritoneum across the terminal ileum resulted in bowel compression.

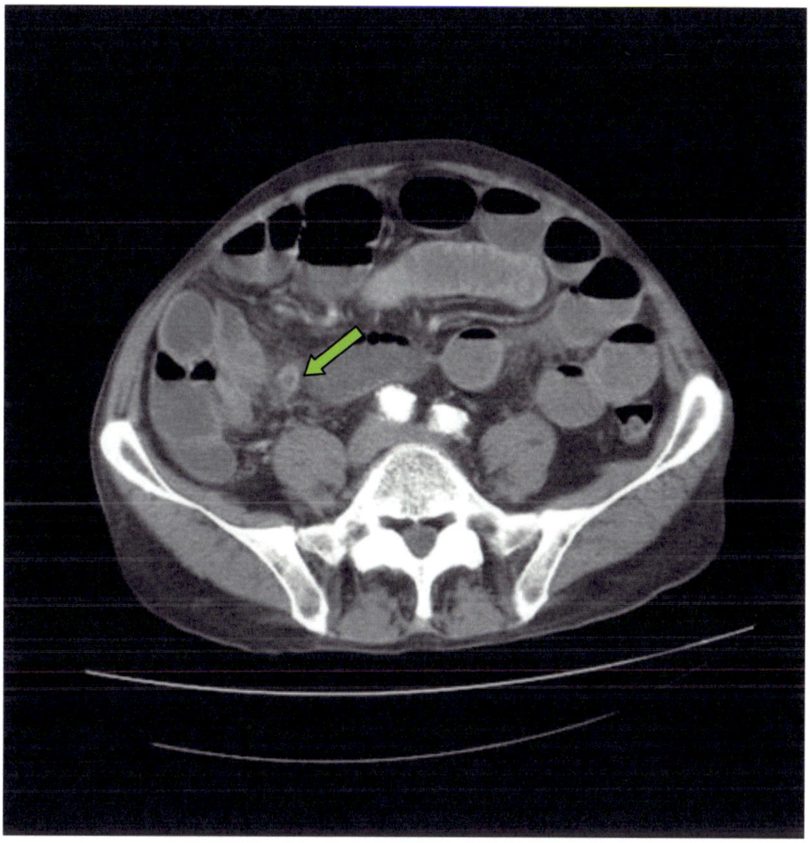

Fig. 3. A computed tomographic image illustrating an inflamed appendix (arrow) with a co-existent small bowel obstruction. (Harrison et al, 2009)

D'Ambrosio et al (2006) report a case of a 71 year old lady who presented with an inflamed tender lump on her right proximal thigh which had been progressively increasing in size over the preceding two weeks. On examination she was noted to have a tender erythematous and indurated mass near her inguinal region and laboratory investigations demonstrated a marked leucocytosis. Subsequent computed tomography demonstrated the inferior portion of the caecum to be thickened and in contact with an inflammatory mass which was contained in a femoral hernia. The patient underwent a laparotomy and right hemicolectomy. The appendix was found to be perforated and abscess formation was also noted and drained at surgery. While inflamed appendices within a hernia is rare, it should be noted that the perforation of the appendix into a limited space prevents the spillage of enteric contents into the abdominal cavity. In this case the perforated appendix was contained within the femoral hernia and so rather than developing diffuse peritonitis, the patient developed superficial signs of erythema, tenderness and induration.

12. Conclusion

Diagnosing appendicitis can pose considerable challenges even to the experienced clinician. A delayed or missed diagnosis can have complications which can result in morbidity and medicolegal claims. To minimise the risks of missing the diagnosis, it is important for clinicians involved in the initial assessment of patients to have a good understanding of factors that can influence the clinical presentation. The clinician should be aware of atypical presentations especially at extremes of age and in pregnancy. No single test nor a combination of tests can distinguish all cases of acute appendicitis from other conditions. An awareness of the limitations of imaging, blood tests and scoring systems is essential. A thorough history and repeated clinical examinations if necessary in conjunction with the results of the appropriate investigations are essential to diagnose acute appendicitis. Sometimes, in equivocal cases, a period of clinical observation is necessary. Despite the advances made in diagnostic modalities, patience may prove to be the most valuable. Often, time and expert clinical review are key to successfully diagnosing acute appendicitis.

13. Acknowledgements

The authors would like to thank Mrs Sindhu Harrison for her help with the artwork for this article.

14. References

Ahmed I, Asgeirsson KS, Beckingham IJ et al (2007). The position of the vermiform appendix at laparoscopy. *Surgical and Radiological Anatomy,* 29(2):165-8.

Akbulut S, Ulku A, Senol A et al (2010). Left-sided appendicitis: review of 95 published cases and a case report. *World Journal of Gastroenterology,* 16(44):5598-602

Al-Salem AH, Qureshi ZS, Qaisarudin S et al (1998). Is acute appendicitis different in patients with sickle cell disease? *Pediatric Surgery International,* 13(4):265-7

Alloo J, Gerstle T, Shilyansky J et al (2004). Appendicitis in children less than 3 years of age: a 28 year review. *Paediatric Surgery International,* 19:777-779

Alvarado A (1986). A practical score for the early diagnosis of acute appendicitis. *Annals of Emergency Medicine,* 15:557-564

Alzaraa A, Chaudhry S (2009). An unusually long appendix in a child: a case report. *Cases Journal,* 11;2:7398.

Andersson R, Hugander A, Thulin A et al (1995). Clusters of acute appendicitis. Further evidence of an infectious aetiology. *International Journal of Epidemiology,* 24:829-833

Andersson RE (2004), Meta-analysis of the clinical and laboratory diagnosis of appendicitis. *British Journal of Surgery,* 91(1):28-37

Andreou P, Blain S, du Boulay EH (1990). A histopathological study of the appendix at autopsy and after surgical resection. *Histopatholoy,* 17:427-431

Arnbjornsson E, Bengmark S (1983). Obstruction of the appendix lumen in relation to pathogenesis of acute appendicitis. *Acta Chirugica Scandinavica,* 149:789-791

Arnbjornsson E, Bengmark S (1984). Role of obstruction in the pathogenesis of acute appendicitis. *American Journal of Surgery,* 147:390-392

Assenza M, Ricci G, Bartolucci P (2005). Mechanical small bowel obstruction due to an inflamed appendix wrapping around the last loop of ileum. *Giornale di Chirugia,* 26(6-7):261-6.

Azodi SO, Sandberg AA, Larsson H (2009). Genetic and environmental influences on the risk of acute appendicitis in twins. *British Journal of Surgery,* 96(11):1336-40

Barker AP, Davey RB (1988). Appendicitis in the first three years of life. *Australian and New Zealand Journal of Surgery,* 58:491-494

Barker JP, Morris J, Nelson M (1986). Vegetable consumption and acute appendicitis in 59 areas in England and Wales. *British Medical Journal,* 292:927-930

Beltrán MA, Almonacid J, Vicencio A et al (2007). Predictive value of white blood cell count and C-reactive protein in children with appendicitis. *Journal of Paediatric Surgery,* 42(7):1208-1214

Binderow SR, Shaked AA (1991). Acute appendicitis in patients with AIDS/HIV infection. *American Journal of Surgery,* 162(1):9-12.

Birnbaum BA, Wilson SR (2000). Appendicitis at the Millennium. *Radiology,* 215:337-48

Blab E, Kohlhuber U, Tillawi S et al (2004). Advancements in the diagnosis of acute appendicitis in children and adolescents. *European Journal of Paediatric Surgery,* 14:404-409

Blumenfeld YJ, Wong AE, Jafari A et al (2011). MR imaging in cases of antenatal suspected appendicitis--a meta-analysis. *Journal of Maternal, Fetal and Neonatal Medicine,* 24(3):485-8.

Burkitt DP (1971). The etiology of appendicitis. *British Journal of Surgery,*58:695-699

Burkitt DP, Walker RP, Painter NS (1972). Effect of dietary fibre on stools and transit times, and its role in the causation of disease. *Lancet,* 2:1408-1412

Carr NJ (2000). The pathology of acute appendicitis. *Annals of Diagnostic Pathology,* 4(1):46-58

Chae HS, Jeon SY, Nam WS (2007). Acute appendicitis caused by colonoscopy. *Korean Journal of Internal Medicine,* 22(4):308-11

Chang AR (1981). An analysis of the pathology of 3003 appendices. *Australian and New Zealand Journal of Surgery,*51:169-178

Choi D, Park H, Lee YR et al (2003). The most useful findings for diagnosing acute appendicitis on contrast enhances helical CT. *Acta Radiologica,* 44:574-82

Chung CH, Ng CP, Lai KK (2000). Delays by patients, emergency physicians and surgeons in the management of acute appendicitis: retrospective study. *Hong Kong Medical Journal,* 6:254-259

Chung JL, Kong MS, Lin SL et al (1996). Diagnostic value of C-reactive protein in children with perforated appendicitis. *European Journal of Paediatrics,* 155:529-531

Codon RE, Telford GL (1991). Appendicitis; In:Townsend CM (eds). Sabiston Text book of Surgery: The biological basis of modern surgical practice. 14th ed, *Philadelphia, Pa:WB Saunders and Co;* pp 884-898

Coggon D, Barker JP, Cruddas et al (1991). Housing and appendicitis in Anglesey. *Journal of Epidemiology and Community Health,* 45:244-246

Collins DC (1932). The Length and Position of the Vermiform Appendix: A Study of 4,680 Specimens. *Annals of Surgery,* 96(6):1044-8

Daehlin L (1982) Acute appendicitis during the first three years of life. *Acta Chirugica Scandinavic,* 148:291-294

D'Ambrosio N, Katz D, Hines J (2006). Perforated appendix within a femoral hernia. *AJR American Journal of Roentgenology,* 186(3):906-7

Devlin B (1971). Midgut malrotation causing intestinal obstruction. *Annals of the Royal College of Surgeons of England,* 48:227-237

Doria AS, Moineddin R, Kellenberger CJ et al (2006). US or CT for diagnosis of appendicitis in children and adults? A meta analysis. *Radiology,* 241:83-94

Dueholm S, Bagi P, Bud M (1989). Laboratory aid in the diagnosis of acute appendicitis. A blinded, prospective trial concerning diagnostic value of leukocyte count, neutrophil differential count, and C-reactive protein. *Diseases of the Colon and Rectum,* 32(10):855-9.

Ergul E (2007). Heredity and familial tendency of acute appendicitis. *Scandinavian Journal of Surgery,* 96(4):290-2

Erkasap S, Ates E, Ustuner Z et al (2000). Diagnostic value of interleukin-6 and C-reactive protein in acute appendicitis. *Swiss Surgery.*6(4):169-72

Fang YJ, Wang HP, Ho CM et al (2009). Barium appendicitis. *Surgery,* 146(5):957-8

Fefferman NR, Roche KJ, Pinkney LP et al (2001). Suspected appendicitis in children: focussed CT technique for evaluation. *Radiology,* 220:691-5

Fraser N, Gannon C, Stringer MD (2004). Appendicular colic and the non-inflamed appendix: fact or fiction? *European Journal of Paediatric Surgery,* 14(1):21-4.

Friedland JA, Siegel MJ (1997). CT appearance of acute appendicitis in childhood. *AJR American Journal of Roentgenology,* 168:439-442

Haaga JR, Lanzieri CF, Gilkeson RC et al (2003). CT and MR imaging of the whole body. 4th edition, St Louis: Mosby: 2061

Harrison S, Mahawar K, Brown D et al (2009). Acute appendicitis presenting as small bowel obstruction: two case reports. *Cases Journal,* Nov 28;2:9106.

Herrinton JL (1991). The vermiform appendix: its surgical history. *Contemporary Surgery,* 39:36-44

Hiraiwa H, Umemoto M, Take H (1995). Prevalence of appendectomy in Japanese families. *Acta Paediatrica Japan,* 37:691-693

Hiu TT, Major KM, Avital I et al (2002). Outcome of elderly patients with appendicitis. *Archives of Surgery,* 135:479-88

Hodjati H, Kazerooni T (2003). Location of the appendix in the gravid patient: a re-evaluation of the established concept. *International Journal of Gynaecology and Obstetrics,* 81(3):245-7

Horton WL (1977). Pathogenesis of acute appendicitis. *British Medical Journal,*2:1672-1673

Horwitz JR, Gursoy M, Jaksic et al (1997). Importance of diarrhoea as a presenting symptom of appendicitis in very young children. *American Journal of Surgery,* 173:80-82

Horzić M, Salamon A, Kopljar M et al (2005). Analysis of scores in diagnosis of acute appendicitis in women. *Collegium Anthropologicum,* 29(1):133-8

Hsu KF, Yu JC, Chan DC et al (2011). Atypical acute appendicitis and its complications: a rare location of the appendix in the periduodenum. *Acta Gastroenterologica Belgica,* 74(1):105

Humes D, Speake WJ, Simpson J (2007). Appendcitis. *Clinical Evidence,* Jul 1;2007. pii: 0408

Jones WG, Barie PS (1988). Urological manifestations of acute appendicitis. *Journal of Urology,* 139(6):1325-1328

Karim OM, Boothroyd AE, Wyllie JH (1990). McBurney's point--fact or fiction? *Annals of the Royal College of Surgeons of England,* 72(5):304-8.

Kessler N, Cyteval C, Gallix B et al (2004). Appendicitis: evaluation of sensitivity, specificity and predictive values of US, Doppler US and laboratory findings. *Radiology,* 230:472-8

Kharbanda AB, Cosme Y, Liu K et al (2011). Discriminative accuracy of novel and traditional biomarkers in children with suspected appendicitis adjusted for duration of abdominal pain. *Academic Emergency Medicine,* 18(6):567-74.

Kilpatrick CC, Monga M (2007). Approach to the acute abdomen in pregnancy. *Obstetric and Gynaecology Clinics of North America,* 34:389-402

Klinger PJ, Smith SL, Abdenstein BJ et al (1997). Management of ingested foreign bodies within the appendix: a case report with review of the literature. *American Journal of Gastroenterology,* 92:2295-2298

Körner H, Söndenaa K, Söreide JA et al (1997). Incidence of Acute Nonperforated and Perforated Appendicitis: Age-specific and Sex-specific Analysis. *World Journal of Surgery,* 21(3):313-317

Kozar RA, Roslyn JL (1999). The appendix. In: Principles of Surgery. 7th International edition, Seymour I Schwartz, (ed); *McGraw-Hill Health Profession Division,* pp 1383-94

Lamps LW (2010). Infectious causes of appendicitis. *Infectious Disease Clinics of North America,* 24(4):995-1018

Larner AJ (1988). The etiology of appendicitis. *British Journal of Hospital Medicine,* 39:540-542

Levine CD, Aizenstein O, Lehavi O et al (2005). Why we miss the diagnosis of appendicitis on abdominal CT: evaluation of imaging features of appendicitis incorrectly diagnosed on CT. *AJR American Journal of Roentgenology,I* 184:855-859

Macklin CP, Radcliffe GS, Merei JM et al (1997). A prospective evaluation of the modified Alvarado score for acute appendicitis in children. *Annals of the Royal College of Surgeons of England,* 79(3):203-5

Malik KA, Khan A, Waheed I (2000). Evaluation of the Alvarado score in diagnosis of acute appendicitis. *Journal of the College of Physicians Surgeons Pakistan,* 10:392-4

Merlin MA, Shah CN, Shiroff AM (2010). Evidence based appendicitis: The initial work up. *Postgraduate Medicine,* 122(3):189-195

Mourad J, Elliol JP, Erikson L et al (2000). Appendicitis in pregnancy: new information that contradicts long held clinical beliefs. *American Journal of Obstetrics and Gynaecology,* 182(5):1027-0

Nayak BS (2010). Why the tip of vermiform appendix has variable position? *Medical Hypotheses,* 75(6):682-683

Ohmann C, Yang Q, Franke C (1995). Diagnostic scores for acute appendicitis. Abdominal Pain Study Group. *European Journal of Surgery,* 161(4):273-81

Old J, Dusing RW, Yap W (2005). Imaging for suspected appendicitis. *American family Physician,* 71(1):71-78

Old O (2011). C-Reactive protein estimation does not improve accuracy in the diagnosis of acute appendicitis in pediatric patients. *International Journal of Surgery,* 9(5):440

Oto A, Srinivasan PN, Ernsl RD et al (2006). Revisiting MRI for appendix location during pregnancy. *AJR American Journal of Roentgenology,* 186(3):883-7

Paajanen H, Mansikka A, Laato M et al (1997). Are serum inflammatory markers age dependent in acute appendicitis? *Journal of the American College of Surgeons,* 184:303-308

Paajanen H, Mansikka A, Laato M et al (2002). Novel serum inflammatory markers in acute appendicitis. *Scandinavian Journal of Clinical Laboratory Investigation,* 62(8):579-84

Paranjape C, Dalia S, Pan J, Horattas M (2007). Appendicitis in the elderly: a change in the laparoscopic era. *Surgical Endoscopy,* 21(5):777-81

Paulson EK, Kalady MF, Pappas TN (2003). Clinical Practice. Suspected appendicitis. *New England Journal of Medicine,* 348:236-242

Pedrosa I, Lafornara M, Pandharipande PV et al (2009). Pregnant patients suspected of having acute appendicitis: effect of MR imaging on negative laparotomy rate and appendiceal perforation rate. *Radiology,* 250(3):749-57.

Peitola H, Ahlqvist J, Rapola J et al (1986). C reactive protein compared with white blood cell count and erythrocyte sedimentation rate in the diagnosis of acute appendicitis in children. *Acta Chirugica Scandianavica,* 152:55-58

Puskar D, Bedalov G, Fridrih S et al (1995). Urinalysis, ultrasound analysis, and renal dynamic scintigraphy in acute appendicitis. *Journal of Urology,* 45(1):108-112

Puylaert JB (1986). Acute appendicitis: US evaluation using graded compression. *Radiology,* 158:355-60

Rao PM, Boland GW (1998a). Imaging of acute right lower abdominal quadrant pain. *Clinical Radiology,* 53:639-49

Rao PM, Rhea JT, Novelline RA et al (1998b). Effect of computed tomography of the appendix on treatment of patients and use of hospital resources. *New England Journal of Medicine,* 338:141-6

Rao PM, Rhea JT, Rao JA et al (1999). Plain abdominal radiography in clinically suspected appendicitis: diagnostic yield, resource use and comparison with CT. *American Journal of Emergency Medicine,* 17:325-328

Raynor MR, Cliff AD, Ord JK (2010). Common acute childhood infections and appendicitis: a historical study of statistical association in 27 English public boarding schools, 1930-1934. *Epidemiology and Infection,* 138(8):1155-65

Rothrock SG, Skeoch G, Rush JJ et al (1991). Clinical features of misdiagnosed appendicitis in children. *Annals of Emergency Medicine,* 20:45-50

Rumack CM, Wilson SR, Charboneau JW et al (1998). Diagnostic ultrasound. 2nd ed. St Louis: Mosby, 1998:303-6

Rusnak RA, Borer JM, Fastow JS et al (1994). Misdiagnosis of acute appendicitis: common features discovered in cases after litigation. *American Journal of Emergency Medicine,* 12:397-402

Sack U, Biereder B, Elouahidi T et al (2006). Diagnostic value of blood inflammatory markers for detection of acute appendicitis in children. *BMC Surgery,* 28;6:15

Sahana's Human Anatomy, Descriptive and Applied (1994). Vol II, Ankur ed, Ankur Publications (AP), pp 362-367

Sanjuán JC, Martín-Parra JI, Seco I et al (1999). C-reactive protein and leukocyte count in the diagnosis of acute appendicitis in children. *Diseases of the Colon and Rectum,* 42(10):1325-1329

Sasso RD, Hanna EA, Moore DL (1970). Leucocyte and neutrophilic counts in acute appendicitis. *American Journal of Surgery,* 120(5):563-566

Schumpelick V, Dreuw B, Ophoff K et al (2000). Appendix and caecum. Embryology, anatomy and surgical applications. *Surgical Clinics of North America,* 80:295-318

Sengupta A, Bax G, Paterson-Brown S (2009). White cell count and C-reactive protein measurement in patients with possible appendicitis. *Annals of the Royal College of Surgeons of England,* 91(2):113-5

Sharma SB, Gupta V, Sharma SC (2005). Acute appendicitis presenting as thigh abscess in a child: a case report..

Sieren LM, Collins JN, Weireter LJ (2010). The incidence of benign and malignant neoplasia presenting as acute appendicitis, *The American Surgeon,* 76(8):808-11

Simpson J, Scholefield JH (2002). Acute appendicitis. *Clinical Evidence,* 20(7):153-157

Sisson RG, Ahlvin RC, Harlow MC (1971). Superficial mucosal ulceration and the pathogenesis of acute appendicitis. *American Journal of Surgery,* 122:378-380

Smith PH (1965). The diagnosis of acute appendicitis. *Post Graduate Medical Journal,* 41:2-5

Sulu B, Gunerhan Y, Palanci Y et al (2010). Epidemiological and demographic features of appendicitis and influences of several environmental factors. *Turkish Journal of Trauma & Emergency Surgery,* 16(1):38-42

Terasawa T, Blackmore CC, Bent S et al (2004). Systematic review: computed tomography and ultrasonography to detect acute appendicitis in adults and adolescents. *Annals of Internal Medicine,* 141(7):537-46

Terry TR, Cook AJ, Talbot A et al (1983). Facial expression in acute appendicitis. *Annals of the Royal College of Surgeons of England,* 65(1):65

Thyagaraj J (2005). Study of the anatomical position of the appendix in normal population and inflamed cases. Accessed June 18th, 2011. Available from : http://119.82.96.198:8080/jspui/bitstream/123456789/1037/1/CDMGENS00045.pdf

Toumi Z, Chan A, Hadfield MB et al (2010). Systematic review of blunt abdominal trauma as a cause of acute appendicitis. *Annals of the Royal College of Surgeons of England,* 92(6):477-482

Tsai SH, Hsu CW, Chen SC (2008). Complicated acute appendicitis in diabetic patients. *American Journal of Surgery,* 196(1):34-9

Vermeulen B, Morabia A, Under PF (1995). Influence of white cell count on surgical decision making in patients with abdominal pain in the right lower quadrant. *European Journal of Surgery,*161(7):483-486

Vissers RJ, Lennarz WB (2010). Pitfalls in appendicitis. *Emergency Medicine Clinics of North America,*28:103-118

Wakeley C (1933). The Position of the Vermiform Appendix as Ascertained by an Analysis of 10,000 Cases. *Journal of Anatomy,* 67(2):277-283

Walker AR, Segal I (1995). Appendicitis: an African perspective. *Journal of the Royal Society of Medicine,* 88:616-619

Walker RP, Segal I (1990). What causes appendicitis? *Journal of Clinical Gastroenterology,* 12:127-129

Wilson EB, Cole JC, Nipper ML et al (2001). Computed tomography and ultrasonography in the diagnosis of appendicitis: when are they indicated? *Archives of Surgery,* 136:670-5

Wise SW, Labuski MR, Kasales CJ et al (2001). Comparative assessment of CT and sonographic techniques for appendiceal imaging. *AJR American Journal of Roentgenology,* 176:933-41

Zimmermann PG (2008). Is it appendicitis? *American Journal of Nursing,* 108(9):27-31

3

Imaging in Suspected Appendicitis

Nadim M. Muallem, Antoine N. Wadih and Maurice C. Haddad
American University of Beirut Medical Center, Department of Diagnostic Radiology, Beirut, Lebanon

1. Introduction

This chapter reviews the imaging modalities available for the diagnosis of appendicitis. The advantages and disadvantages of each technique and the impact of pre-operative imaging on the management of appendicitis as well cost- effectiveness are discussed.

2. Epidemiology

Appendicitis is a common problem encountered in acute care departments and represents approximately one fourth of all acute abdominal emergencies [1]. Addiss et al [2], estimated that approximately 250,000 cases of appendicitis occur annually in the United States alone. In a population of about 300 million, this translates into 1 case per 1200 individuals per year. The highest incidence of appendicitis was found in those aged 10-19 years with males having higher rates of appendicitis than females for all age groups. The lifetime risk of appendicitis is 8.6% for males and 6.7% for females whereas the lifetime risk of appendectomy is higher, estimated at 12.0% for males and 23.1% for females [2]. This suggests that more appendectomies are performed than required. Note that these figures were based on data collected during 1979-1984 at a time when cross-sectional imaging technology was only burgeoning, but it illustrates well the concern practitioners had about the morbidity and mortality of a ruptured or perforated appendicitis. The mortality rate of a complicated appendicitis had reached 3% and about 47% of patients experienced significant morbidity [3], which led to the accepted general notion that a negative appendectomy rate of 20% was acceptable with its much lower morbidity to balance the higher risks associated with perforation. Overall, an estimated 36 incidental procedures are performed to prevent one future case of appendicitis. Currently, negative appendectomy rates are much less, because of the incorporation of imaging tests in the pre-operative work-up.

In patients presenting to the emergency room with right iliac fossa pain, appendicitis remains the most frequent diagnosis accounting for 39% of patients, whilst less frequent causes include: non-specific abdominal pain (26%), gynecological (22%), and miscellaneous causes (14%) [4].

Given its high prevalence, the accurate diagnosis of appendicitis is therefore essential in any emergency setting in order to provide the most adequate management. The ideal diagnostic test or process, one with a high sensitivity and specificity, would be one that minimizes the rates of missed appendicitis, but also one that minimizes the need for unnecessary appendectomies.

3. Clinical diagnosis

The clinical diagnosis of appendicitis is suspected on the basis of history, physical examination and laboratory tests. A clinical scoring system may help and one was first developed by Alvarado [5] (see appropriate chapters). In the Alvarado system a low score of 1 to 4 suggests that there is only a low probability of appendicitis and some patients may be discharged without further investigation though some should be considered for imaging. It can be argued that all those with an Alvarado score of 5 to 7 should have imaging performed. In those with Alvarado scores of 8 to 10 there is a very high probability for appendicitis and appendectomy should be performed promptly without further studies.

The standard Alvarado scoring is useful in areas with limited resources and no imaging diagnostic tools. It may even help in avoiding unnecessary testing and eventually unnecessary exposure to ionizing radiation in clear cut cases with typical presentations and clinical findings of appendicitis. However, the standard Alvarado score has inadequate predictive values especially in children [6],[7], and results in a relatively high negative appendectomy rate of 8.8% [8].

Laboratory blood testing has been a staple in the evaluation of any clinically suspected infection; it even figures in the predictive scoring system of Alvarado. However, more recent studies suggest that WBC count is a poor predictor of the severity of the appendicitis [9].

Laparoscopy is a useful diagnostic and potentially therapeutic tool for evaluating patients with right lower abdominal pain especially in women and can be an alternative to active clinical observation [10].

4. Diagnostic imaging

The diagnosis of appendicitis should be prompt and accurate, and dependence on imaging techniques has become necessary. The risks of delay in the management of appendicitis secondary to waiting for imaging are largely outweighed by the benefits of the additional information provided by the imaging tests. Recent data show that the temporal components associated with perforated appendicitis are the duration of pre-hospital symptoms rather than the in-hospital delays to surgery [4]. Recently, a clear evidence-based guideline from the Dutch College of Surgeons recommends that appendectomy should not be carried out without prior imaging [11].

In this section, we review the most commonly available imaging techniques and their application to the diagnosis of appendicitis with emphasis on appropriateness, advantages, disadvantages and contraindications.

4.1 Conventional radiography

The traditional imaging techniques include conventional plain abdominal radiographs (PAR) and barium enema. PAR may show an appendicolith (Fig. 1) which is only present in 15% of patients with appendicitis. Importantly, those without appendicitis may have an incidental appendicolith identified on PAR or on CT scan (Fig. 2), with an incidence estimated at 2.6% in children. Appendicitis has been seen to develop in 5.8% to 6.7% of those with an appendicolith, which is little different than the average lifetime risk. Therefore, an incidental appendicolith may be a marker of increased but low risk for developing appendicitis when compared to the normal population and it is not an indication for prophylactic appendectomy in children and adults [12], [13].

The presence of air-fluid levels in the right lower quadrant or a "sentinel loop" may suggest a localized paralytic ileus or mechanical obstruction. Free peritoneal or extraluminal air can indicate a perforated appendicitis. Loss of the right psoas margin or displacement of the bowel loops in the right lower quadrant may be seen with abscess or phlegmon formation. However, these are non-specific features.

The diagnosis of appendicitis by barium enema depends mainly on the identification of indirect signs including non-filling of the appendix with barium sulfate or the presence of an extrinsic impression on the caecum by an appendiceal abscess.

Both the PAR and barium enema are insensitive methods for diagnosing appendicitis but in the absence of more advanced facilities, they are simple and inexpensive and may provide some useful information. Advanced cross-sectional imaging modalities have largely replaced PAR and barium enema in the diagnosis of appendicitis because of their limited diagnostic value [14].

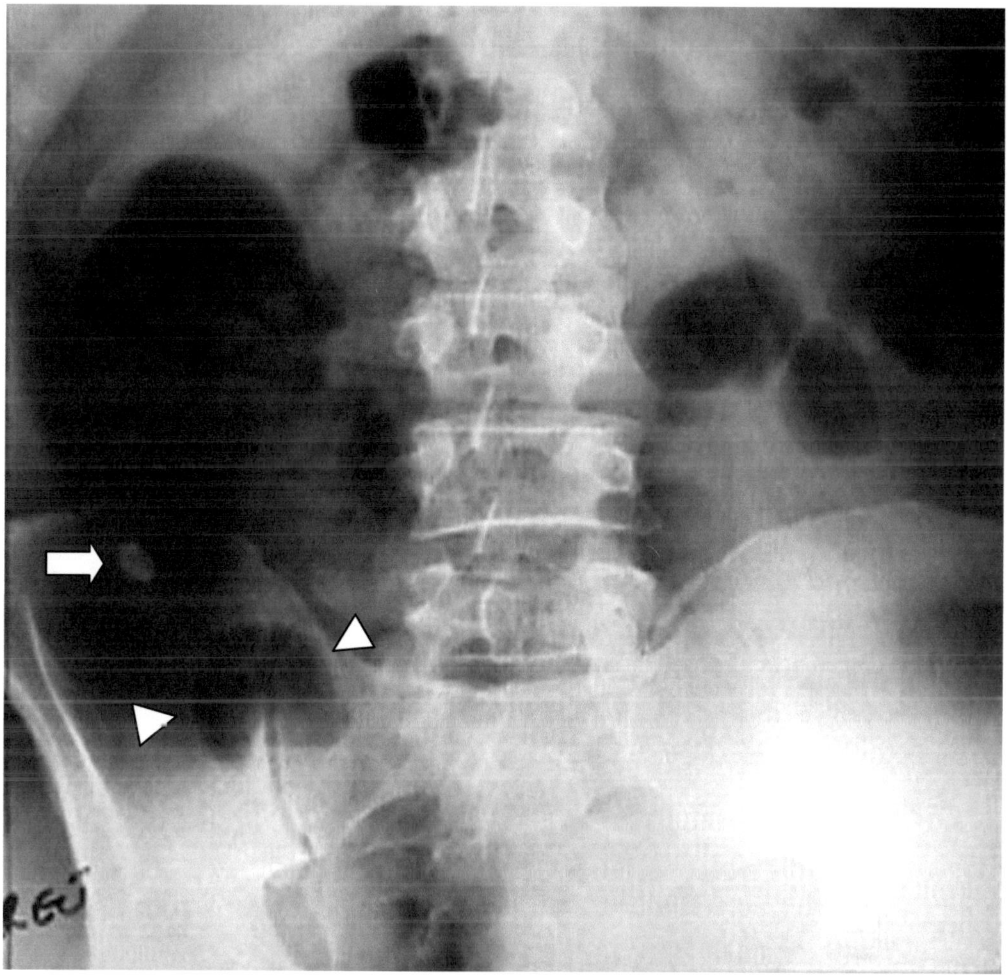

Fig. 1. Plain abdominal radiograph demonstrating the presence of an appendicolith (arrow) and a sentinel loop (arrowheads) in the right lower quadrant.

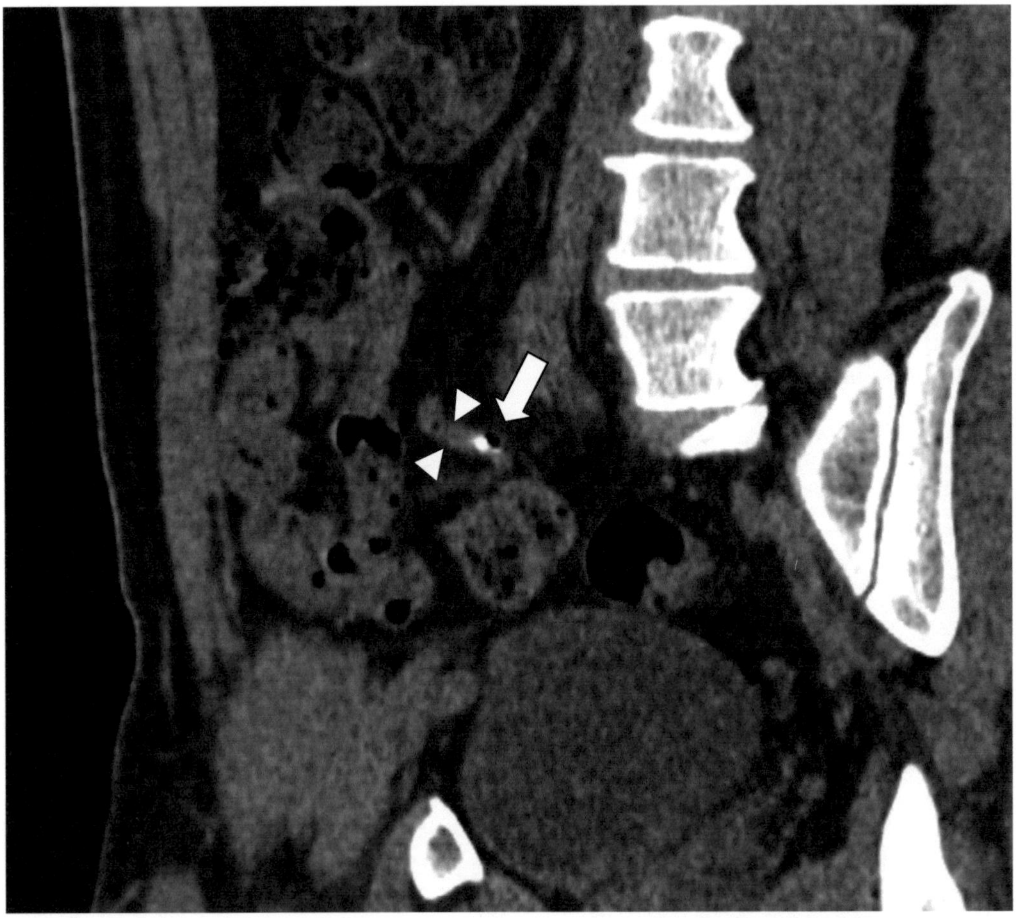

Fig. 2. Incidental appendicolith (white arrow) seen on a non-enhanced MDCT of the abdomen. This patient presented for routine evaluation and had no signs or symptoms of appendicitis. Notice the normal looking appendix (arrowheads) and lack of periappendiceal inflammation.

4.2 Cross-sectional imaging

The most widely used cross-sectional imaging techniques for the diagnosis of appendicitis are graded compression color Doppler ultrasound (CDUS) which is a non-irradiating technique and multi-detector CT scan (MDCT). Each has its particular advantages and disadvantages. MRI has been gaining popularity with its shorter acquisition times and with resolution approaching that of CT imaging without the burden of ionizing radiation.

4.2.1 Ultrasound US

Graded compression sonography using a linear high frequency 5-12 MHz transducer is a non-invasive low cost technique which is particularly suitable for children, young and pregnant women with suspected appendicitis. However, sonography has limitations especially in the obese where tissue penetration is reduced and in the presence of a retrocecal appendix surrounded by bowel gas which prevents sound transmission. US allows visualization of a normal appendix in approximately 4% - 12% of patients without appendicitis as opposed to 43% to 75% with more advanced modalities such as MDCT [14], [15], [16]. Finally, sonography is essentially operator-dependent and requires years of formative training. Qualified technologists are not always available and the sensitivity of the examination is directly affected by the operator's competence, therefore, it has to be performed by experienced sonographers.

On real-time graded compression sonography, the identification of a non-compressible, thickened appendix greater than 6-7 mm in diameter is diagnostic of appendicitis (Fig. 3a, 3b). Other associated findings that can be determined on ultrasound are the presence of a hyperechoic appendicolith with posterior acoustic shadowing, or the presence of anechoic fluid or an abscess in the right lower quadrant (Fig. 4). Similar to the sonographic Murphy's sign in the diagnosis of cholecystitis, a sonographic "McBurney's" sign can be elicited by compressing the visualized inflamed appendix using the ultrasound probe which further enhances the diagnostic value of the ultrasound examination.

Color Doppler sonography permits the detection of increased blood flow in the wall of the inflamed appendix (Fig. 3c) and the absence of blood flow in the thickened appendiceal wall of the gangrenous appendix.

Real-time ultrasound elastography can be helpful in the depiction of the severity of inflammation [17].

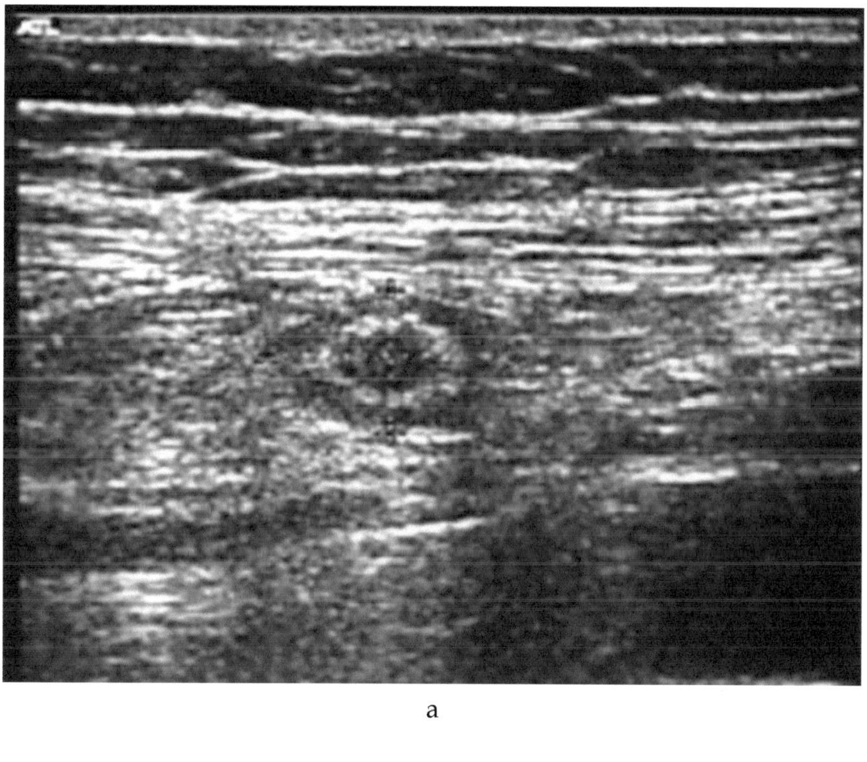

a

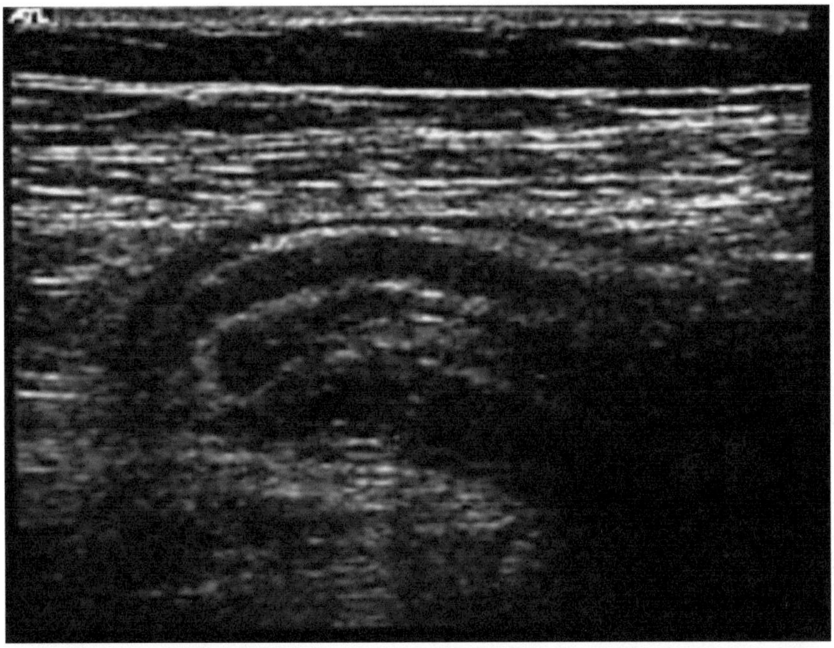

b

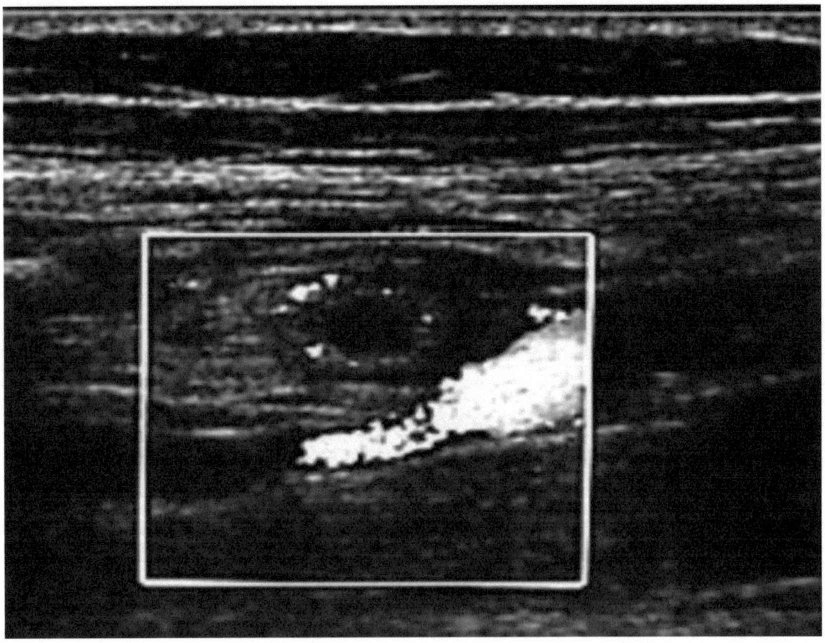

c

Fig. 3. Graded compression sonography images in transverse (a) and longitudinal (b) sections of an enlarged, non-compressible appendix (cursors) compatible with non-complicated appendicitis. Color Doppler flow image (c) demonstrated increased blood flow in the wall of the inflamed appendix due to hyperemia.

Because of its diagnostic limitations, if sonography is not capable of demonstrating a normal appendix or the sonographic diagnosis of appendicitis is equivocal, indeterminate or inconclusive, further evaluation preferably by more advanced cross-sectional imaging is required, such as an emergency MRI (in pediatric, young or pregnant patients). If MRI is not available, a contrast enhanced low dose MDCT with lower mA and kV exposure factors to minimize radiation is an option.

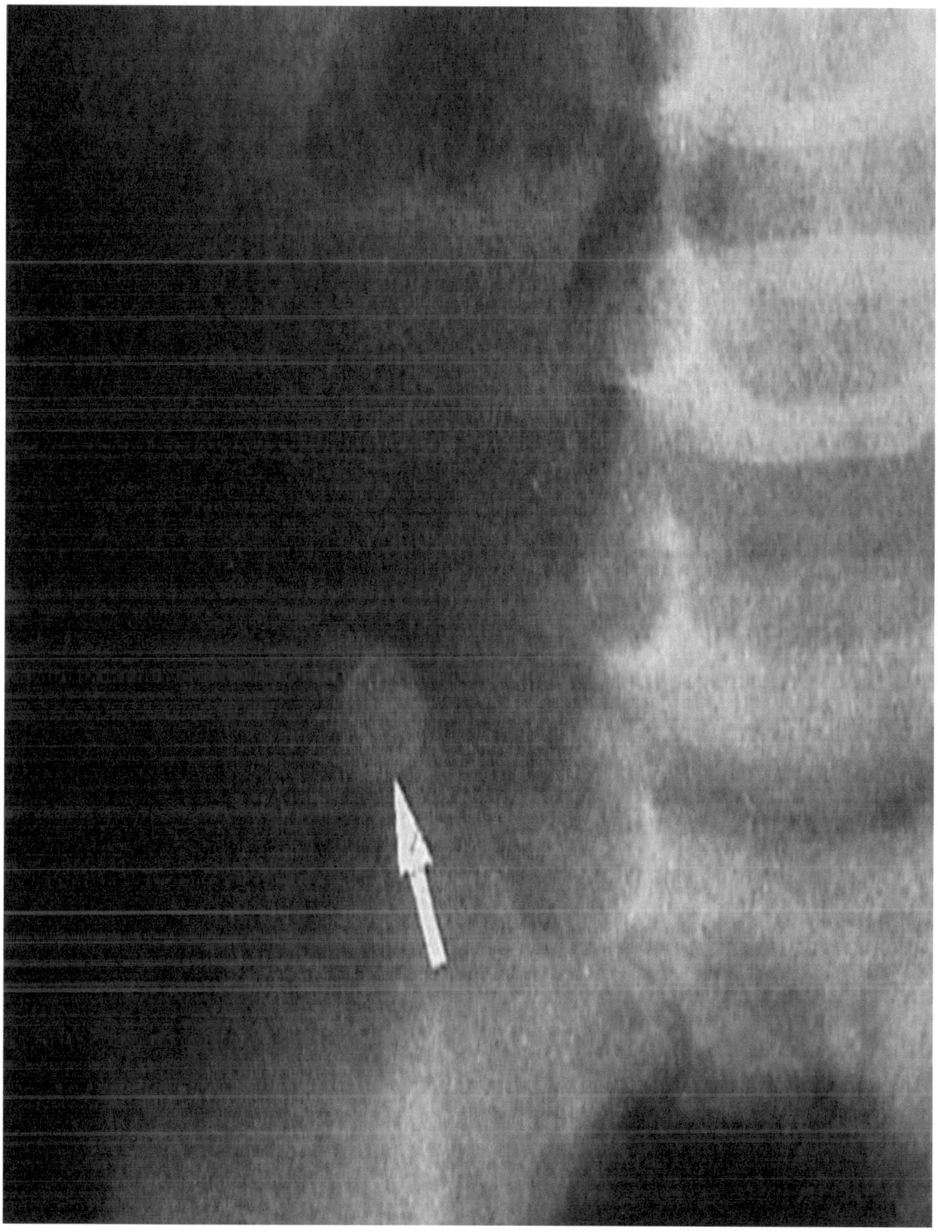

a

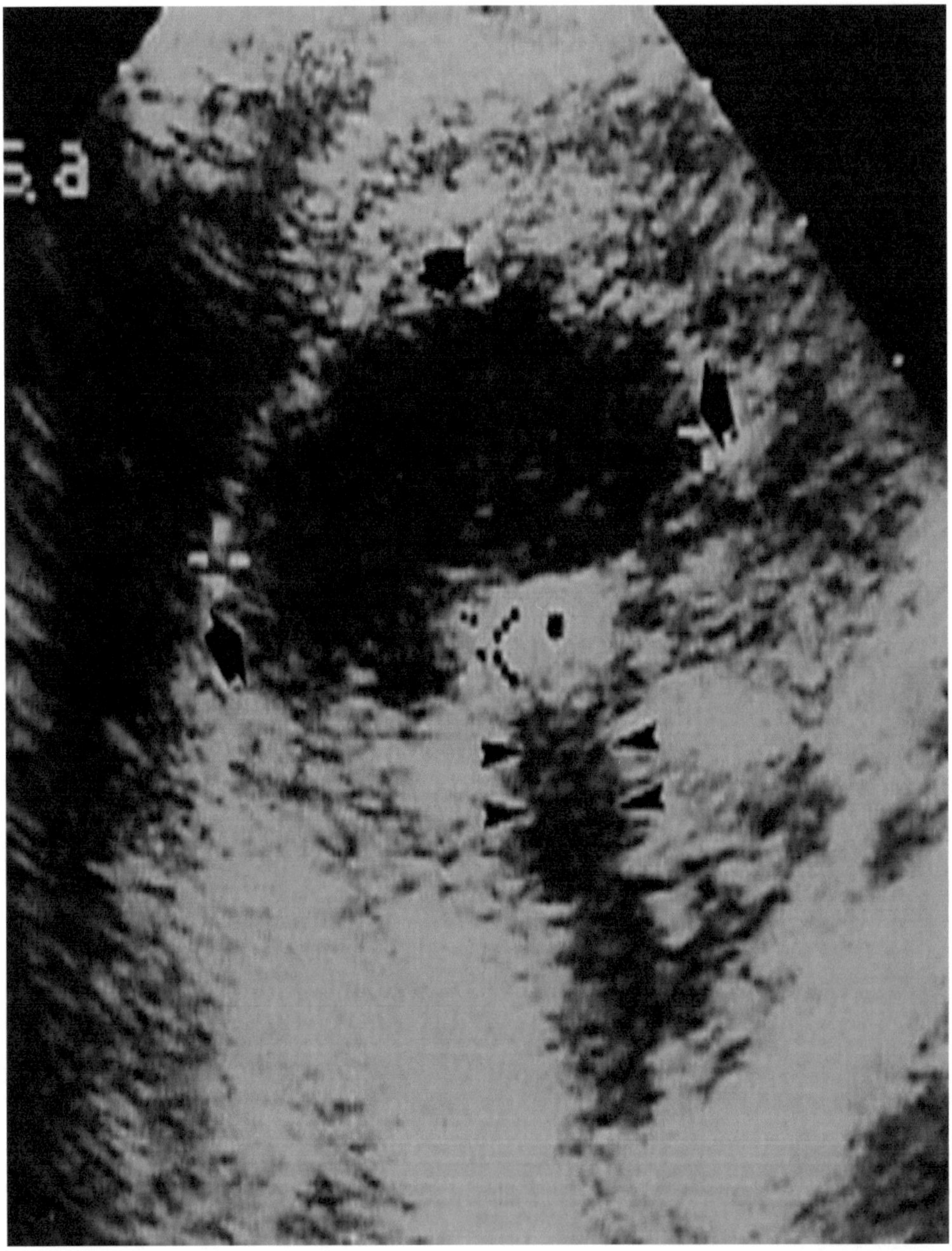

b

Fig. 4. Plain abdominal radiograph (a) and focal right lower quadrant ultrasound (b) images in a child with an appendiceal abscess showing the presence of an appendicolith (white arrow) on the plain abdominal radiograph, which demonstrates increased echogenicity and posterior acoustic shadowing on ultrasound (black arrowhead). The abscess is also seen on ultrasound as an overlying hypoechoic fluid collection containing debris (black arrows).

4.2.2 Multi-Detector Computed Tomography (MDCT)

Multi-detector CT (MDCT) is a fast scanning method which costs more than sonography and uses ionizing radiation. It is because of its exceptional higher diagnostic accuracy, speed of image acquisition and high resolution that MDCT has emerged in many centers as the primary imaging modality for pediatric and non-pregnant adult patients with suspected appendicitis. Table 1 lists the main differences between MDCT and ultrasound for the diagnosis of appendicitis.

Ultrasound	MDCT
Low cost	Higher cost
No radiation (use in children & women)	High radiation dose (caution in children & women, use of low dose MDCT)
Widely available	Not widely available
Operator-dependent	Not operator-dependent
Lower overall reported sensitivity & accuracy	Higher overall reported sensitivity & accuracy
Visualization of a normal appendix in 4%-12% of patients without appendicitis	Visualization of a normal appendix in 43% to 75% of patients without appendicitis

From: Haddad MC, et al. *LMJ* 2003; 51(1):211 5

Table 1. Listed differences between ultrasound and MDCT

Imaging findings on MDCT

On a contrast enhanced MDCT scan with intravenous and oral or rectal contrast, a normal appendix is identified at the cecal pole below the ileo-cecal valve, it appears filled with air and contrast material. Its caliber should be normally less than 7 mm, with intact periappendicular mesenteric fat (Fig. 5). However, a normal appendix may reach 11 mm in maximal diameter on a contrast enhanced MDCT scan with rectal contrast because of a better distention of the colon than with oral contrast [18], [19]. Non-filling of a thickened appendix with enhancement of its wall and streaking of the periappendiceal fat are major and direct diagnostic signs of a non-complicated appendicitis (Fig. 6, 7), whilst an appendicitis complicated by perforation will show periappendiceal abscess formation on MDCT (Fig. 8). An appendicolith may or may not be seen and is usually found on MDCT much more frequently than on conventional radiographs. Secondary or indirect signs of appendicitis which may provide clues to the diagnosis include inflammatory changes and fat streaking around the cecal pole, a fluid collection in the right lower quadrant and small bowel obstruction.

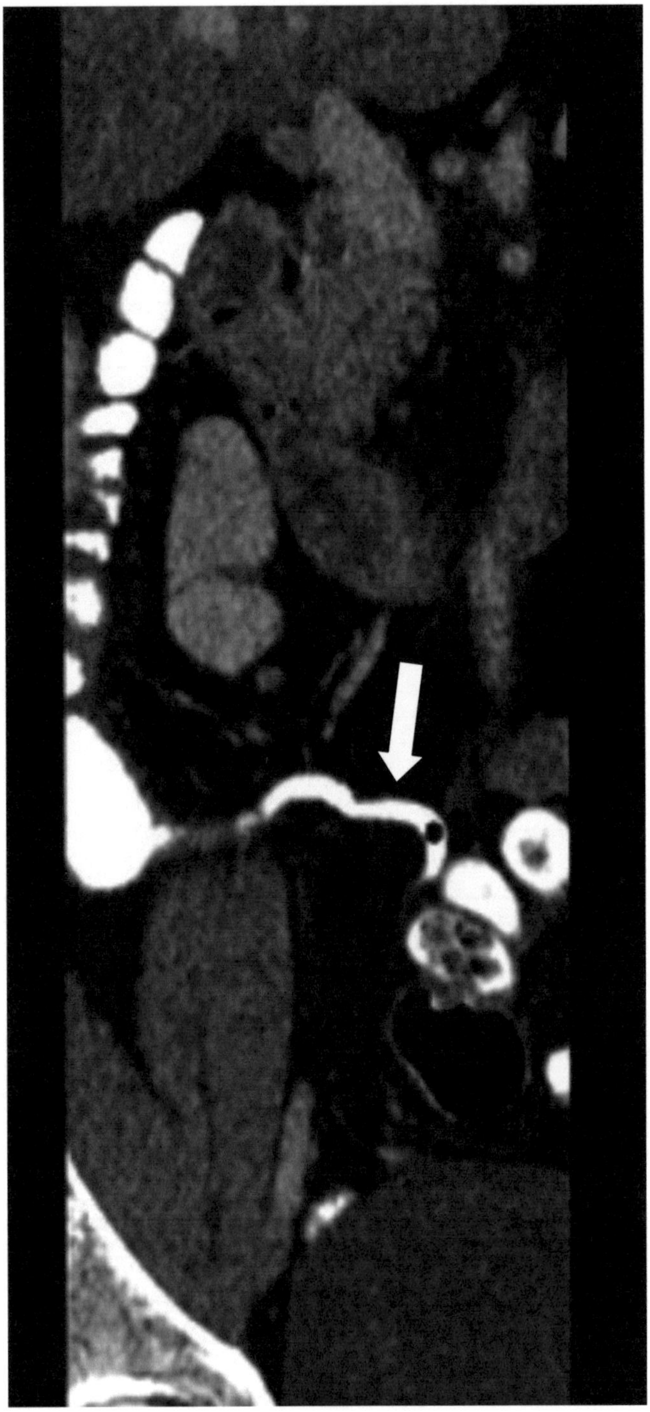

Fig. 5. Coronal image of a MDCT scan with intravenous and rectal contrast enema. The appendix is shown filled with contrast (white arrow) and has a normal caliber (6mm). The surrounding mesenteric fat is intact.

In a study by Nikolaidis et al. [20], non-visualization of the appendix on MDCT with intravenous and oral contrast was encountered in 15% of adults and in 30% of children. The main cause was the paucity of intra-abdominal fat which deprives the radiologist from the negative contrast that fat provides. However, in the absence of a distinctly visualized appendix and secondary inflammatory changes, the incidence of appendicitis was found to be low, estimated at 2%.

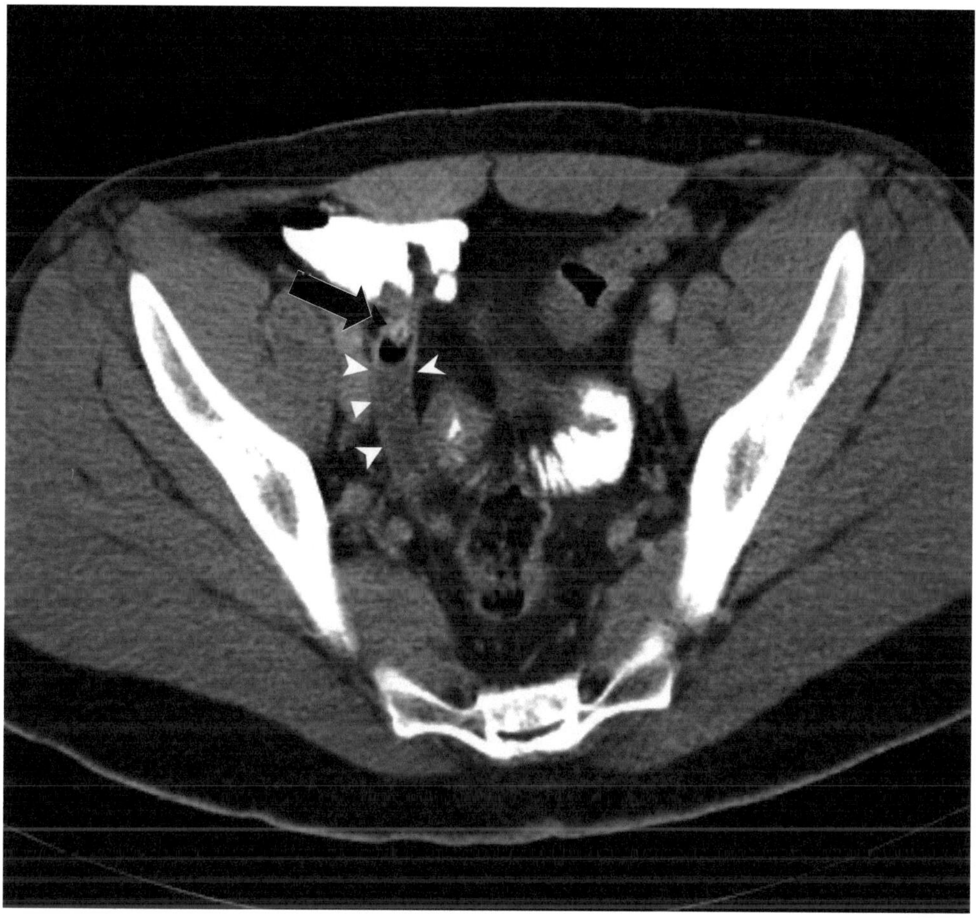

Fig. 6. MDCT scan with intravenous and oral contrast in a 29-year-old man with right lower quadrant pain, vomiting, and low-grade fever. The appendix (white arrowheads) is fluid filled, shows an increased caliber (> 7mm), and is not opacified by contrast despite adequate filling of the cecum consistent with non-complicated appendicitis. An appendicolith (*black arrow*) is identified in its proximal segment.

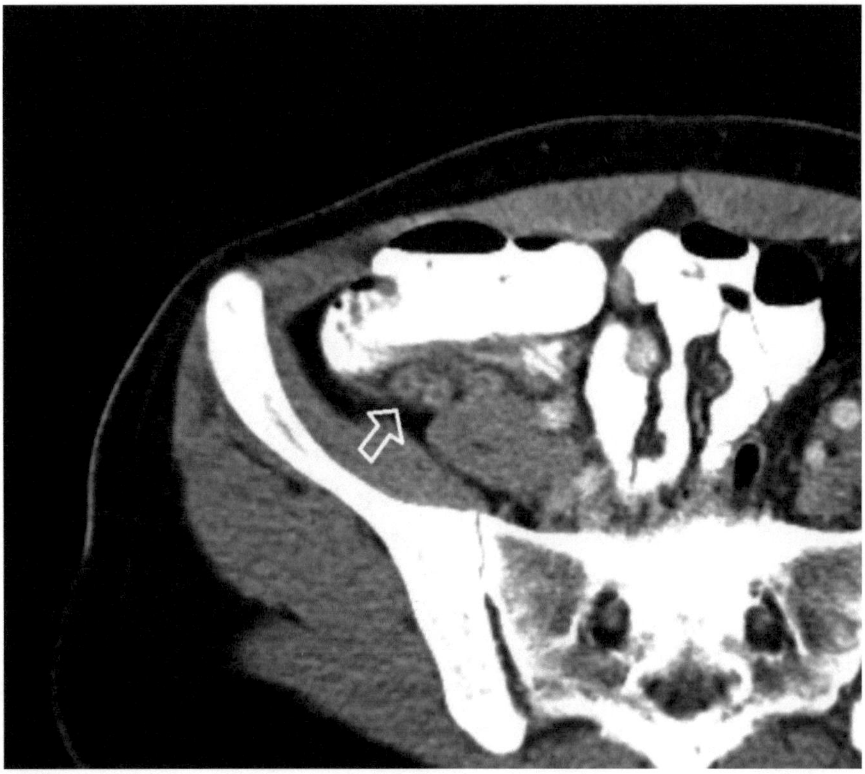

Fig. 7. MDCT with intravenous and oral contrast axial image demonstrating a retrocecal appendix (*white arrow*) that is not opacified with contrast with wall enhancement and streaking of the surrounding mesenteric fat consistent with non-complicated appendicitis.

CT imaging protocols

There are a variety of different imaging and contrast protocols for the diagnosis of appendicitis. It has been the experience at our institution that the highest diagnostic value can be obtained from a contrast enhanced MDCT scan with an intravenous contrast bolus and a rectal contrast enema. 25 ml (Telebrix 350 mgI/ml, Guerbet) of water-soluble iodinated contrast diluted in 1.5 L of warm water is given as a rectal enema in an adult in the right decubitus position to properly opacify the cecum. Contrast enhanced MDCT with rectal contrast enema has yielded an accuracy of 94.7% in the diagnosis of appendicitis [18]. The advantages of a MDCT with intravenous and rectal contrast enema include high diagnostic accuracy, particularly in the thin or constipated patient where visualization of the appendix can be limited. A rectal contrast enema serves to distend and opacify the appendix if it is normal and has a patent lumen. Non opacification of the appendix despite adequate filling of the cecum is a highly sensitive, specific and reproducible diagnostic sign of appendicitis [18]. It is a relatively fast technique and it takes about 5-10 minutes more than a non-enhanced MDCT scan in order to account for the time needed for the administration of the enema. The disadvantage of MDCT with a rectal contrast enema is that some patients may experience discomfort, intolerance and abdominal cramps during the administration of the enema. It is therefore recommended to use warm water for the enema and a slow enema infusion rate as well as spasmolytics if needed.

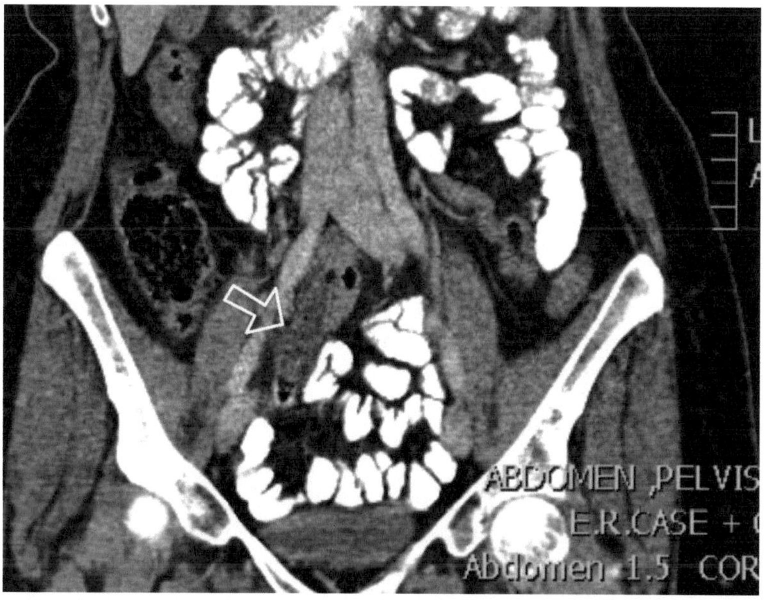

a

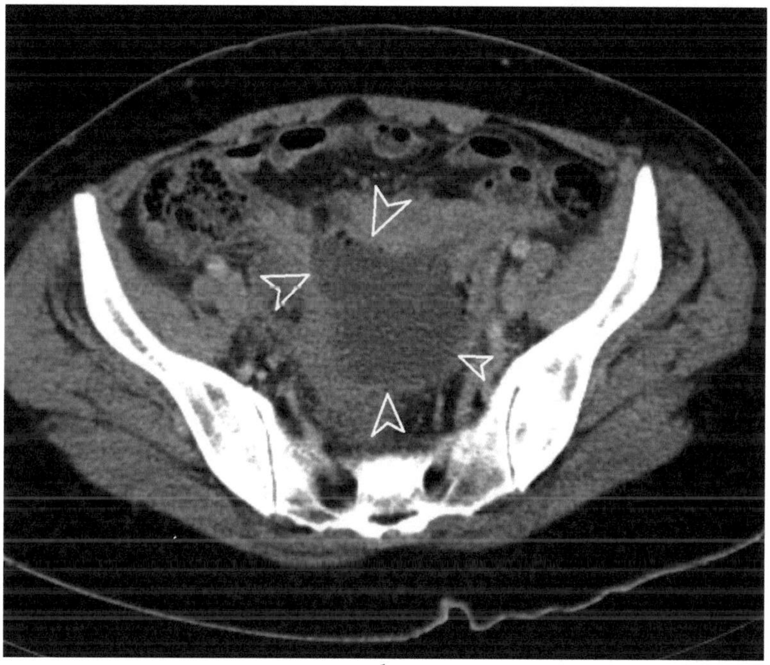

b

Fig. 8. MDCT scan with intravenous and oral contrast images of a patient in whom appendicitis was missed on initial presentation and later returned with a ruptured appendicitis and pelvic abscess formation. Initial exam (a) revealed a fluid filled blind-ended tubular structure (arrow) with extensive surrounding fat streaking consistent with the inflamed appendix. On the patient's second presentation (b), the appendix had ruptured and produced a large pelvic abscess (arrowheads) containing tiny pockets of gas.

Alternatively, contrast enhanced MDCT with intravenous and oral contrast administration for bowel opacification is a more commonly used technique. It is generally more accepted by patients than rectal contrast enema, however, it's main disadvantage compared to the MDCT with rectal contrast enema is a prolonged waiting time as mentioned previously, mainly because of the contrast transit time to reach the cecum (60 to 120 minutes) in order to properly opacify the terminal ileum and possibly the appendix.

Furthermore and because of its progression through the entire small bowel, the amount of contrast that eventually reaches the cecum does not provide sufficient luminal distention as compared to the rectal contrast enema study. Therefore distention and opacification of the appendix, even when normal, is not always guaranteed with oral contrast MDCT studies.

Also, many patients presenting to the emergency department with suspected appendicitis have nausea and vomiting which precludes the drinking of the 1.5 L of oral contrast.

The use of IV contrast is advocated in both rectal and oral contrast MDCT studies as it provides additional diagnostic clues that may indicate the presence of appendicitis such as appendiceal wall enhancement which also represents a major criterion or diagnostic sign.

Finally, a non-enhanced or plain MDCT scan may be used if there is a contraindication for the usage of iodinated contrast material such as contrast-induced nephropathy in patients with renal function impairment, or a positive history for severe allergic reactions to contrast media. A non-enhanced MDCT scan remains the fastest study that can be performed with short image acquisition time while still maintaining a high diagnostic accuracy without fear of adverse reactions or patient intolerance.

It is important to emphasize, however, that the routine use of MDCT imaging, despite its high diagnostic accuracy, carries the burden of increased exposure to ionizing radiation. Care should be taken not to expose pediatric and pregnant women without proper justification and discussion with the patients or surrogates about the risks of the examination versus the benefits.

4.2.3 Magnetic Resonance Imaging (MRI)

MRI is a non-irradiating imaging technique but is not as widely or readily available as ultrasound and MDCT. It is more expensive and the examination itself takes a longer time to perform, and image quality has a higher chance of becoming degraded by motion artifacts [21].

Because of major concern about risks and hazards from exposure to high radiation doses and potential allergic and toxic effects of intravenous contrast material associated with MDCT, MRI is increasingly becoming the study of choice to evaluate children and pregnant women with suspected appendicitis and non-diagnostic ultrasound results. Pregnant patients can be accepted to undergo MR scans at any trimester or stage of pregnancy, however, MR contrast agents should not be administered to pregnant patients because of their potential teratogenic effects [22]. Most studies reported the use of T1, T2 and T2 fat saturation sequences with axial and coronal acquisitions, with or without additional T1 post contrast image in the absence of any contraindication.

On MRI (Fig. 9), a thickened appendix of more than 7 mm in diameter, an appendiceal wall thicker than 2 mm, signs of inflammatory changes surrounding the appendix or presence of a pelvic abscess are diagnostic signs of appendicitis [21]. A meta-analysis of recently published data regarding the utility of MRI in pregnant women with suspected appendicitis performed by Blumenfeld and colleagues showed high diagnostic accuracies of MRI in the diagnosis of appendicitis [23].

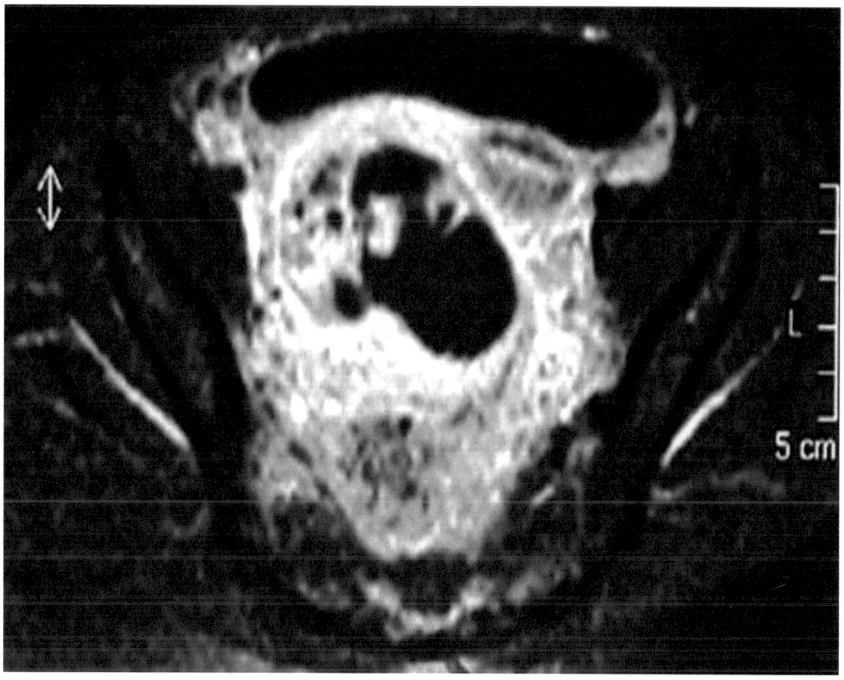

a

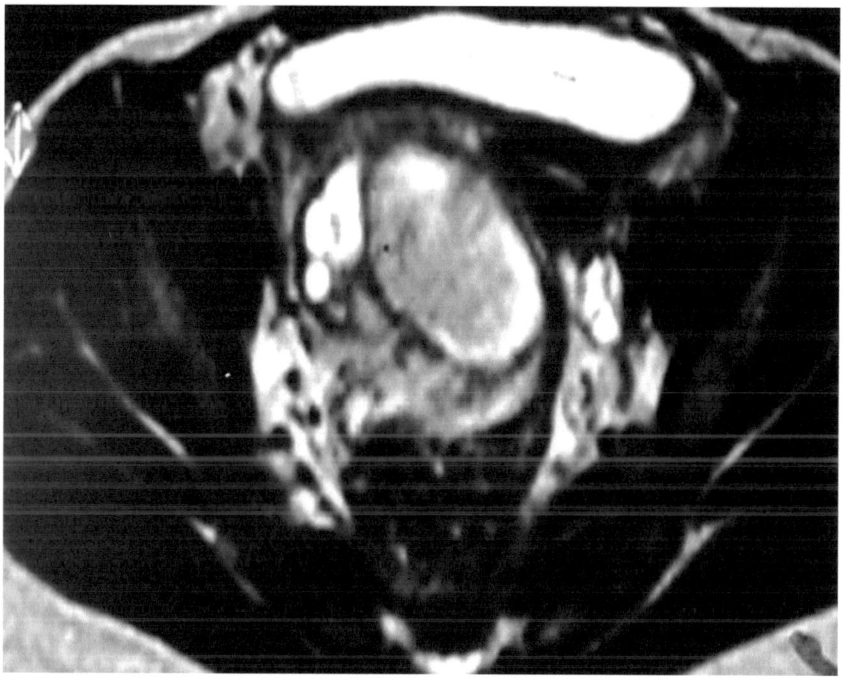

b

Fig. 9. T2-weighted MR images (a and b) demonstrating an abscess formation in the pelvis secondary to a ruptured or perforated appendicitis in a child.

4.3 Scintigraphy

Scintigraphy using technetium-99m labeled leukocytes (Tc-99m HMPAO) or technetium-99m monoclonal antibodies-leukoscan (LeuTech anti-CD 15) allow detection of appendicitis with a sensitivity ranging between 81% and 100% and a reported specificity ranging between 82% and 100% [12]. The scintigraphic examinations should be interpreted with caution because focally increased uptake of the radiotracer in the right lower quadrant can indicate an inflammatory source that may be due to appendicitis as well as other inflammatory conditions such as diverticulitis and Crohn's disease. The major disadvantages of scintigraphy are cost, exposure of patients to ionizing radiation, limited availability of the radiotracer and a long scanning time.
The utility of 18F-FDG PET-CT imaging in the diagnosis of appendicitis was highlighted by researchers in a few case reports [24], [25], [26]. Its performance compared to conventional MDCT scan is yet to be determined, and availability of the radiotracer also limits its regular use in most centers.

5. Differential diagnosis

There are many conditions that may mimic appendicitis and one of the reasons why MDCT scan has gained such an increasing popularity over recent years is because of its ability to detect and differentiate other causes of right lower quadrant pain which occur in approximately 32% of patients investigated for suspected appendicitis [27], [28]. It is important to keep in mind these alternative diagnostic possibilities or differential diagnoses when evaluating patients with right lower quadrant pain, as their treatment options differ from each other and from that of appendicitis.
These clinical mimickers include:

- Mesenteric adenitis
- Crohn's disease
- Primary epiploic appendagitis
- Neutropenic typhlitis in cancer and transplant patients on immunosuppression
- Cecal diverticulitis
- Familial Mediterranean fever
- Omental torsion
- Lupus peritonitis
- Bowel perforation without evidence of a pneumoperitoneum
- Torsion of a Meckel's diverticulum
- Ureteric colic
- Gynecological emergencies such as ovarian torsion, pelvic inflammatory disease, uterine fibroids, etc…

Some of these conditions may be surgical, but on the other hand it is of utmost importance to recognize the non-surgical conditions at imaging such as mesenteric adenitis or epiploic appendagitis among others, thus avoiding unnecessary surgery. Color Doppler ultrasound and MDCT can readily exclude appendicitis and differentiate it from these mimickers by the identification or visualization of a normal appendix.

6. Treatment

Differentiation of complicated from uncomplicated appendicitis may be of greater importance in the future as several studies are now suggesting differing treatment options.

In uncomplicated appendicitis, laparoscopic appendectomy is currently the standard treatment but non-operative management with antibiotics alone may be a justifiable alternative [29], [30].

For appendicitis complicated by perforation and abscess formation, MDCT scan can help guide percutaneous catheter drainage (Fig. 10) followed by interval appendectomy [31], [32].

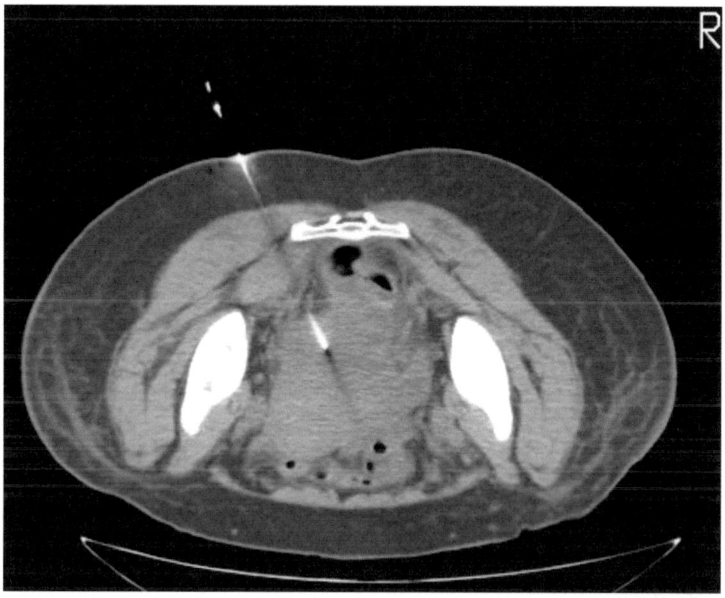

a

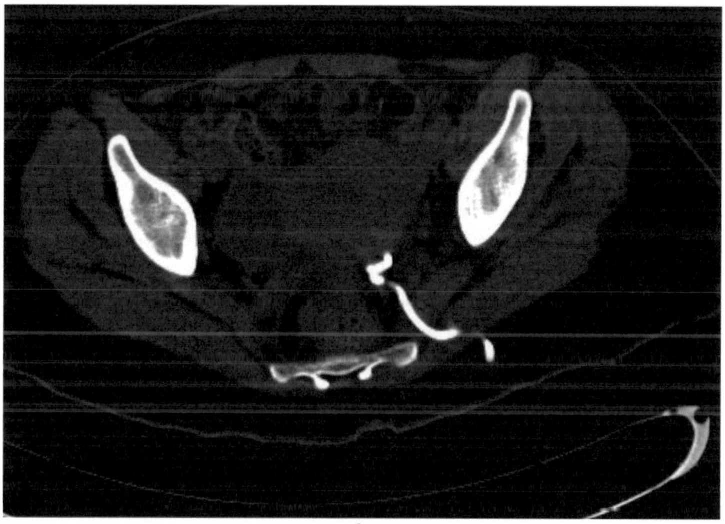

b

Fig. 10. CT-guided percutaneous catheter drainage of a pelvic abscess secondary to a ruptured appendicitis. (a) CT-guidance for a percutaneous transgluteal approach needle and catheter insertion. (b) Follow-up MDCT image showing complete healing of the pelvic abscess. Patient underwent subsequent elective and interval appendectomy shortly afterward.

7. Cost-effectiveness

Imaging provides a quick and accurate diagnosis of appendicitis, which has several clinical and economical implications.

- It allows an early diagnosis of appendicitis and so in some may reduce the risk of perforation with its associated morbidity and prolonged hospitalization time.
- Its routine use results in a reduction in the number of patients admitted to the hospital for clinical observation with a reduction in cost.
- It identifies alternative diagnoses namely non-surgical acute abdominal and pelvic emergencies, therefore avoiding unnecessary operations and reducing cost.
- It significantly decreases the negative appendectomy rate which is used in several hospitals as a Performance Indicator (PI) for quality assurance and accreditation. Routine pre-operative imaging for suspected appendicitis has significantly reduced the negative appendectomy rate (NAR) to 4% at our institution compared to a previous NAR of 16% during the era of clinical diagnosis when used alone without pre-operative imaging [33]. This is of particular concern since some third party payers may not cover the costs of removal of a histologically normal appendix at surgery.

8. Conclusion

There is an increasing consensus for routine pre-operative imaging in patients with suspected appendicitis. Ultrasound is the imaging modality of first choice in children and pregnant women because of concerns about exposure to ionizing radiation and secondary carcinogenic and teratogenic potential risks. If the ultrasound examination is non-diagnostic, then MRI is the next choice. Multi-detector CT remains the preferred imaging modality in adults because of its higher diagnostic accuracy. Imaging has proven to have a great impact on clinical outcome and cost-effectiveness in patients presenting to the emergency room with suspected appendicitis.

9. References

[1] Federle MP. Focused appendix CT technique: a commentary. Radiology 1997 Jan;202: 20-1.

[2] Addiss DG, Shaffer N, Fowler BS, et al. The epidemiology of appendicitis and appendectomy in the United States. Am J Epidemiol 1990;132:910–25.

[3] Rybkin AV, Thoeni RF. Current concepts in imaging of appendicitis. Radiol Clin North Am 2007;45:411–22.

[4] McCartan DP, Fleming FJ, Grace PA. The management of right iliac fossa pain - is timing everything? Surgeon. 2010 Aug;8(4):211-7.

[5] Alvarado A. A practical score for the early diagnosis of acute appendicitis. Ann Emerg Med. 1986 May;15(5):557-64.

[6] Schneider C, Kharbanda A, Bachur R. Evaluating appendicitis scoring systems using a prospective pediatric cohort. Ann Emerg Med. 2007 Jun;49(6):778-84.

[7] Mandeville K, Pottker T, Bulloch B. Using appendicitis scores in the pediatric ED. Am J Emerg Med. 2010 Jul 30. [Ahead of print]

[8] Bhatt M, Joseph L, Ducharme FM, Dougherty G, McGillivray D. Prospective validation of the pediatric appendicitis score in a Canadian pediatric emergency department. Acad Emerg Med. 2009 Jul;16(7):591-6.
[9] Coleman C, Thompson JE Jr, Bennion RS, Schmit PJ. White blood cell count is a poor predictor of severity of disease in the diagnosis of appendicitis. Am Surg. 1998 Oct;64(10):983-5.
[10] Lim GH, Shabbir A, So JB. Diagnostic laparoscopy in the evaluation of right lower abdominal pain: a one-year audit. Singapore Med J. 2008 Jun;49(6):451-3.
[11] Bakker OJ, Go PM, Puylaert JB, Kazemier G, Heij HA. Guideline on diagnosis and treatment of acute appendicitis: imaging prior to appendectomy is recommended. Ned Tijdschr Geneeskd. 2010;154:A303.
[12] Rollins MD, Andolsek W, Scaife ER, Meyers RL, Duke TH, Lilyquist M, Barnhart DC. Prophylactic appendectomy: unnecessary in children with incidental appendicoliths detected by computed tomographic scan. J Pediatr Surg. 2010 Dec;45(12):2377-80.
[13] Rabinowitz CB, Egglin TK, Beland MD, Mayo-Smith WW. Outcomes in 74 patients with an appendicolith who did not undergo surgery: is follow-up imaging necessary? Emerg Radiol. 2007 Jul;14(3):161-5.
[14] Haddad MC, Azzi MC, Hourani MH. Current diagnosis of acute appendicitis. J Med Liban. 2003 Oct-Dec;51(4):211-5.
[15] Rao PM, Rhea JT, Novelline RA. Helical CT of appendicitis and diverticulitis. Radiol Clin North Am. 1999 Sep;37(5):895-910.
[16] Lehmann D, Uebel P, Weiss H, Fiedler L, Bersch W. Sonographic representation of the normal and acute inflamed appendix in patients with right-sided abdominal pain. Ultraschall Med. 2000 Jun;21(3):101-6.
[17] Kapoor A, Kapoor A, Mahajan G. Real-time elastography in acute appendicitis. J Ultrasound Med. 2010 Jun;29(6):871-7.
[18] Naffaa LN, Ishak GE, Haddad MC. The value of contrast-enhanced helical CT scan with rectal contrast enema in the diagnosis of acute appendicitis. Clin Imaging. 2005 Jul-Aug;29(4):255-8.
[19] Applegate KE, Sivit CJ, Myers MT, Pschesang B. Using helical CT to diagnosis acute appendicitis in children: spectrum of findings. AJR Am J Roentgenol. 2001 Feb;176(2):501-5.
[20] Nikolaidis P, Hwang CM, Miller FH, Papanicolaou N. The nonvisualized appendix: incidence of acute appendicitis when secondary inflammatory changes are absent. AJR Am J Roentgenol. 2004 Oct;183(4):889-92.
[21] Parks NA, Schroeppel TJ. Update on imaging for acute appendicitis. Surg Clin North Am. 2011 Feb;91(1):141-54.
[22] Kanal E, Barkovich AJ, Bell C, et al. ACR guidance document for safe MR practices: 2007. AJR Am J Roentgenol. 2007 Jun;188(6):1447-74
[23] Blumenfeld YJ, Wong AE, Jafari A, Barth RA, El-Sayed YY. MR imaging in cases of antenatal suspected appendicitis--a meta-analysis. J Matern Fetal Neonatal Med. 2011 Mar;24(3):485-8.
[24] Moghadam-Kia S, Nawaz A, Newberg A, Basu S, Alavi A, Torigian DA. Utility of 18F-FDG-PET/CT imaging in the diagnosis of appendicitis. Hell J Nucl Med. 2009 Sep-Dec;12(3):281-2.

[25] Koff SG, Sterbis JR, Davison JM, Montilla-Soler JL. A unique presentation of appendicitis: F-18 FDG PET/CT. Clin Nucl Med. 2006 Nov;31(11):704-6.

[26] Ogawa S, Itabashi M, Kameoka S. Significance of FDG-PET in Identification of Diseases of the Appendix - Based on Experience of Two Cases Falsely Positive for FDG Accumulation. Case Rep Gastroenterol. 2009 Apr 29;3(1):125-130.

[27] Lane MJ, Mindelzun RE. Appendicitis and its mimickers. Semin Ultrasound CT MR. 1999 Apr;20(2):77-85.

[28] Karam AR, Birjawi GA, Sidani CA, Haddad MC. Alternative diagnoses of acute appendicitis on helical CT with intravenous and rectal contrast. Clin Imaging. 2007 Mar-Apr;31(2):77-86.

[29] Mason RJ. Surgery for appendicitis: is it necessary? Surg Infect (Larchmt). 2008 Aug;9(4):481-8.

[30] Sakorafas GH, Mastoraki A, Lappas C, Sampanis D, Danias N, Smyrniotis V. Conservative treatment of acute appendicitis: heresy or an effective and acceptable alternative to surgery? Eur J Gastroenterol Hepatol. 2011 Feb;23(2):121-7.

[31] Friedell ML, Perez-Izquierdo M. Is there a role for interval appendectomy in the management of acute appendicitis? Am Surg. 2000 Dec;66(12):1158-62.

[32] St Peter SD, Aguayo P, Fraser JD, Keckler SJ, Sharp SW, Leys CM, Murphy JP, Snyder CL, Sharp RJ, Andrews WS, Holcomb GW 3rd, Ostlie DJ. Initial laparoscopic appendectomy versus initial nonoperative management and interval appendectomy for perforated appendicitis with abscess: a prospective, randomized trial. J Pediatr Surg. 2010 Jan;45(1):236-40.

[33] Birjawi GA, Nassar LJ, Atweh LA, Akel S, Haddad MC. Emergency abdominal radiology: the acute abdomen. J Med Liban. 2009 Jul-Sep;57(3):178-212.

4

Clinical Scoring Systems in the Management of Suspected Appendicitis in Children

Graham Thompson
Pediatric Emergency Medicine
University of Calgary, Alberta Children's Hospital
Canada

1. Introduction

Abdominal pain is a common problem in children presenting to the Emergency Department (ED) and though the differential diagnosis is expansive, appendicitis is the most common surgical emergency of childhood. While many children present with classical findings of right lower quadrant (RLQ) pain associated with nausea or vomiting and fever, subtle features and difficult examinations can make identifying appendicitis in a child challenging, leaving Health Care Providers struggling to distinguish this surgical emergency from less urgent conditions. Appendicitis is a progressive condition making early recognition essential in limiting morbidity and mortality. While some suggest Diagnostic Imaging (DI) as a routine screen for all children with abdominal pain, ED wait times, fiscal restraints and increasing concern related to radiation exposure require a more prudent, selective approach to identifying the child with suspected appendicitis. Clinical Scoring Systems (CSSs) have been developed to assist clinicians in appropriately stratifying a child's clinical risk of having appendicitis. This chapter reviews the literature and reports on the experience of a tertiary care Pediatric Emergency Department (PED) in incorporating a clinical score into a Clinical Pathway in order to stratify children into High/Moderate/Low risk for appendicitis, thus guiding management and departmental patient flow.

2. What are Clinical Scoring Systems?

An increase in the use of Clinical Prediction Rules (CPRs) to improve diagnostic accuracy has occurred over the last 2 decades. CPRs are tools that use specific criteria in order to establish probabilities of outcomes or to assist in management decisions. Some researchers have distinguished 3 types of CPRs; Diagnostic CPRs which focus on factors related to arriving at a clinical diagnosis; Prognostic CPRs which predict outcomes; and Prescriptive CPRs which provide recommendations for clinical intervention.(Beattie & Nelson, 2006) CPRs have been defined as decision-making tools that include 3 or more variables obtained from the history, physical examination or basic diagnostic tests in order to assist the clinician in decision making.(Laupacis, Sekar, & I. G. Stiell, 1997)

The format of a CPR can be variable, depending on the purpose. Some require fulfillment of a complete set of criteria in order to direct management. Others assign values to weighted criteria, the summation of which provides a score. These are often known as Clinical Scoring Systems (CSSs). Even within CSSs, several categories can be determined. Some CSSs are dichotomous, utilizing a cutoff value above which an action is recommended or an outcome is expected. For example, surgical intervention may be recommended for a certain validated score over 6. Others CSSs lean more toward a continuous nature to provide graded risk stratification. A simple example may stratify a patient to low risk of a disease process for scores of 1-2, moderate risk for scores of 3-5 and high risk for scores of 6-7.

While many CSSs exist, not all have been appropriately developed or evaluated. In the process of evaluation, one must consider several factors including the internal validity, accuracy, external validity, sensibility and potential impact (Beattie & Nelson, 2006). Table 1 details some factors to consider when assessing a Clinical Scoring System.

McGinn et al have proposed a 4-level hierarchy to assist health care providers in determining the strength of CPRs and CSSs. Those that have been rigorously tested, including impact analysis, are deemed Level 1, while those that have simply been derived but not tested are Level 4 (McGinn et al., 2000). Ian Stiell, well known for the Ottawa Ankle Rules and the Canadian CT Head Rules (I. G. Stiell et al., 1992)(I. G. Stiell et al., 1993)(I. Stiell, 2001)(I. G. Stiell et al., 2001), created a checklist for assessing the developmental rigor of CPRs, including evaluation of clinical need, derivation methodology, prospective validation, successful implementation into practice, cost-effectiveness and dissemination strategies. (Stiell 1999).

Assessment Criterion	**Questions to Ask when evaluating a Clinical Scoring System**
Internal Validity	How was the Score derived? How well defined are the criterion? What is the inter- and intra- rater reliability of the Score? How was the Score Validated? Has the Score been evaluated for Impact?
Accuracy	What are the sensitivity, specificity, likelihood ratios and predictive values of the Score?
External Validity	Is the Score generalizable to my patient population?
Sensibility	How many criteria are included in the Score? How accessible are the criteria elements? Are the criteria time-sensitive? How easy is the Score to calculate? Do I need computer assistance? Can all key stakeholders accurately and consistently apply the Score? (Are responses reproducible?)
Potential Impact	Will implementation of the Score improve my diagnostic accuracy? How will patient flow in my health care environment be impacted by the Score? Will implementation of the Score be consistent with other departmental processes? How will other key stakeholders be affected by the implementation of the Score?

Table 1. Factors for determining the appropriateness of a Clinical Scoring System

3. Why use Clinical Scoring Systems?

Making wise, educated decisions is the cornerstone of good medical practice and often involves estimating the probability of an event. Inherent to all medical decisions is an assessment of potential risk and benefit. Risk tolerance within a clinical setting is dependent on the key stakeholders involved, for example the health care providers, the patients, the general public, the health care organization and policy makers. For a clinician, factors such as personality traits, quality and quantity of practice, experience with recent adverse events or near misses, fears of litigation and external stressful events may impact risk tolerance.

Risk assessment requires at least some basic knowledge of statistics, though mastery is far from needed. While terms such as sensitivity and specificity are familiar to many medical staff they are not as useful as other concepts. An understanding of Pre- and Post- Test likelihoods, Positive- and Negative- Predictive Values (PPV, NPV), Positive- and Negative-Likelihood Ratios (PLR, NLR) and Accuracy impact on the interpretation of results.

There are significant variations in clinical practice and outcomes, at national, regional and even local levels in a number of conditions and appendicitis is amongst them. A number of studies have demonstrated practice variation, as well as the impact of variation on clinical outcome measures (Chang, Ng, Y.-C. Chen, J.-C. Chen, & Yen, 2010)(Goldman et al., 2009)(Plint et al., 2004)(Richer et al., 2010)(Jain, Elon, Johnson, Frank, & Deguzman, 2010). While practice variation results in patient outcome differences, standardization of practice based on the best evidence can result in improved care (Eitel, Rudkin, Malvehy, Killeen, & Pines, 2010). Numerous studies have demonstrated the efficacy of Evidence Based Clinical Algorithms (EBCA) such as pathways and protocols in reducing delays in time-sensitive medication administration, reducing unwarranted radiation exposure and reducing mortality (Rivers et al., 2001)(Francis 2010, Osmond 2010,). Integrating CSSs into EBCA is key to standardizing patient care in an effort to improve global and individual health outcomes.

4. The literature search strategy

To obtain complete information related to CSSs for suspected appendicitis in children, a formal literature review of common scientific databases was performed by the Health Information Network Calgary, University of Calgary, Alberta, Canada. Multiple databases were searched including Medline, Embase, Cochrane, PubMed, CINAHL Plus and Academic Search Complete. The following terms were utilized in the search: appendicitis, acute appendicitis, clinical decision rule, clinical prediction rule, prediction, score, and risk stratification. Search strategies limited the results to those published between 1980 and 2011 and included all children aged 0 – 18 years (infant, preschool, school aged, adolescent, all child).

Abstracts of the above search strategy were reviewed, refining the final manuscript database to those relevant to the current topic. Two hundred sixty six references were reviewed. Thirty-six articles were retrieved for inclusion in this review. Reference lists of these manuscripts were examined and any additional citations relevant to the topic were added.

5. Clinical Scoring Systems for suspected appendicitis in children

Over the last 3 decades, a number of CSSs have been developed to assist the clinician in assessing patients presenting with abdominal pain and suspected appendicitis. Several of these scores were specifically derived for children, while others were developed for adults or mixed populations and subsequently validated in children. The best known, such as the Alvardo Score and the Pediatric Appendicitis score, have been studied at length. Lesser known scores such as Kharbanda's Low Risk Score, the Lindberg Score, and the Ohmann Sore, among others, are listed in Table 2. Most Scoring Systems include a combination of Historical, Clinical and Laboratory measures. Each of these scores will be reviewed in detail.

Alvarado Score (MANTRELS)
Pediatric Appendicitis Score (Samuel)
Low Risk for Appendicitis Score (Kharbanda)
Lintula Score
Eskelinen Score
Fenyo - Lindberg Score
Ohmann Score
Christian Score
RIPASA Score

Table 2. Clinical Scoring Systems used in the Diagnosis of Appendicitis in children

Care is needed when evaluating studies of CSSs. Several studies include children and adults and some have few children. Populations may also differ; some studies include all-comers to the ED with abdominal pain whilst others include only those with suspected appendicitis, still others include those in whom a surgical consult was obtained and finally, some are limited to those children who had an appendectomy. Additionally, the medical specialty, level of training and experience of the staff performing Score assessments may also have a significant impact on generalizability (Emergency Physician vs. Surgeon, Senior Trainee vs. Attending Staff). Those studies that enroll prospectively are obviously more robust than retrospective analyses. And finally, some studies use modifications to a Score criteria (e.g. dropping a criteria) or to the threshold level (e.g. standard Alvarado Score threshold for probable appendicitis is ≥7, but some studies use a cutoff of 6).
In light of some of these potential biases, Ohmann et al re-evaluated data from 10 published CSSs for appendicitis to determine their performance in meeting predefined quality criteria. Subsequently, they prospectively collected data on 1254 patients with acute abdominal pain from 6 different sites in order to evaluate the same Scores. The predefined quality criteria included a) initial negative appendectomy rate < 15%; b) potential perforation rate < 35%; c) initial missed perforation rate < 15% and d) missed appendicitis rate < 5%. Four of the original derivation studies met at least one quality criteria, however, when applied to the prospective evaluation, none of the 10 Scores were successful in meeting the predefined quality criteria. Ohmann et al concluded that significant bias existed in the derivation of the Scores, as mentioned in the paragraph above. (Ohmann, Yang, & Franke, 1995)

5.1 The Alvarado Score (MANTRELS)

In 1986, Alvarado published what is now one of the most well-known and studied appendicitis scores (Alvarado, 1986). This retrospective study of 305 patients admitted for suspected appendicitis evaluated common clinical and laboratory findings in relation to pathologically proven acute appendicitis. 277 patients were eligible for analysis.

Eight criteria were chosen for inclusion in the diagnostic score, weighted to represent joint probability of disease. The Diagnostic criteria for the Alvarado Score are shown in Table 3. Right Lower Quadrant (RLQ) Pain and a Left Shift were found to be the most prevalent, thus receiving 2 points each, while each of the remaining criteria were attributed 1 point. This initial study included both adults and children, with an age range of 4 to 80 years (mean 25.3). An Alvarado Score of ≥7 was considered high risk for appendicitis. Though not explicitly stated in the study, this threshold value had a sensitivity of 81% and a specificity of 74%. Several elements of the score have been criticised, particularly the threshold for fever (37.3 C) and the availability of peripheral cell count differentials at some health centres, prompting some investigators to modify the score (see below).

Alvarado Score		**Pediatric Appendicitis Score**	
Diagnostic Criteria	**Value**	**Diagnostic Criteria**	**Value**
Migration of pain to RLQ	1	Migration of Pain	1
Anorexia/Acetone in urine (i.e. ketones)	1	Anorexia	1
Nausea-Vomiting	1	Nausea/Emesis	1
Tenderness in RLQ	2	Tenderness in RLQ	2
Rebound Pain	1	Cough/Percussion Tenderness	2
Elevation of Temperature (≥37.3 C)	1	Pyrexia (not defined)	1
Leukocytosis (> 10 000)	2	Leukocytosis (> 10 000)	1
Shift to Left (> 75%)	1	Neutrophilia	1
Total Score	**10**	**Total Score**	**10**

Table 3. Comparison of Diagnostic Criteria between the Alvarado Score (MANTRELS) and the Pediatric Appendicitis Score (Samuel Score)

Numerous studies have examined the Alvarado Score, particularly in children. (Table 4) Bond et al prospectively studied 187 children aged 2 - 17 years with suspected appendicitis, of which 143 were admitted. Using Alvarado's cutoff score of 7 to indicate the need for surgery, the authors found a sensitivity and specificity of 90% and 72% respectively, with a negative appendectomy rate of 17%. Lower cutoff scores (5 or 6) demonstrated improved sensitivity, but corresponding reductions in specificity, as expected. Subgroup analysis showed the score to be least accurate in preschool children, corresponding to the clinical experience of many health care providers, though overall numbers in this age group were limited. The authors concluded that the Alvarado Score failed to achieve their predetermined standard for accuracy, however, this was set quite high at 99.5% sensitivity. (Bond, Tully, Chan, & Bradley, 1990)

A retrospective study of children under 14 years by Hsiao et al confirmed Alvarado's data showing that RLQ tenderness and a left shift were the most prevalent signs in those with pathologically proven appendicitis. Children with Alvarado Scores ≥7 were statistically more likely to have appendicitis than controls. Overall sensitivity and specificity for an Alvarado Score >=7 were 60% and 61% respectively. (Hsiao, Lin, & D.-F. Chen, 2005)

Study	Year	Population	Ages	Design	T+	F+	F-	T-	Sens	Spec	PPV	NPV	Acc	Notes
Alvarado	1986	305 suspected appendicitis 277 included	4 to 80 years	Retrospective	184	13	43	37	81%	74%	93%	46%	80%	Derivation Study
Bond	1990	189 suspected appendicitis 143 included	2 to 17 years	Prospective	103	21	12	52	90%	71%	83%	81%	82%	
Owen	1992	215 suspected appendicitis 70 children	Not defined	Prospective	40	5	3	22	93%	81%	89%	88%	89%	Sub-group analysis
Kalan	1994	49 suspected appendicitis 11 children	Not defined	Prospective	11	0	0	0	100%	N/A	100%	N/A	100%	Modified Alvarado - No Left Shift
Macklin	1997	118 suspected appendicitis	4 to 14 years	Prospective	29	17	9	63	76%	79%	63%	88%	78%	Modified Alvarado - No Left Shift
Hsiao	2005	222 suspected appendicitis	< 14 years	Retrospective	66	45	43	68	61%	60%	59%	61%	60%	
Schneider	2007	821 suspected appendicitis 588 included	3 to 21 years	Prospective	142	75	55	316	72%	81%	65%	85%	78%	Alvarado /PAS comparison
Shreef	2010	350 suspected appendicitis	8 to 14 years	Prospective	114	37	18	181	86%	83%	75%	91%	84%	Based on threshold = 7 Paper reports threshold = 6
Escriba	2011	112 suspected appendicitis 99 included	4 to 18 years	Prospective	?	?	?	?	90%	91%	88%	93%	?	Alvarado/ PAS comparison Threshold used was 6
Rezak	2011	61 suspected appendicitis 59 included	3 to 16 years	Retrospective	?	?	?	?	92%	82%	?	?	92%	Alvarado/ PAS comparison
Chong	2011	200 suspected appendicitis 192 included	Adults & children, not defined	Prospective	69	11	32	80	68%	87%	86%	71%	86%	Alvarado /RIPASA comparison
Mandeville	2011	487 diagnosed appendicitis 287 enrolled	4 to 16 years	Prospective	?	?	?	?	76%	72%	76%	72%	?	In Press

T+ True Positive, F+ False Positive, F- False Negative, T- True Negative, Sens Sensitivity, Spec Specificity, PPV Positive Predictive Value, NPV Negative Predictive Value, Acc Accuracy, ? data not provided, N/A not applicable

Table 4. Summary of Studies Evaluating the Alvarado Score in the Pediatric Population

A higher sensitivity and specificity was found by Rezak et al in their retrospective study (92% and 82% respectively). Sixty-one children aged 3 to 16 years with suspected appendicitis had CT evaluation. This study suggested a 27% reduction in CT scanning would occur had children with scores >7 been managed directly by appendectomy without

CT evaluation. High sensitivity and specificity were maintained, at 100% and 97% respectively, suggesting that surgical intervention was best suited to children with an Alvarado Score of 8-10, while those with scores of 5-7 be further evaluated with imaging studies (Rezak, Abbas, Ajemian, Dudrick, & Kwasnik, 2011).

In a mixed pediatric-adult population, Owen et al prospectively evaluated 215 patients, 70 of whom were children. In this pediatric subgroup analysis, sensitivity and specificity were 93% and 81% (Owen 1992).

Shreef et al recently performed a dual-centre prospective study, reviewing 350 children aged 8 to 14 years. Interestingly, their reported statistical analysis was based on an Alvarado threshold of 6, and was based upon 2 different outcomes; 1) performance of appendectomy and 2) histology. Using the standard threshold of 7 and including all comers related to histologic diagnosis, the sensitivity and specificity were 86% and 83% respectively (Shreef, Waly, Abd-Elrahman, & Abd Elhafez, 2010).

Several attempts have been made to modify the Alvarado Score to improve its accuracy. Macklin et al sought to simplify the Alvarado Score by eliminating the criteria for left shift (Modified Score total 9), as done by Kalan in a mixed adult/pediatric study. Children aged 4-14 years were enrolled, demonstrating sensitivity and specificity of 76.3% and 78.8% respectively using a cutoff score of 7 or higher to predict histological appendicitis. Kalan's study was limited to 11 children, all of which had modified Alvarado Scores >=7 and corresponding appendicitis. Obviously these numbers are too small to draw any conclusions (Macklin, Radcliffe, Merei, & Stringer, 1997)(Kalan 1994).

Sooriakumaran et al further modified the score by decreasing the value of leukocytosis, to make a total score of 8. This score was then compared to clinical assessment by Emergency Physicians, and found wanting. However, one must be cautious, as only 3 children were included (!) , and, due to the change in total score, the threshold value was tested at 5 (Sooriakumaran, Lovell, & Brown, 2005).

Significant changes to the Alvarado Score were suggested by Impellizzeri et al. who studied 156 children aged 2-17 years, replacing anorexia with an elevated fibrinogen level (>400mg/dL), changing migration of pain to length of pain (although not defined), combining RLQ pain and rebound into one criteria, and decreasing the temperature cutoff to 37 C. Of note, the diagnosis of appendicitis was made on surgical report, not pathologic diagnosis. The authors suggest the above modifications would have decreased admission rates by 15% (Impellizzeri et al., 2002).

5.2 The Pediatric Appendicitis Score (Samuel Score)

Madan Samuel introduced the Pediatric Appendicitis Score (PAS) in 2002. A theoretical advantage to the PAS exists for 2 reason; 1) data was prospectively collected, and 2) the score was specifically derived in a population of children (aged 4 - 15 years). The PAS has been subject to multiple subsequent validation and comparison studies.

Evaluating 1170 children with suspected appendicitis, Samuel compared historical, clinical and laboratory features in children with appendicitis (n=734) and those without appendicitis (n=436). Using stepwise multiple linear regression, 8 variables were included in a diagnostic model out of 10 points, with greater weight attributed to RLQ pain and maneuvers eliciting rebound tenderness (cough/percussion). Diagnostic criteria for the PAS are shown in Table 3. Samuel concludes that a score of 6 or greater shows a high probability of acute appendicitis.(Samuel, 2002)

Unlike the Alvarado Score, there have been no attempts to modify the PAS. However, multiple studies have sought to prove its validity (Summary provided in Table 5). Two very high quality prospective trials have recently been completed. Goldman et al expanded the original age group by including 849 children aged 1 to 17 years, 123 of whom had histological appendicitis. Sensitivity and Specificity were 72% and 94% respectively. The Receiver Operating Curve (ROC) demonstrated high sensitivity with an Area Under the Curve (AUC) of 0.948. Goldman suggest increasing the threshold score to 7, and which would give a negative appendectomy rate of 4%.(Goldman et al., 2008)

A similar study was published by Bhatt et al in 2009. Of the 246 children included in the study, 95 had surgical intervention. Using the standard PAS threshold of 6, the authors demonstrated a high sensitivity (93%), but only a moderate specificity (69%). Bhatt found an AUC that was slightly less in the study by Goldman at 0.895. In this study population, the negative appendectomy rate would have approached 38%. The authors concluded that a single threshold point would not be clinically relevant, but rather the PAS was useful in risk stratification into 3 groups; a) safe to discharge, b) requires further investigation through DI studies or c) requires direct surgical consultation. (Bhatt, Joseph, Ducharme, Dougherty, & McGillivray, 2009)

A retrospective study by Goulder et al analyzed 56 children aged 4 to 15 years found less favorable results. Sensitivity remained high at 87%, but specificity was significantly lower than the previously described studies at 59%. Surgical intervention based on a threshold of 6 would have resulted in a negative appendectomy rate of 17%(Goulder & Simpson, 2008).

Interestingly, a recent publication by Shera et al compared the Alvarado Score to what they considered a new modified score by replacing RLQ rebound tenderness with RLQ cough/percussion/hopping tenderness and weighing this element higher in value (2) while demoting leukocytosis to a value of 1. This "new" modified score, however, seems to have the exact criteria of the PAS (Samuel combined cough/percussion tenderness with hopping tenderness because of good correlation and also promoted this elements value), and therefore could be considered in the PAS group (Shera, Nizami, Malik, Naikoo, & Wani, 2010).

5.3 Comparison of the Alvarado Score and the Pediatric Appendicitis Score

Upon reviewing Table 3 one will notice the similarities between the Alvarado Score and the PAS. However, several differences exist between the two. These include the following:

1. The Alvarado Score was derived in a mixed pediatric/adult population (aged 4 - 80 years) and subsequently validated in children. The PAS was derived in children (aged 4 - 15 years).
2. The Alvarado Score was derived retrospectively and subsequently validated both retrospectively and prospectively. The PAS was derived prospectively and has been validated as such.
3. The Alvarado Score specifically defined elevated temperature as ≥37.3 C, while the PAS does not define pyrexia.
4. The Alvarado Score specifically defined neutrophilia as > 75%, while the PAS does not define neutrophilia (similarly most subsequent studies utilize > 75%).
5. The weighted criteria differ. Alvarado emphases leukocytosis, while Samuel places higher value on rebound tenderness.

Given the above differences, can one choose which score is better? Three well-designed prospective studies have performed head-to-head comparison of the Alvarado Score and the PAS.

Schneider et al enrolled 755 children aged 3 to 21 years who were evaluated by their surgical team for suspected appendicitis. Alvarado Scores and PAS were calculated on 588 participants with complete data. Overall, the PAS was more sensitive (82% vs. 72%) while the Alvarado Score was more specific (81% vs. 65%) in this population. Negative- and Positive- Predictive values were similar between groups (85 vs. 88% and 65 vs. 54% for Alvarado vs. PAS respectively). However, the Alvarado Score had a better Positive Likelihood ratio (3.8 vs. 2.4). ROC curves were similar between the two scores. Unfortunately, this study included patients up to 21 years of age, which may have improved the diagnostic accuracy of the score in this population, though the number of patients over 17 years was not large. Interestingly, the Positive Predictive Value of the Alvarado Score in children < 10 years was diminished (65% vs. 58%) (Schneider, A. Kharbanda, & R. Bachur, 2007).

Study	Year	Population	Ages	Design	T+	F+	F-	T-	Sens	Spec	PPV	NPV	Acc	Notes
Samuel	2002	1170 suspected appendicitis	4 to 15 years	Prospective	734	33	0	403	100%	92%	96%	100%	97%	Derivation Study
Schneider	2007	821 suspected appendicitis 588 included	3 to 21 years	Prospective	162	136	35	255	82%	65%	54%	88%	71%	Alvarado/PAS comparison
Goulder	2008	60 suspected appendicitis 56 included	4 to 15 years	Retrospective	34	7	5	10	87%	59%	83%	67%	79%	
Goldman	2008	1060 abdo pain 849 included	1 to 17 years	Prospective	89	44	34	682	72%	94%	67%	95%	91%	Calculations based on threshold = 6
Bhatt	2009	275 convenience	4 to 18 years	Prospective	77	50	6	113	93%	69%	61%	95%	77%	
Escriba	2011	112 suspected appendicitis 99 included	4 to 18 years	Prospective	?	?	?	?	88%	98%	97%	92%	?	Alvarado/PAS comparison
Adibe	2011	112 suspected appendicitis	1 to 18 years	Prospective	56	4	27	25	67%	86%	93%	48%	72%	
Mandeville	2011	487 diagnosed appendicitis 287 included	4 to 16 years	Prospective	?	?	?	?	88%	50%	67%	79%	?	Alvarado/PAS comparison In Press

T+ True Positive, F+ False Positive, F- False Negative, T- True Negative, Sens Sensitivity, Spec Specificity, PPV Positive Predictive Value, NPV Negative Predictive Value, Acc Accuracy, ? data not provided, N/A not applicable

Table 5. Summary of Studies Evaluating the Pediatric Appendicitis Score

More recently, Escriba et al evaluated 112 children aged 4 - 18 years, with 99 meeting the inclusion criteria. The authors published sensitivity and specificity for all cut-off values for both the Alvarado and the PAS, and favored using a value of 6-points for both tests (the Alvarado Score most commonly uses 7). In keeping with the traditional threshold values,

the Alvarado Score had a sensitivity and specificity of 74% and 98%; respective values for the PAS were 88% and 98%. ROC curves for both Scores were similar (0.96 vs. 0.97) (Escribá, Gamell, Fernández, Quintillá, & Cubells, 2011).
Using a slightly different approach, Mandeville enrolled 287 of 487 children aged 4 to 16 years with a clinical diagnosis of appendicitis in whom 155 had pathologically proven appendicitis. Similar to Schneider's results, the PAS was more sensitive (88% vs. 76%) while the Alvarado Score was more specific (72% vs. 50%). ROC curves were once again similar, yet somewhat lower than the two studies described above (PAS - 0.78, Alvarado - 0.78). When stratified by sex, both Scores had slightly improved sensitivities in boys (Mandeville, Pottker, & Bulloch, 2010). The authors of these three prospective comparison studies concluded that there was insufficient evidence to favor one CSS over the other. Caution was stressed, suggesting that neither score was sensitive nor specific enough to be used as a stand-alone diagnostic test; further investigations such as Computed Tomography (CT) or Ultrasonography (US) were encouraged to complete the evaluation for intermediate-risk children.
The Alvarado Score and the PAS both make use of several key features of CSSs. The criteria are easy to elicit, each criteria is dichotomous (Yes/No), and the Score is easy to calculate. Overall, the PAS appears to be a more sensitive tool, while the Alvarado Score is more specific.

5.4 The Low Risk for Appendicitis Score (Kharbanda)

Increased ED wait times, hospital over-crowding and concerns related to radiation exposure from imaging studies have put pressure on clinicians to quickly and accurately decide which children with abdominal pain should be admitted and observed or discharged without a CT evaluation. Kharbanda et al derived and validated a score to do just that; identify children at low risk for appendicitis.
Kharbana et al prospectively enrolled 767 children aged 3 to 18 years with suspected appendicitis who were evaluated by a surgeon. Of these 767, 601 were included (425 derivation set, 176 validation set). Using logistic regression 6 weighted predictors of appendicitis were determined for a total score of 14. (Table 6) Children with a score of <=5 were highly unlikely to have appendicitis (sensitivity 99%, NPV 98%, NLR 0.032 during derivation, 96%, 96% and 0.102 for validation set)

Diagnostic Criteria	Value
Absolute Neutrophil Count >6.75	6
Rebound pain or pain with percussion	2
Unable to walk, or walks with a limp	1
Nausea	2
History of migration of pain to RLQ	1
History of focal RLQ pain	2
Total	**14**

Table 6. Diagnostic Criteria of Kharbanda's Low Risk Score

In addition to creating the Low Risk Score, the Kharbanda study was novel in that it created a low risk decision tree using recursive partitioning. During derivation, the rule was perfectly sensitive, with a NPV of 98% and a NLR of 0. Validation demonstrated a sensitivity of 98%, NPV of 98% and NLR of 0.058. The Low Risk decision tree in shown in Figure 1 (A. B. Kharbanda, Taylor, Fishman, & R. G. Bachur, 2005).

Practically speaking, Kharbanda's Low Risk Score helps to answer the age old question "Can I safely send this child home?"

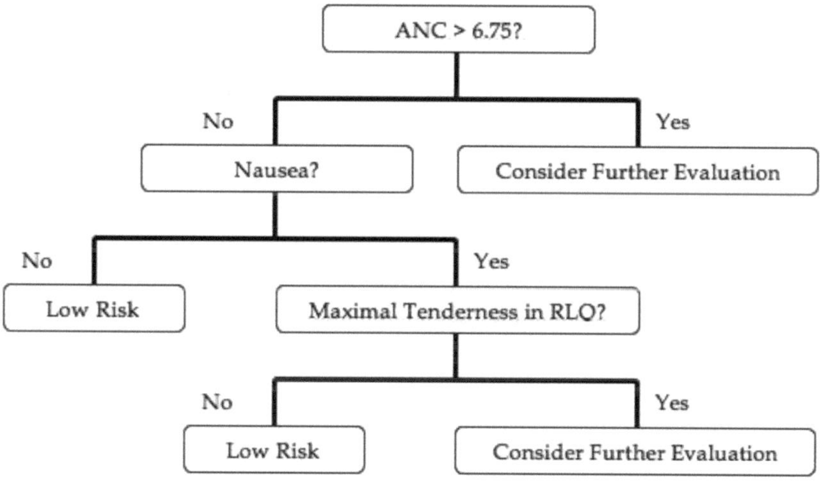

ANC – Absolute Neutrophil Count. RLQ – Right Lower Quadrant

Fig. 1. Decision Tree for identifying children at Low Risk for Appendicitis (Kharbanda)

5.5 The Lintula Score

The Lintula Score relies on clinical data alone. There are no laboratory results required. Using a nice 2-phased approach, Lintula et al first prospectively evaluated 35 clinical variables to derive a score in 127 children aged 4 to 15 years (Score criteria are found in Table 7). Subsequent prospective validation of the score was performed on a similar sample of 109 children. The Lintula Score has a maximum value of 32. A high risk threshold was established at >=21, while low risk was <=15 (Lintula, Pesonen, Kokki, Vanamo, & Eskelinen, 2005).

Four years later, Lintula tested the score in a prospective randomized parallel design. Children aged 4 to 15 years randomized to assessment by score had surgical intervention based on the score result while intervention for those randomized to "no-score" was based on overall clinical and laboratory assessments by the surgeon. Assessments were made at three-hour intervals until a decision to operate or discharge home was established. Of note, imaging studies were not used in either group. Use of the Lintula Score resulted in a significantly higher accuracy (92% vs. 80%) and a lower rate of negative appendectomies. The 2 groups showed no significant difference in sensitivity, however specificity was improved in the Lintula Score group (88% vs. 67%) (Lintula, Kokki, Kettunen, & Eskelinen, 2009).

Diagnostic Criteria	Response	Value
Gender	Male	2
	Female	0
Intensity of Pain	Severe	2
	Mild to moderate	0
Relocation of Pain	Yes	4
	No	0
Vomiting	Yes	2
	No	0
Pain in the RLQ	Yes	4
	No	0
Fever ≥37.5	Yes	3
	No	0
Guarding	Yes	4
	No	0
Bowel Sounds	Absent, tinkling, high-pitched	4
	Normal	0
Rebound Tenderness	Yes	7
	No	0
Total Score		32

Table 7. Diagnostic Criteria for the Lintula Score

5.6 The Eskelinen Score

The Eskelinen Score is relatively complex to perform, (requiring factor multiplication) and was originally designed for use within a computer program. Table 8 details the criteria and design.

Zielke et al compared the Eskelinen and Ohmann Scores using a pooled database of a total of 5 prospective studies. 2359 patients aged 0 to 95 years with suspected appendicitis were analyzed, of which 2209 were included. 845 of these underwent a laparotomy, with histological diagnosis confirmed in 662. Sensitivity, Specificity, PPV, NPV and accuracy were 70%, 92%, 73%, 90% and 87% (Zielke 2001).

Diagnostic Criteria	Presence/Absence	Multiplication Factor	Final Value
Tenderness in RLQ	Yes - 2, No - 1	11.41	
Rigidity	Yes - 2, No - 1	6.62	
WBC > 10 000	Yes - 2, No - 1	5.88	
Rebound Tenderness	Yes - 2, No - 1	4.25	
Pain in RLQ at Presentation	Yes - 2, No - 1	3.51	
Duration of pain > 48 hours	Yes - 2, No - 1	2.13	
		Total Score:	**/67.6**

Table 8. Factorial Multiplication Design of the Eskelinen Score

Taking advantage of the complete pooled database of Zielke (2359 patients), Sitter et al used a higher predetermined threshold score of 55 to determine a sensitivity, specificity, PPV, NPV and accuracy of 79%, 85%, 68%, 91% and 84%. The corresponding AUC of the ROC was 0.91. The authors further calculated these statistical variables using thresholds ranging from 50 to 60, and determined 57 to be the most favorable in their population. (Sitter, Hoffmann, Hassan, & Zielke, 2004)

5.7 The Fenyo-Lindberg Score

This score appears to be one of the most complex, incorporating criteria with multiple levels of response that both add to and subtract from the total score. (Diagnostic Criteria found in Table 9) In 1987, Fenyo prospectively evaluated 259 adult patients with suspected appendicitis. The resulting score was further validated in 830 patients, of which 256 had proven appendicitis. Sensitivity, Specificity, PPV and NPV were 90%, 91%, 83% and 95% respectively. (Fenyo 1987)

Fenyo and Lindberg prospectively validated their score in 1167 patients with suspected appendicitis. Of these, 392 had histologically proven appendicitis. Using the standard threshold score of -2 to predict appendicitis, the sensitivity was 73% and specificity was 87%, notably less than in the original study. Of note, this study made use of 2 different settings, a district and a university hospital. 30% of the patients included from the University hospital were children (age unknown) (Fenyö, Lindberg, Blind, Enochsson, & Oberg, 1997).

Diagnostic Criteria	Response	Value
Sex	Male	+8
	Female	-8
WBC	≥14	+10
	9.0 - 13.9	+2
	≤8.9	-15
Duration of Pain (hours)	<24	+3
	24 - 48	0
	>48	-12
Progression of Pain	Yes	+3
	No	-4
Relocation of pain	Yes	+7
	No	-9
Vomiting	Yes	+7
	No	-5
Aggravation by coughing	Yes	+4
	No	-11
Rebound Tenderness	Yes	+5
	No	-10
Rigidity	Yes	+15
	No	-4
Tenderness outside RLQ	Yes	-6
	No	+4
Constant		-10

Table 9. Diagnostic Criteria of the Fenyo-Lindberg Score

Once again, modification to a CSS was studied. The following changes were made by Dado et al: a) increased WBC cut-off values (<12, 12-20, >20), b) altered values of migratory pain (Yes +4, No -11), c) insertion of elevated temperature >37.5 C (Yes +7, No -9), and d) removal of aggravation by coughing. 197 children aged 2 to 17 years were retrospectively stratified into 3 risk groups using the modified Lindberg Score. Sensitivity and Specificity were 86% and 87%, with an excellent PPV of 96%, but only a modest NPV at 69%(Dado et al., 2000).

5.8 The Ohmann Score

In 1999, Ohmann prospectively validated his own score in a multi-centre, multi-phase trial (Diagnostic Criteria are found in Table 10). Subjects evaluated during phase 1 (n=870) received surgical intervention based on surgeon assessment, while those in phase 2 (n= 614) received computer-assisted diagnostic support using the Ohmann Score. Children less then 6 were excluded from the study, overall pediatric numbers were not published. The authors found a statistically significant improvement in specificity, PPV and accuracy in the phase 2 Score group, along with a decrease in the number of delayed diagnoses (defined as appendectomy on the second day after admission or later) (Ohmann 1999).

Several studies have evaluated the Ohmann Score. In a large study of 2359 subjects (age 0 - 95 years) Zielke compared the score to clinical assessments. Overall accuracy using the Ohmann Score was found to be better than junior surgical staff, with a sensitivity, specificity, PPV, NPV and accuracy of 63%, 93%, 77%, 86% and 84%. However, it was not found to be better than senior surgical staff assessments. (Zielke et al., 1999) Data from this population was further used to compare CSS's, Ohmann Scores, Eskelinen Scores and Ultrasonography with similar statistical results. (Zielke 2001)

Diagnostic Criteria	Value
Tenderness in the RLQ	4.5
Rebound Tenderness	2.5
No Micturation Difficulties	2.0
Steady Pain	2.0
WBC > 10	1.5
Age < 50	1.5
Relocation of pain to RLQ	1.0
Rigidity	1.0
Maximum Total Score	**16**

Table 10. Diagnostic Criteria of the Ohmann Score

5.9 The Christian Score

Probably the simplest of the group, the Christian Score uses a mere 5 criteria (Diagnostic Criteria are found in Table 11). The case group of 58 subjects with suspected appendectomy had surgical intervention if >=4 criteria were met. Fifty-nine appendectomy controls had intervention based solely on surgical staff assessment. Ages ranged from 7 to 56 years. The negative appendectomy rate was significantly less in the Score group than that of the controls (6.5% vs. 17%). This is a rather simple score, which unfortunately does not to appear to have been validated or assessed in a pediatric specific population, but probably should be (Christian 1992).

Abdominal pain on history, occurring within 48 hours of presentation
Vomiting - one or more episode
RLQ tenderness on examination
Low grade fever - defined as <=38.8 C
Polymorphonuclear leukocytosis - define as WBC > 10 000 AND neutrophils > 75%

Table 11. Diagnostic Criteria for the Christian Score

5.10 The RIPASA Score

What is probably the newest member to the group of appendicitis scores is the RIPASA Score, named after its hospital of origin in Brunei. A mixed population of 400 adults and children who had an appendectomy were retrospectively identified, the records of 312 were used to derive the score. Individual criteria were weighted (0.5, 1, 2) based on probabilities and a panel of staff surgeons. The resulting maximal RIPASA score is 16 (diagnostic criteria are found in Table 12); a threshold of 7.5 proving a sensitivity of 88% and specificity of 67% PPV and NPV were 93% and 53%, while accuracy was 81%. Using the score, an absolute reduction in negative appendectomies of 9% would have occurred. (Chong 2010)

Diagnostic Criteria	**Value**
Sex	1.0 - Male 0.5 - Female
Age	1.0 - < 39.9 years 0.5 - > 40 years
RLQ pain	0.5
Migration of RLQ pain	0.5
Anorexia	1.0
Nausea & Vomiting	1.0
Duration of Symptoms	1.0 - < 48 hours 0.5 - > 48 hours
RLQ tenderness	1.0
RLQ guarding	2.0
Rebound tenderness	1.0
Rovsig Sign	2.0
Fever (not defined)	1.0
Raised WBC (not defined)	1.0
Negative Urinalysis (no blood, neutrophils, bacteria)	1.0
Foreign National registration Identity Card	1.0

Table 12. Diagnostic Criteria for RIPASA Score

Chong et al continued to evaluate their new score by prospectively enrolling 200 adults and children in a comparison of the RIPASA and Alvarado Scores. In this group of patients, the RIPASA was statistically superior to the Alvarado Score in Sensitivity (98% vs. 68%), NPV (97% vs. 71%) and accuracy (92% vs. 87%). Specificity, PPV and negative appendectomy rates were similar between the 2 scores. (Chong 2011)

5.11 Other Scores

Several other CSSs have been developed for patients with suspected appendicitis, but do not appear to have been formally evaluated in children and as a result are not further discussed in this chapter. Some of these include the Teicher Score, Arnbjornsson Score, Izbicki Score, and DeDombal Score.

6. Clinical Scoring Systems in practice: Experience of the Alberta Children's Hospital Pediatric Appendicitis Pathway

The real test of a CSS is whether it works in practice. Here I report our experience at the Alberta Children's Hospital (ACH) during a Quality Improvement process from 2006-2011. The Alberta Children's Hospital is a tertiary referral centre for children aged 0 - 18 years, serving a population of approximately 1.8 million in southern Alberta, western Saskatchewan and eastern British Columbia, the 3 western-most provinces of Canada. The Pediatric Emergency Department (PED) at ACH has an annual census of approximately 60 000 visits, and the surgical staff perform approximately 350 acute appendectomies each year.

Following several highly publicized adverse outcomes surrounding appendicitis in both children and adults in the former Calgary Health Region (now Alberta Health Services - Calgary and Area), a formal safety review was conducted. Early diagnosis and standardization of care were determined to be of utmost importance. As a result, Clinical Pathways were developed for both adults and children.

Early diagnosis remains a significant challenge for the pediatrician. After reviewing the literature related to CSSs, the ACH Pediatric Appendicitis Committee agreed to incorporate a score into the pathway development to assist in standardization of assessment, investigation and inter-disciplinary communication. The Alvarado Score and PAS were felt to have similar qualities and to be the most thoroughly evaluated of the CSSs in children with acceptable performance for risk stratification. Since a number of staff groups are employed in both pediatric and adult hospital settings one consistent CSS was felt to be optimal. The Alvarado Score was incorporated into both the adult and pediatric Appendicitis Pathways for the region.

The Pediatric Appendicitis Pathway (Figure 2) uses the Alvarado Score in 2 different ways; the first is a novel departmental flow advancement through a screening tool that initiates Advanced Nursing Directives (ANDs); the second, is a risk stratification tool for physician decision making. Since ED assessment and management are a team effort, we felt it was vital for both nursing and medical staff to use an assessment tool with common features.

6.1 Incorporating Clinical Scoring Systems into Advanced Nursing Directives

Advanced Nursing Directives are used in the ACH PED to improve patient flow and reduce waiting times. ANDs are not simple nursing protocols for administering antipyretics for children with fever or non-steroidal anti-inflammatory drugs for musculo-skeletal pain. Nor are they meant to formally diagnose disease. Rather they are a recognition that skilled nurses are able to identify certain common disease processes (in this case appendicitis), that some of these disease presentations have common investigations and/or management processes, and that empowering pediatric emergency nurses in the frontline can expedite patient care. The purpose of an AND, therefore, is 1) to assist pediatric emergency nurses in identifying children who would likely need further investigation and (2) to empower pediatric emergency nurses to initiate investigations and management before pediatric emergency physician assessment (deForest & Thompson, 2010). (Thompson 2010a)

A number of ED practices, such as initiating intravenous access and fluid management, are commonly performed by nurses caring for adults but are less widely performed in children. Pediatric centres rightly try to limit potentially painful procedures unless they are absolutely required and our AND aims to do precisely this. The important components of any AND include standardized assessment measures using set criteria, a defined care plan if criteria are met, and the option to seek assistance when necessary. Validated CSSs are ideal for integration into an AND.

It must be recognized that different clinical settings may be more appropriate for the use of ANDs. For some health care centres, implementing ANDs into departmental flow may stretch beyond normal nursing practice. For others, it may simply be a matter of formally documenting a process already in place.

The Alvarado Score utilizes both clinical and laboratory variables but at the initial assessment triage of a child with abdominal pain laboratory results are rarely available. Our AND (Figure 3) uses a modification of the original score, leaving out laboratory criteria, and increasing the cutoff value of elevated temperature from 37.3 C to 38.0 C (as a fever is defined as temperature > 38 C in our department). The remaining historical and clinical variables are evaluated by the nursing staff and recorded as a dichotomous variable, either Yes or No. If overall AND criteria are met, the nursing staff are empowered to initiate intravenous access, obtain blood and urine samples for laboratory assessment and give a bolus of crystalloid fluid. These processes occur prior to physician assessment. The objectives of the AND are to identify children with suspected appendicitis earlier in their health care visit, to decrease the time to obtain laboratory results, to identify potential confounding diagnoses early on (i.e. urinary tract infection, pregnancy) and to prepare the child for potential diagnostic imaging.

Preliminary data demonstrates accuracy of our nurses in predicting appendectomy using the AND is similar to the previously published data from the Alvarado Score studies discussed above (Sensitivity 72%, Specificity 72%, NPV 91%, PPV 40%, accuracy 72%. (Thompson 2010b)

6.2 Incorporating the Alvarado Score for medical decision making in the ACH PED

It is well recognized that some children presenting to the ED clearly require surgery for acute appendicitis. However, over the last 2 decades, there has become increased reliance on Diagnostic Imaging modalities (DI) to confirm or rule out appendicitis and potentially provide alternate diagnoses (particularly in post-menarchal girls). Given the availability of DI including Ultrasonography (U/S) and Computed Tomography (CT), and the relatively high sensitivity and specificity of these tests, they are often requested by the surgical team in order to improve diagnostic accuracy and decrease the rate of negative appendectomy. However, given recent concerns related to radiation exposure in children (Brenner & Hall, 2007), as well as overcrowding in many EDs and DI departments leading to delays in imaging acquisition, a more responsible approach to risk stratification is required.

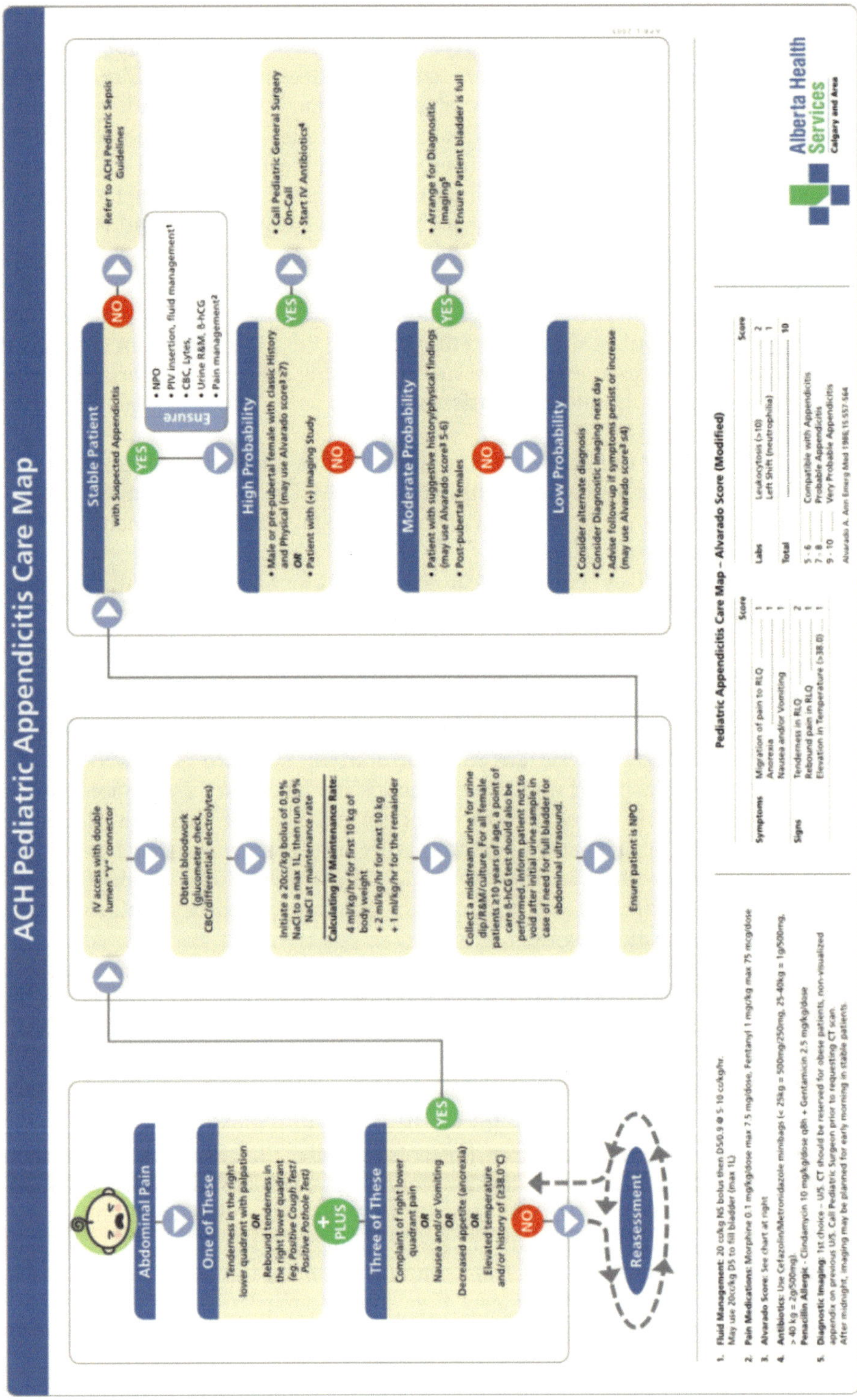

Fig. 2. The Alberta Children's Hospital Appendicits Pathway

Patient Information Label

Nursing Protocol for the Child with Suspected Appendicitis

Purpose: For Emergency Nursing staff to initiate investigations and treatment for the patient presenting in the Emergency Department with signs and symptoms of ap pendicitis prior to an assessment by an Emergency Physician.

For this protocol to be initiated:

The patient **must have ONE** of the following clinical signs:	YES	NO
• Any tenderness in the right lower quadrant with palpation by examiner **OR** • Rebound tenderness in the right lower quadrant (eg. Positive Jump Test/Positive Pothole Test)		! !

The patient **must also have 3 OR MORE** of the following screening criteria:	YES	NO
• Any complaint of right lower quadrant pain by patient	!	!
• Nausea and/or vomiting	!	!
• Decreased appetite (anorexia)	!	!
• Elevated temperature and/or history of (" 38.0°C)	!	!

Does this patient meet the above clinical criteria? ! YES ! NO

If a patient meets the above screening criteria, an Emergency Depar tment Nurse is able to perform the following procedures prior to Emergency Department Physician assessment/orders:

- IV access with double lumen "Y" connector
- Obtain bloodwork (glucometer check, CBC/differential, electrolytes)
- Initiate a 20cc/kg bolus of 0.9% NaCl (maximum 1 litre), then run 0.9% NaCl at maintenance rate:

Calculating IV Maintenance Rate:	**Example Calculation for patient weighing 27kg:**
4 ml/kg/hr for first 10 kg of body weight	4mlx10kg= 40ml/kg/hr
+ 2 ml/kg/hr for next 10 kg	+2mlx10kg= 20ml/kg/hr
+ 1 ml/kg/hr for the remainder	+1mlx7kg= 7ml/kg/hr = 67ml/kg/hr maintenance rate

- Collect a midstream urine for urine dip/R&M, send for culture if urine dip is positive. For all female patients " 10 years of age, a point of care #-HCG test should also be performed. Inform patient not to void after initial urine sample in case of need for full bladder for abdominal ultrasound.
- Ensure patient is NPO

A maximum of 2 IV attempts will be made prior to the Physician's assessment. The Nurse will communicate with the Charge Nurse to ensure that the patient is prioritized appropriately prior to initiation of this protocol.

Fig. 3. Alberta Children's Hospital Advanced Nursing Directive for children with suspected appendicitis

High risk patients (Alvarado Score ≥7) are evaluated by the surgical team after consultation by the ED staff without the need for imaging. Similarly, children at low risk for appendicitis with an Alvarado Score of ≤4, are evaluated by the ED staff for alternate diagnoses or managed with watchful waiting in the home setting, to return should the child's condition worsen. Those children at moderate risk for appendicitis (Alvarado 5-6) or those with high risk for alternate diagnoses (post-menarchal females) are most likely to benefit from imaging studies.

Our post - implementation data has shown that over 40% of appendectomy patients went to the Operating Room (OR) without any imaging studies, a reflection of high risk stratification related to incorporating the Alvarado Score into our pathway. (Thompson 2010c)

7. Implementation and measurement

While it is well known that incorporating carefully developed CSSs into practice improves patient care and departmental processes, the optimal method of implementation is yet to be determined. Many local, national and international medical organizations have developed strategies related to implementation science and knowledge management/translation. Cognitive, social, motivational and organization factors all influence knowledge uptake and use (Gaddis, Greenwald, & Huckson, 2007).

Realistically, it is difficult to achieve 100% uptake of CSSs. Careful planning, with input from all key stakeholders is vital. Introducing new system processes for the care of the child with suspected appendicitis has a multidisciplinary impact. It is highly advisable to solicit representative input from Emergency Medicine, Surgery, Nursing, Diagnostic Imaging, Infectious Disease, Anesthesia, Pharmacy as well as unit managers of Emergency Department, Operating Room, and clinical wards. In order to optimize the potential buy-in from these key stakeholders, departmental leaders would be wise to identify specific outcomes measures ("key wins") geared to each discipline that they will target, for example reduced ED and post-operative lengths of stay.

Donabedian identifies 3 quality measurement pillars. These include structural measures (factors that are present prior to a client visit), process measures (factors occurring during the client visit) and outcome measures (factors occurring after the client visit). Ideally, these outcomes are easily measurable, and within attainable reach (Donabedian, 1992)(Schiff & Rucker, 2001).

The statistical Methods for measuring change related to implementation of CSSs are beyond the scope of this chapter. Interested readers are encouraged to review the literature on Quality Assessment and Measurement.

8. Conclusions

Due to the often-difficult task of the early identification of appendicitis in children, the development of CSSs has increased over the last 3 decades. While most clinicians caring for children with suspected appendicitis are well versed in regard to the Alvarado Score and the Pediatric Appendicitis Score, many other models have been developed. Overall, these scores have been shown to improve clinical and process outcomes including reduced negative appendectomy rates, reduced radiation exposure from unwarranted DI studies, and reduced missed diagnoses. However, one must remain optimistically cautious; to date these Scores have yet to demonstrate a sensitivity or specificity sufficient enough to recommend their use beyond a calculated risk stratification (low, moderate or high).

Even with the abundance of literature regarding CSSs related to appendicitis in children, the need for well-designed, prospective studies to further validate the scores, evaluate implementation strategies and assess impact provides ample opportunity for future research.

Due to the vast number of CSSs and the significant variability in the quality and quantity of validation studies, implementing Clinical Scores into practice can be challenging for individual clinicians. Departmental leaders should therefore carefully consider incorporating CSSs into locally driven Evidence Based Clinical Algorithms.

9. Acknowledgments

The author would like to acknowledge the significant contributions of Mr. Spencer Stevens, Information Services Assistant, Health Information Network Calgary/Alberta Children's Hospital Knowledge Centre and Ms. Luisa Steen, Administrative Assistant, Division of Pediatric Emergency Medicine, Alberta Children's Hospital.

10. References

Alvarado, A. (1986). A practical score for the early diagnosis of acute appendicitis *Annals of Emergency Medicine*, *15*(5), 557-564.

Beattie, P., & Nelson, R. (2006). Clinical prediction rules: what are they and what do they tell us *The Australian journal of physiotherapy*, *52*(3), 157-163.

Bhatt, M., Joseph, L., Ducharme, F. M., Dougherty, G., & McGillivray, D. (2009). Prospective validation of the pediatric appendicitis score in a Canadian pediatric emergency department *Academic emergency medicine : official journal of the Society for Academic Emergency Medicine*, *16*(7), 591-596. doi:10.1111/j.1553-2712.2009.00445.x

Bond, G. R., Tully, S. B., Chan, L. S., & Bradley, R. L. (1990). Use of the MANTRELS score in childhood appendicitis: a prospective study of 187 children with abdominal pain *Annals of Emergency Medicine*, *19*(9), 1014-1018.

Brenner, D. J., & Hall, E. J. (2007). Computed tomography--an increasing source of radiation exposure *The New England journal of medicine*, *357*(22), 2277-2284. doi:10.1056/NEJMra072149

Chang, Y.-C., Ng, C.-J., Chen, Y.-C., Chen, J.-C., & Yen, D. H. T. (2010). Practice variation in the management for nontraumatic pediatric patients in the ED *The American Journal of Emergency Medicine*, *28*(3), 275-283. doi:10.1016/j.ajem.2008.11.021

Dado, G., Anania, G., Baccarani, U., Marcotti, E., Donini, A., Risaliti, A., Pasqualucci, A., et al. (2000). Application of a clinical score for the diagnosis of acute appendicitis in childhood: a retrospective analysis of 197 patients *Journal of Pediatric Surgery*, *35*(9), 1320-1322. doi:10.1053/jpsu.2000.9316

deForest, E. K., & Thompson, G. C. (2010). Implementation of an advanced nursing directive for suspected appendicitis to empower pediatric emergency nurses *Journal of emergency nursing: JEN : official publication of the Emergency Department Nurses Association*, *36*(3), 277-281. doi:10.1016/j.jen.2010.02.015

Donabedian, A. (1992). Quality assurance. Structure, process and outcome *Nursing standard (Royal College of Nursing (Great Britain) : 1987)*, *7*(11 Suppl QA), 4-5.

Eitel, D. R., Rudkin, S. E., Malvehy, M. A., Killeen, J. P., & Pines, J. M. (2010). Improving Service Quality by Understanding Emergency Department Flow: A White Paper and Position Statement Prepared For the American Academy of Emergency Medicine. *The Journal of emergency medicine*, *38*(1), 70-79. Elsevier Inc. doi:10.1016/j.jemermed.2008.03.038

Escribá, A., Gamell, A. M., Fernández, Y., Quintillá, J. M., & Cubells, C. L. (2011). Prospective validation of two systems of classification for the diagnosis of acute appendicitis *Pediatric emergency care*, *27*(3), 165-169. doi:10.1097/PEC.0b013e31820d6460

Fenyö, G., Lindberg, G., Blind, P., Enochsson, L., & Oberg, A. (1997). Diagnostic decision support in suspected acute appendicitis: validation of a simplified scoring system *The European journal of surgery = Acta chirurgica, 163*(11), 831–838.

Gaddis, G. M., Greenwald, P., & Huckson, S. (2007). Toward improved implementation of evidence-based clinical algorithms: clinical practice guidelines, clinical decision rules, and clinical pathways *Academic emergency medicine : official journal of the Society for Academic Emergency Medicine, 14*(11), 1015–1022. doi:10.1197/j.aem.2007.07.010

Goldman, R. D., Carter, S., Stephens, D., Antoon, R., Mounstephen, W., & Langer, J. C. (2008). Prospective validation of the pediatric appendicitis score. *The Journal of Pediatrics, 153*(2), 278–282. doi:10.1016/j.jpeds.2008.01.033

Goldman, R. D., Scolnik, D., Chauvin-Kimoff, L., Farion, K. J., Ali, S., Lynch, T., Gouin, S., et al. (2009). Practice variations in the treatment of febrile infants among pediatric emergency physicians *PEDIATRICS, 124*(2), 439–445. doi:10.1542/peds.2007-3736

Goulder, F., & Simpson, T. (2008). Pediatric appendicitis score: A retrospective analysis *Journal of Indian Association of Pediatric Surgeons, 13*(4), 125–127. doi:10.4103/0971-9261.44761

Hsiao, K.-H., Lin, L.-H., & Chen, D.-F. (2005). Application of the MANTRELS scoring system in the diagnosis of acute appendicitis in children *Acta paediatrica Taiwanica = Taiwan er ke yi xue hui za zhi, 46*(3), 128–131.

Impellizzeri, P., Centonze, A., Antonuccio, P., Turiaco, N., Cifalà, S., Basile, M., Argento, S., et al. (2002). Utility of a scoring system in the diagnosis of acute appendicitis in pediatric age. A retrospective study *Minerva chirurgica, 57*(3), 341–346.

Jain, S., Elon, L. K., Johnson, B. A., Frank, G., & Deguzman, M. (2010). Physician practice variation in the pediatric emergency department and its impact on resource use and quality of care *Pediatric emergency care, 26*(12), 902–908. doi:10.1097/PEC.0b013e3181fe9108

Kharbanda, A. B., Taylor, G. A., Fishman, S. J., & Bachur, R. G. (2005). A clinical decision rule to identify children at low risk for appendicitis *PEDIATRICS, 116*(3), 709–716. doi:10.1542/peds.2005-0094

Laupacis, A., Sekar, N., & Stiell, I. G. (1997). Clinical prediction rules. A review and suggested modifications of methodological standards *JAMA: The Journal of the American Medical Association, 277*(6), 488–494.

Lintula, H., Kokki, H., Kettunen, R., & Eskelinen, M. (2009). Appendicitis score for children with suspected appendicitis. A randomized clinical trial *Langenbeck's Archives of Surgery, 394*(6), 999–1004. doi:10.1007/s00423-008-0425-0

Lintula, H., Pesonen, E., Kokki, H., Vanamo, K., & Eskelinen, M. (2005). A diagnostic score for children with suspected appendicitis *Langenbeck's Archives of Surgery, 390*(2), 164–170. doi:10.1007/s00423-005-0545-8

Macklin, C. P., Radcliffe, G. S., Merei, J. M., & Stringer, M. D. (1997). A prospective evaluation of the modified Alvarado score for acute appendicitis in children *Annals of the Royal College of Surgeons of England, 79*(3), 203–205.

Mandeville, K., Pottker, T., & Bulloch, B. (2010). Using appendicitis scores in the pediatric ED. *American Journal of Emergency Medicine*, 1–6. Elsevier B.V. doi:10.1016/j.ajem.2010.04.018

McGinn, T. G., Guyatt, G. H., Wyer, P. C., Naylor, C. D., Stiell, I. G., & Richardson, W. S. (2000). Users' guides to the medical literature: XXII: how to use articles about clinical decision rules. Evidence-Based Medicine Working Group *JAMA: The Journal of the American Medical Association, 284*(1), 79–84.

Ohmann, C., Yang, Q., & Franke, C. (1995). Diagnostic scores for acute appendicitis. Abdominal Pain Study Group *The European journal of surgery = Acta chirurgica, 161*(4), 273–281.

Plint, A. C., Johnson, D. W., Wiebe, N., Bulloch, B., Pusic, M., Joubert, G., Pianosi, P., et al. (2004). Practice variation among pediatric emergency departments in the treatment of bronchiolitis *Academic emergency medicine : official journal of the Society for Academic Emergency Medicine, 11*(4), 353–360.

Rezak, A., Abbas, H. M. A., Ajemian, M. S., Dudrick, S. J., & Kwasnik, E. M. (2011). Decreased use of computed tomography with a modified clinical scoring system in diagnosis of pediatric acute appendicitis *Archives of surgery (Chicago, Ill : 1960), 146*(1), 64–67. doi:10.1001/archsurg.2010.297

Richer, L. P., Laycock, K., Millar, K., Fitzpatrick, E., Khangura, S., Bhatt, M., Guimont, C., et al. (2010). Treatment of children with migraine in emergency departments: national practice variation study *PEDIATRICS, 126*(1), e150–5. doi:10.1542/peds.2009-2337

Rivers, E., Nguyen, B., Havstad, S., Ressler, J., Muzzin, A., Knoblich, B., Peterson, E., et al. (2001). Early goal-directed therapy in the treatment of severe sepsis and septic shock. *The New England journal of medicine, 345*(19), 1368–1377.

Samuel, M. (2002). Pediatric appendicitis score *Journal of Pediatric Surgery, 37*(6), 877–881.

Schiff, G. D., & Rucker, T. D. (2001). Beyond structure-process-outcome: Donabedian's seven pillars and eleven buttresses of quality *The Joint Commission journal on quality improvement, 27*(3), 169–174.

Schneider, C., Kharbanda, A., & Bachur, R. (2007). Evaluating appendicitis scoring systems using a prospective pediatric cohort *Annals of Emergency Medicine, 49*(6), 778–84, 784.e1. doi:10.1016/j.annemergmed.2006.12.016

Shera, A. H., Nizami, F. A., Malik, A. A., Naikoo, Z. A., & Wani, M. A. (2010). Clinical Scoring System for Diagnosis of Acute Appendicitis in Children. *Indian journal of pediatrics, 78*(3), 287–290. doi:10.1007/s12098-010-0285-9

Shreef, K., Waly, A., Abd-Elrahman, S., & Abd Elhafez, M. (2010). Alvarado score as an admission criterion in children with pain in right iliac fossa. *African Journal of Paediatric Surgery, 7*(3), 163. doi:10.4103/0189-6725.70417

Sitter, H., Hoffmann, S., Hassan, I., & Zielke, A. (2004). Diagnostic score in appendicitis. Validation of a diagnostic score (Eskelinen score) in patients in whom acute appendicitis is suspected *Langenbeck's Archives of Surgery, 389*(3), 213–218. doi:10.1007/s00423-003-0436-9

Sooriakumaran, P., Lovell, D., & Brown, R. (2005). A comparison of clinical judgment vs the modified Alvarado score in acute appendicitis *International journal of surgery (London, England), 3*(1), 49–52. doi:10.1016/j.ijsu.2005.03.009

Stiell, I. (2001). Canadian CT head rule study for patients with minor head injury: methodology for phase II (validation and economic analysis). *Annals of Emergency Medicine, 38*(3), 317–322. doi:10.1067/mem.2001.116795

Stiell, I. G., Greenberg, G. H., McKnight, R. D., Nair, R. C., McDowell, I., & Worthington, J. R. (1992). A study to develop clinical decision rules for the use of radiography in acute ankle injuries *Annals of Emergency Medicine, 21*(4), 384-390.

Stiell, I. G., Greenberg, G. H., McKnight, R. D., Nair, R. C., McDowell, I., Reardon, M., Stewart, J. P., et al. (1993). Decision rules for the use of radiography in acute ankle injuries. Refinement and prospective validation *JAMA: The Journal of the American Medical Association, 269*(9), 1127-1132.

Stiell, I. G., Wells, G. A., Vandemheen, K. L., Clement, C. M., Lesiuk, H., de Maio, V. J., Laupacis, A., et al. (2001). The Canadian C-spine rule for radiography in alert and stable trauma patients. *JAMA: The Journal of the American Medical Association, 286*(15), 1841-1848.

Thompson GC, deForest EK, Eccles R, Ensuring Diagnostic Accuracy in Pediatric Emergency Medicine, Clinical Pediatric Emergency Medicine 2011 12(2):121.

Thompson GC, Stang A, deForest E, Eccles R. Can Pediatric Emergency Nurses Use a Modified Alvarado Score to Accurately Predict Appendecomy? Academic Emergency Medicine 17(5):s118

Thompson GC, Stang A, deForest E, Boag G, Eccles R. Utilization of Diagnostic Imaging after Implementation of a Clinical Pathway for Suspected Pediatric Appendicitis Paediatrics and Child Health 2010 15suppl:31A.

Zielke, A., Sitter, H., Rampp, T. A., Schäfer, E., Hasse, C., Lorenz, W., & Rothmund, M. (1999). [Validation of a diagnostic scoring system (Ohmann score) in acute appendicitis] *Der Chirurg; Zeitschrift für alle Gebiete der operativen Medizen, 70*(7), 777-83; discussion 784.

5

Recent Trends in the Treatment of the Appendicular Mass

Arshad M. Malik and Noshad Ahmad Shaikh
Liaquat University of Medical and Health Sciences, Janshoro (Sindh) Pakistan

1. Introduction

An appendicular mass is one of the common complications seen in patients presenting a few days late after the onset of acute appendicitis. There is no consensus on the optimum treatment of this potentially dangerous condition. The ideal treatment of acute appendicitis is considered to be appendectomy failing which a number of complications, including an appendicular mass, usually result (Margaret Farquharson and Brendan Moran 2007). This usually follows a late presentation or a failure of diagnosis at presentation. Sadly, when the diagnosis has been missed at first presentation to a physician the history is often found to have been quite unremarkable and the error considered avaoidable Traditionally acute appendicitis was principally diagnosed on repeated physical examinations after active observation, without much reliance on laboratory investigations. Greater reliance on putatively objective tools for the diagnosis can delay the diagnosis and has changed the outlook for some patients (Muhammad Shoiab et al 2010). Delayed diagnosis changes the uncomplicated simple acute appendicitis into complicated appendicitis (Chan L et al 2011). A reluctance for surgery is common in third world where most of the population live below the poverty line and a single member may generate the income for the whole family. For this reason time off work can be difficult for some. Another important factor is a general fear of surgery amongst much of the population. Additional factors that contribute to the development of an appendicular mass include lack of health facilities in remote under-resourced areas. In some rural areas general practitioners often keep the patient on symptomatic therapy rather than referring to a higher level hospital.

The appendicular mass is reported to be more common among males who are elderly (Okafor etal 2003) and have different pathogenesis, clinical course and outcome (Gurleyik G and Gurleyik E2003). The mass usually forms in the right iliac fossa after 48-72 hours after the first symptoms of acute appendicitis.The mass develops when appendicitis is caused by obstruction of the lumen and there is an ensuing danger of perforation of the appendix following ischemic necrosis and gangrene of the appendicular wall (Norman S William, Christopher JK Bulstrode and P Ronan O' Connel 2008). As a natural protective mechanism, the omentum and small bowel wrap up the inflamed appendix in an attempt to prevent infection from spreading by isolating the inflamed organ from rest of the abdominal cavity. There may have been an evolutionary advantage that selected this kind of defensive mechanism.

The patient usually presents with a tender mass in the right iliac fossa associated with fever, malaise and anorexia. This walling off mechanism may fail and generalized peritonitis may ensue. This is more often seen when there is obstruction of the appendicular lumen by a faecolith, an immunocompromized patient, the extremes of age, diabetes Mellitus and when the inflamed appendix is lying freely in the pelvis beyond the ability of the omentum to wrap the inflamed organ (Norman S. Williams et al 2008).

1.1 Pathogenesis of the appendicular mass

The appendicular mass usually develops following an attack of acute appendicitis and ranges from a phlegmon to an abscess formation and is usually palpable as a tender mass in the right iliac fossa (Brown CV et al 2003). As described above it usually develops in patients presenting later in the course of acute appendicitis where there is a natural walling off of the inflamed appendix by omentum and coils of small bowel in the vicinity of appendix. Initially this mass is composed of a confused mixture of inflamed appendix these organs and granulation tissue (Brian W.Ellis and Simon -Paterson-Brown 2000). If the barriers work and the inflamed appendix does not perforate a clinically palpable tender mass develops in the right iliac fossa within 48 hours. If the barriers cannot wall off the inflammatiom or the appendix perforates an appendicular abscess may develop. Another term for the mass is phlegmon.
The mass poses a dilemma to the surgeon as to the optimum treatment since there are more than one schools of thought and different modes of treatment are suggested.

1.2 Treatment options for the appendicular mass

The treatment of the appendicular mass is controversial and perhaps confusing as there is no consensus about the optimum approach. Currently there are four modes of treatment practiced all over the world with a very clear distinction between two of these schools of thought.

1. The conventional mode of management includes an initial conservative treatment assuming the patient is well and settles, followed by an interval appendectomy after a period of 6-8 weeks.
2. A totally conservative treatment without interval appendectomy. This approach was introduced after the need for an interval appendectomy was questioned in a number of reports.
3. An early and aggressive approach favouring early appendectomy in appendicular mass.
4. Laparoscopic management of the appendicular mass is the most recent advancement in the treatment of appendicular mass.

All four modalities are practiced and since there are advocates and critics of every technique, we need to explore each in detail.

2. Coventional treatment: The Ochsner-Sherren regime

Traditionally it was believed that surgery during the phase of acute appendicitis with a mass was potentially dangerous and could lead to life threatening complications because of oedema and the fragility of important structures like the terminal ileum and caecum. The surgeon may do more harm than good considering the fact that the problem was contained and resolution might follow. The Ochsner-Sherren regime was popularised by Oschner (Oschner AJ 1901) The concept has enjoyed a unique position over many years as the standard treatment for the appendicular mass.
The essential components are now are as follws:

- Nursing the patient in a popped -up position encouraging gravitational flow of any exudates towards the pelvis.

- Nothing is to be given by mouth for an initial 24-48 hours while the patient is kept on intravenous fluids
- Intravenous antibiotics are administered with regular monitoring of vital sign a as well as measurement of the size of the mass.
- If the patient's general condition improves, the size of the mass reduces and the fever and anorexia subside, the patient is usually allowed liquids orally and then diet. If this is tolerated discharge home is considered. After six weeks an interval appendectomy is performed.
- On the other hand, if the condition of the patient deteriorates, the size of the mass increases, pulse rate increases or general peritonitis develops or the patient becomes septic then the conservative management is curtailed and the patient is considered for operation.

Failure of the conservative regime is reported in 2-3% and urgent exploration is considered essential.

2.1 Advocates of the conventional treatment

This is the most commonly practiced treatment for an appendicular mass without abscess formation (Price MR 1996). It is favoured because it can avoid the potential hazards of damage to the caecum and the development of faecal fistula (Nitecki S 1993) ,(Norman S William). Surgeon preference remains a common reason (Kim JK 2010). The conservative approach is considered to be associated with a substantially low rate of complications (Tingstedt B 2002) and is safe (Kumar S and Jain S 2004). The rate of success is reported to range between 88-95% (safirUllah 2007). Interval appendicectmy is considered essential believing that the rate of recurrence of appendicitis and mass formation is high after conservative treatment and resolution of the mass (Friedell ML and Perez-Izquierdo M 2000). Another reason for aninterval appendectomy is the conformation of the diagnosis as it is possible to miss other pathology like ileocaecal tuberculosis or malignancy. These conditions mimic acute appendicitis and conservative therapy alone should be considered cautiously (E.S Garba 2008) (Garg P et al 1997).

2.2 Critics of conventional treatment

Critics report poor patient compliance, a requirement for re-admission, and sometimes difficulty in finding the appendix at the interval appendectomy or undue bleeding (Malik et al 2008). It is also reported that about 10% of patients need exploration due to deterioration on a conservative regimen (Olika D 2000). In the Third World patients frequently do not attend for an interval appendectomy if they have been pain free and asymptomatic. The recurrence rate is reported to be as low as 5-20% (Tekin A 2008, Adala SA 1996) and importantly the recurrent disease is milder than the primary acute appendicitis (Dixon MR 2003). The effectiveness of the immediate conservative therapy is a proven and acceptable mode of treating the mass but the need of interval appendectomy is questioned and it may not be cost effective(Hung-Wen Lai 2005).

2.3 Conservative treatment without interval appendiciectomy

It is argued that interval appendectomy is unnecessary after successful conservative management of an appendicular mass (Anna Kaminski et al 2005). This approach can be applied in selected patients who do not develop recurrent symptoms(Garba ES et al 2008).

Conservative treatment alone will suffice in 80% of patients. The greatest risk of developing recurrent appendicitis after successful conservative management is during the first 6 months (Hoffmann j et al 1984) and there is a minimal chance of developing symptoms after 2 years. Interval appendectomy is considered by some to be a difficult operation and sometimes the fibrotic appendix may not be found on operation (Deakin DE et al 2007). This has led to the concept of a "wait and watch policy" after successful conservative management and has been found to be cost effective (Hung-Wen lai et al 2005). The advocates of this approach may go as far as to propose that recurrent disease is also amenable to conservative treatment and is cost effective (Willemsen PJ et al 2002).

3. Early appendectomy in appendicular mass

Many surgeons will perform an appendectomy if a small mass is felt under a general anaesthetic but a minority will wake the patient and continue with a non-operative approach. It is crucial that the patient understands this option if it is a possibility when they go to theatre. Thus, early appendectomy is widely performed but not when the mass is substantial and felt pre-operatively.

This author argues that during the early phase of the appendicular mass surgery is not as hazardous, as it once was. The key to early surgery is good resuscitation, expert anaesthesia, broad spectrum antibiotics and an experienced surgeon (De U et al 2002). This approach obviates the need of re-admission, cures the problem totally, and there is an opportunity to reach to a conclusive diagnosis at an early stage. A number of studies consider this approach to be safe, economical and time saving, facilitating an early return to work (Sardar Ali et al 2010). The experience of the surgeon plays a vital role.

4. Authors study

We conducted a study of 176 patients with an appendicular mass who were managed in two groups of equal size. In this study the patients chose their own group. One group was operated immediately on admission after relevant investigations and work up while the other group had conservative management and an interval appendectomy after 6-8 weeks. The outcome measures included operative difficulties, total operating time, operative and post-operative complications, total duration in hospital, and the willingness for interval appendectomy.

The patients had a history of pain around the peri umbilical region at the start and then localized to right iliac fossa. Most of them reported to general practitioners who either advised them some symptomatic treatment or appendectomy. Due to various reasons many of them declined operative treatment and returned back with an established appendicular mass in a few days. All relevant investigations were performed and patients were categoriszed on their own will into two groups. The procedures were explained to both groups of patients explaining benefits and drawbacks of each technique.

4.1 Results

- Most of the patients who were treated successfully on an initial conservative treatment either did not return or were not willing for an operation unless there were recurrent attacks of acute appendicitis.

- We found immediate operation to be relatively easy compared to interval appendectomy. There were more complications in the the interval appendectomy group.

Some of the results appear below. Our results favour early appendectomy in line with the findings of others (Asal Y Izzidien Al-Samarrai 1995) (Friedell ML 2000) (Sardar Ali And Rafique Hm).

To date the authors have extended the previous study to a total of 1356 patients divided into two groups as in the earlier study. The results are similar.

We now conclude that the best way of managing the appendicular mass is immediate operation as it saves time, ensures total recovery during the initial admission and excludes other pathology. There is a great satisfaction to the patient that the actual problem is completely cured while if appendectomy is delayed for 6-8 weeks, the patients compliance is poor and there can be mild pain for which patients usually do not seek medical advice.

In Third World countries like Pakistan and India, where the majority of the population are living below the poverty line early intervention is a better option as it proves to be cost effective.

Variable	Type of Treatment (n = 130)		P value
	Immediate appendectomy n (88)	Interval appendectomy n (42)	
Operative findings:			
Simple mass	64(72.7%)	3(7.14%)	< 0.001*
Perforated appendix	8(9.1%)	0	
Loculated collection of pus	7(8.0%)	0	
Appendicular abscess	4(4.5%)	0	
Firm Adhesions	5(5.7%)	33(78.57%)	

N= Numer of patients

Table 1. Operative findings

Variable	Type of Treatment (n = 130)		P value
	Immediate appendectomy n (88)	Interval appendectomy n (42)	
Difficulty in localization of appendix	12(13.63%)	28(66.66)	0.001*
Difficulty in adhesiolysis	23(26.1%)	32(76.19%)	
Minor trauma to bowel	13(14.8%)	2(2.3%)	
Bleeding	11(12.5%)	9(21.42%)	

N= Number of patients

Table 2. Operative problems.

Variable	Type of Treatment (n = 130)		P value
	Immediate appemdectomy n (88)	Interval appendectomy n (42)	
Post-operative complications:			
Wound sepsis	14(15.9%)	6(6.8%)	0.12
Partial wound dehiscence	4(4.5%)	2(2.3%)	
Residual abscess	1(1.1%)	0	

Table 3. Post-operative complications.

Variable	Type of Treatment (n = 130)		P value
	Immediate appendectomy n (88)	Interval appendectomy n (42)	
Total operative time:			
30-60 Minutes	69(78.40%)	8(19.04%)	
60-90 Minutes	13(14.77%)	31(73.80%)	< 0.001*
90-120 Minutes	6(6.81%)	2(76.19%)	
>120 Minutes	Nil	1(2.38%)	

Table 4. Total operative time.

Outcome of total patients managed conservatively followed by interval appendectomy

	Outcome	No: of Patients	Percentage (%)
1.	Sucessfull mass resolution	75	85.22
2.	Converted to appendectomy	13	14.77
3.	Refused interval appendectomy	21	23.86
4.	Lost to follow up	11	12.5
5.	Underwent interval appendectomy	42	47.72

Table 5. Break up of patients in Conservative group.

Laparoscopic appendectomy has recently gained popularity as an alternative to open appendectomy but is still in the evolving stage. A number of studies have proposed this to be a safe and cost effective method of treating acute appendicitis. Despite rising popularity of this method in acute appendicitis, its role is not really established so far in appendicular mass and a consensus is yet to be developed. However, a number of reports are published claiming its role in the treatment of appendicular mass (Vishwanath V et al 2011). It is also considered to be safe and the patient is cured at the first admission obviating the need for re-admission (sanapathi S et al 2002). Although technically demanding, it is yet considered a safe option of management in children presenting with appendicular mass (Goh BK et al 2005). As claimed by Garg Cp et al 2009, the technique of laparoscopic surgery in appendicular mass can be as safe as open techniques but it has an additional advantage of being cost effective and is cosmetically more acceptable to patients specially the females. Despite all the reports favouring laparoscopic approach to appendicular mass, the role of this technique is yet to be established as there are no randomized control studies substantiating adequately to this recent advancement in the management of appendicular mass.

5. References

Adala SA. Appendiceal mass: Interval appendectomy should not be the rule. Br J Clin Prac 1996;50:16

Al - Samarrai A. Surgery for appendicular mass. Saudi J Gastroenterol 1995;1:43-6.

Arshad M, Aziz LA, Qasim M, Talpur KA.Early appendectomy in appendicular mass.A liaquat University hospital experience. J Ayub Med Coll Abbottabad 2008;20(1):70-2.

Brian W. Ellis,Simon Paterson-Brown. In Acute appendicitis in Hamilton Baily's emergency surgery,13th Edn,2000, Published by Arnold; 399-410.

Brown CV, Abrishami M, Muller M, Velmahos GC. Appendicular Abscess:Immediate operation or percutaneous drainage? Am Surg 2003; 69:829-32?

Chan L, Shin LK, Pai RK, Jeffery RB. Pathologic continuum of acute appendicitis: Sonographic findings and clinical management implications. Ultrasound Q 2011; 27(2):71-9.

De U ,Ghosh S. Acute appendectomy for appendicular mass. A study of 87 patients. Ceylon Med J 2002;47(4):117-8.

Deakin DE, Ahmed I. Interval appendectomy after resolution of the mass.Is it necessary? The surgeon 2007; 5(1): 45-50.

Dixon MR, Hauoos JS, Park IU. An assessment of the severity of recurrent appendicitis. Am J Surg 2003; 186:718-722?

E.S Garba & A. Ahmed. Management of appendiceal mass. Ann Afr Med 2008; 7(4): 200-204.

Friedell ML & Perez-Izquierdo M. Is there a role for interval appendectomy in the management of acute appendicitis? Am Surg 2000; 68:1158-1162?

Garg P, Dass BK,Bansaal AR, Chitkara N. comparative evaluation of conservative management versus early surgical intervention in appendicular mass- A clinical study. J Indian Med Assoc 1997; 95(6):179-80.

Garg CP, Vaidya BB, Chengalath MM. Efficacy of laparoscopy in complicated appendicitis. Int J Surg 2009; 7(3):250-2.

Goh BK, Chui CH, Yap TL, Low Y, Lama TK, Alkouder G, Prasad S, Jacobson AS. Is early appendectomy feasible in children with acute appendicitis presenting with an appendicular mass? A propective study. J Pediatr Surg 2005; 40(7):1134-7.

Gurleyik G, Gurleyik E. Age-related clinical features in older patients with acute appendicitis. Eur J Emerg Med 2003; 10(3):200-203.

Hoffmann J, Lindhard A,Jensen H. Appendix mass: conservative management without interval appendectomy. Am j Surg; 148:379-82.

Hung-Wen Lai, Che-Chuan Loong, Chew-Wun Wu, Wing-Yui Lui. Watchful waiting versus interval appendectomy for patients who recovered from acute appendicitis with tumor formation: A cost-effective analysis. J Chin Med Assc 2005;68(9): 431-34.

Kaminski A, Liu IA, Applebaum, Lee SL, Haigh PI. Routine interval appendectomy is not justified after initial non-operative treatment of acute appendicitis. Arch Surg 2005; 140: 897-901.

Kim JK, Ryoos S, Oh HK, Kim JS, Shin R, Choe EK, Jeong SY, Park KJ. Management of appendicitis with abscess or mass. J Korean Soc Coloproctol 2010; 26(6): 413-9.

Kumar S,Jain S. Treatment of appendiceal mass: Prospective randomized control trial. Indian J Gastro Enterol 2004; 23(5):165-7.

Margaret Farquharson (Author), Brendan Moran (Author).Operations on appendix. *InFarquharson's Textbook of Operative General Surgery, 9th Edition*A Hodder Arnold Publication

Muhammad Shoib Hanif, Tufail Hussain Tahir, Irfan Ali sheikh, Muhammad Zaman Ranjha. Acute appendicitis: gaining time in mass casualty scenario. Pak Armed Forces J Med 2010; 3 23-25.

Nitecki S, Assalia A & Schein M. Contemporary management of appendiceal mass. Br J Surg 1993; 80:18-20.

Norman S.William, Christopher J.K.Bulstrode, P Ronan O' Connel in Vermiform appendix in Short practice Of surgery, 25th ed, 2008, Edward Arnold publisher Ltd 1205-1217.

Oscner AJ. The cause of diffuse peritonitis complicating appendicitis and its prevention. JAMA 1901; 26:1747-1754.

Okafor PL, Orakwe JC, Chianakawana GU. Management of appendiceal mass in a peripheral hospital in Nigeria: review of thirty cases. World J Surg 2003; 27(7): 800-3.

Olika D, Yamini D, Udani VM, et al.Non-Operative management of perforated appendicitis without peri-appendiceal -mass. Am J Surg 2000; 179:177-81?

Price MR, Hasse GM, Satorelli KH, Meagher DP Jr. Recurrent appendicitis after initial conservative treatment of appendiceal abscess. J paediatr Surg 1996; 31:291-4.

Rintoul RF. Operations on appendix . In Farquharsonson's Text book of Surgery, 9th Ed, Edward Arnold publishers Ltd, 2005, 378-390.

Sardar Ali, Rafique HM. Early exploration versus conservative management. Professional Med J 2010; 17(2):180-4.

Ssfirullah et al. Conservative treatment of appendicular mass without interval appendectomy. JPMI 2007; 21(1):55-59.

Takin A, Kurtoglu HC, Can I, Oztan S. Routine interval appendectomy is unnecessary after conservative treatment of appendiceal mass. Colorectal Dis 2008; 10: 465-8.

Tingstedt B, Bexe-Lindskog F,Ekelund M, Anderson R. management of appendiceal masses.Eur J Surg 2002;168(11):579-82.

Vishwanath V Shindholimath, K Thinakaran, T Narayana rao, Yenni Veerabhadappa Veerappa. Laparoscopic management of appendicular mass. J Min Access Surg 2011; 7(2):136040.

Willemsen PJ, Hoorntie LE, Eddes EH, Ploeg RJ. The need for interval appendectomy after resolution of an appendiceal mass questioned. Dig Surg 2002; 19(3):216-20.

6

What Is the Role of Conservative Antibiotic Treatment in Early Appendicitis?

Inchien Chamisa
Mediclinic Medforum Private Hospital, Pretoria, South Africa

1. Introduction

Acute appendicitis remains a common surgical condition and appendicectomy remains the mainstay of treatment for over 130 years. The first appendicectomy was performed by A. Groves more than a century ago. Following the publication of R. Fitz's classical (1) paper in 1886 on 247 patients with perforated appendicitis, early appendicectomy has been advocated as the standard treatment for early appendicitis. Later, in 1889 McBurney (1) published his study of eight patients with acute appendicitis and further recommended early appendicectomy as optimal management. Since then early appendicectomy has been widely accepted as the best treatment for early appendicitis. (1, 2).
However, as the diagnosis of acute appendicitis remains largely a clinical one, diagnostic uncertainty may lead to a delay in treatment or negative surgical exploration, both adding to the morbidity associated with this condition. While antibiotics are indicated in patients with signs of peritonism, their current role in the routine management of early acute non-perforated appendicitis remains debatable.
Over the past two decades, three randomised controlled trials have been published comparing the efficacy of antibiotics alone with that of surgery for selected and unselected patients with that of surgery for acute appendicitis (3, 4, and 5). It is the aim of this chapter to give a critical analysis of the existing data regarding the non-surgical management of acute appendicitis with special reference to the efficacy, long-term outcome and the selection of patients for conservative treatment.

2. Pathophysiology of acute appendicitis

To appreciate the potential role of the conservative approach in the management of acute appendicitis it is essential to have an understanding of the basic patho-physiology of the condition. Acute inflammation of the appendix is associated with obstruction of the appendiceal lumen in 50 to 80% of patients. The majority are attributed to hyperplasia of sub-mucosal lymphoid follicles and this is commonly seen in children. Other causes include faecolith, parasitic infections (e.g. schistosoma), gallstones, carcinoid tumours and carcinoma of the caecum. As the mucinous secretions accumulate in the lumen, the intra-luminal pressure rises and this is sufficient to cause collapse of the draining veins. Once obstruction and ischaemia sets in, this facilitates bacterial proliferation with further inflammatory oedema and exudation, compromising the blood supply. On the other hand, a minority of acute appendicitis have no demonstrable luminal obstruction and the pathogenesis of inflammation in this subgroup is largely unknown.

During the early stages, only scanty neutrophilic exudate is evident throughout the mucosa, sub-mucosa and muscularis propria. This results in congestion of the sub-serosal vessels. This stage signifies early acute appendicitis. Later on, prominent neutrophilic exudate forms a fibrino-purulent reaction over the serosa. Further inflammation results in formation of abscesses in the wall together with ulceration and foci of necrosis in the wall resulting in acute suppurative appendicitis. This then progresses to larger areas of haemorrhagic ulceration of the mucosa and gangrenous necrosis through the wall extending to the serosa. This is the acute gangrenous appendicitis stage which rapidly progresses to rupture and suppurative peritonitis. The histological pathognomonic features of acute appendicitis are neutrophilic infiltration of the muscularis, usually accompanied with ulceration and neutrophils in the mucosa.

It is interesting to note that Luckmann et al (6, 7) has proposed that the entities of perforated and non-perforated appendicitis are two distinct and different conditions. These authors believe that one form of appendicitis results in early perforation whereas the other one does not perforate and may resolve spontaneously. This begs the question, how do we distinguish these two clinical entities and do they demand the same management?

3. The concept of conservative management

The complications of acute appendicitis can be severe and include perforation, generalised peritonitis and intra-abdominal abscesses. Up to 15-30% of patients operated for suspected appendicitis are found to have a normal appendix on histological examination (8). Since appendicectomy is associated with complications (e.g. wound infections, adhesive small bowel obstruction, pneumonia, hernias) the possibility of non-surgical treatment has been proposed since the middle of the 20th century. The first report of choosing the conservative management of acute appendicitis over an operation was presented in the British Medical Journal in1945 by McPherson and Kinmonth (9). Then in 1959 Coldrey (2) studied and reported on 471 unselected patients who had antibiotic treatment alone with acceptable mortality and morbidity rates. In 1977 a study was published from China which described 425 patients managed with a combination of antibiotics and traditional Chinese medicine and at follow up a recurrence of 7% was found (10). The conservative treatment with antibiotics was described in nine USA submariners in 1990 with encouraging results but this was in a situation where surgery was not safely available. (11)

4. Background

Diagnostic un-certainty in those with suspected appendicitis may result in delayed treatment or negative explorations sometimes associated with complications. Population-based studies have shown that there are significant long-term risks associated with surgical explorations for appendicitis (12). The risk of small bowel obstruction needing surgical intervention has been shown to be around 1.3% by 30 years. (13) It is of interest that a negative appendicectomy has been shown to have more complications compared with a positive appendicectomy especially the risk of small bowel obstruction (14). It is because of these concerns that in recent years there has been a heightened interest in the use of antibiotic therapy as the primary treatment for patients with uncomplicated appendicitis. It

is still uncertain as to what extend these promising results of conservative management of acute appendicitis are in unselected populations.
Traditionally, patients with no overt clinical signs such as right iliac fossa guarding and peritonism are monitored and re-assessed for any changes in clinical signs with or without commencing antibiotic therapy. The place of routine antibiotic treatment in patients presenting with acute non-perforated appendicitis is still a debatable issue. Other studies have concluded that antibiotic therapy reduces the rate of wound and intra-abdominal sepsis following surgery (15, 16).

5. Conservative management compared with appendicectomy

Appendicectomy has been regarded as the principal procedure for patients presenting with acute appendicitis since the first appendicectomy was performed by A. Grooves more than 130 years ago. The mortality rate for emergency appendicectomy ranges from 0.07 % to 0.7% in patients without perforation and 0.5% to 2.4% in those with (6). The chances of death in patients undergoing an emergency appendicectomy for acute appendicitis is up to seven times that of the general population of the same age and gender (17). The post-operative morbidity following emergency appendicectomy is 10 to 19% in those without perforation and reaches 12 to 30 % in patients with a perforation (18). It has been shown that the operative morbidity following appendicectomy for a normal appendix in patients with suspected acute appendicitis is similar to that in patients with non-perforated appendicitis (19).

6. Financial costs

Over and above the human costs of operative morbidity and mortality, there is a significant financial burden associated with appendicectomy. The overall cost of appendicitis in the United States in 1997 was estimated as one million hospital days and $3 billion in hospital charges, of which postoperative morbidity accounted for 50% of the charges (17) The costs are expected to rise further with the advent and popularity of laparoscopic appendicectomy.

7. Antibiotic resistance

The availability of monotherapy for effective treatment of intra-abdominal infection has made triple-regimen antibiotics almost obsolete. Furthermore, new effective oral antibiotics are now available which allow treatment of serious infections on an outpatient basis. Because of these advances in antibiotic therapy, surgeons have considered the possibility of treating acute appendicitis with antibiotics alone with the hope of replacing urgent appendectomy in a selected group of patients.
Despite the recent improvements in medical technology, the perforation rate for acute appendicitis has remained almost unchanged since the 1980s, ranging from 20 to 30%. This apparent constant perforation rate supports Lachmann's hypothesis that perforated and non-perforated appendicitis represent two different disease processes.
There is sonographic evidence in the literature supporting the spontaneous resolution of acute appendicitis (20) managed conservatively. The widely believed theory of disease progression from mucosa to serosa to perforation may not apply in all cases of acute appendicitis as supported by Lachmann and colleagues.

This chapter includes all the randomised controlled trials and other studies on which patients over 18 years with suspected acute appendicitis were randomised to antibiotic therapy alone or surgery at initial presentation. The primary outcome measures of most of these randomised controlled trials was complications such as reoperation, tra-abdominal abscess, small bowel obstruction, wound dehiscence, incisional hernia, deep venous thrombosis, pulmonary embolism, cardiac complications and the need for ileo-caecal resection. The minor complications included prolonged post-operative recovery, urinary dysfunction, anaesthesia-related complications, diarrhoea, clostridium difficile infection, fungal infection and wound sepsis. Secondary outcome measures included duration of hospital stay and re-admission rates.

8. Efficacy

It is important to bear in mind that the conservative management of acute appendicitis has several safety implications which need to be taken into consideration. The act of delaying surgical intervention may increase the risk of appendiceal perforation, intra-abdominal abscesses and localised or generalised peritonitis. On the other hand, appendicectomy is associated with significant morbidity which includes wound sepsis, incisional hernias and adhesive small bowel obstruction.

Several recent literature reports which include randomised controlled studies, meta-analyses and prospective studies comparing conservative management and appendicectomy for acute appendicitis in selected patients have concluded that the former is effective with a reported success rate ranging from 68% to 95% (21, 3). In a randomised clinical trial by Hansson et al (3), the authors found efficacy in the study group according to intention to treat to be 48 % (97 of 202). Out of 119 patients who received antibiotics, eleven (9.2%) had an appendicectomy owing to clinical progression of the disease within 24-36hours. They found that of the 250 patients who had surgical exploration, 223 (89.2 %) had confirmed appendicitis or another surgical condition. From this they concluded that the primary treatment efficacy was 90.8 per cent for antibiotic therapy compared to 89.2 per cent for those who underwent surgical exploration. However, they found out that after 1 year follow-up, antibiotic treatment efficacy decreased to 78.2 % mainly due to recurrences. The efficacy was significantly lower than in the surgery group ($P<0.05$). The minor complications were similar for both groups while major complications were threefold higher in the appendicectomy patients ($p<0.05$). Of the operated patients, 2.9% needed a second operation, 3% had abscesses, 2.4% postoperative small bowel obstruction, wound rupture (1.8%), pulmonary embolism (0.6%), postoperative cardiac dysfunction (0.6%) and 1.2% needed ileo-caecal resection. Anaesthesia-related complications were 1.2% and the wound infection rate 7.6%. Their readmission rate was 15 (13.9 %) after a median of 1 year. A third of these admissions appeared within 10 days of hospital discharge and the other two-thirds between 3 and 16 months after discharge.

In a prospective randomised controlled study by Styrud et al, (4) antibiotic therapy alone was found to be sufficient in the majority of patients with acute appendicitis with only 12% of patients from the antibiotic group requiring surgery within the next 24 hrs. Out of 128 patients managed conservatively, 17 (12%) went on to have surgery within 24 hours. After one year, the recurrence rate was 15% (16 patients) and they found out many of these patients requested conservative management the second time around.

In a series of five patients reported by Wiegering et al, the authors concluded that conservative management of acute appendicitis is safe and that it should be considered in patients with neutropaenia who are otherwise clinically stable (22).

Efficiency can be measured by comparing the recurrence or readmission rates of patients managed conservatively to that of complications after appendicectomy. Recurrence rates reported in the literature range from 3 to 25% within the first year (4). In a recent met-analysis by Varadhan et al, they reported recurrent rates of 15% in the first year following conservative management on antibiotics (21). It is interesting to note that the perforation rate in patients admitted with a recurrence was not higher compared to those who underwent initial appendicectomy. It is not surprising that the investigators who reported a higher recurrence rate following conservative treatment have advocated that this approach should be considered in patients with a high risk for post-operative complications.

In a meta-analysis by Varadhan et al., out of 350 patients randomised to the antibiotic group, 238 (65%) were managed successfully on antibiotics alone with 38 recurrences (21). After 1 year follow up, 200 patients from the antibiotic group remained asymptomatic.

A metanalysis of RCTs showed a trend for reduced complications for antibiotic therapy [RR (95% CI): 0.43 (0.16, 1.18)] with no difference between antibiotic therapy and surgery for length of hospital stay.

In a study by Eriksson et al, 40 patients with a sonographic diagnosis of acute appendicitis were randomised to either appendicectomy or antibiotics only therapy (5). They concluded that patients who received nonsurgical treatment did as well as the patients who underwent an appendicectomy.

The conservative management of acute appendicitis has safety implications which should be considered in decision making. This form of treatment has attracted the attention of clinicians because of the growing body of evidence that it eliminates the surgical and anaesthesia-related complications associated with appendicectomy. Possible complications following surgery include accidental enterotomies, post-operative haematomas, colonic fistula, surgical site infection, intra-abdominal abscess, paralytic ileus, adhesive small bowel obstruction and incisional hernias with the possible need for a second operation. The rate of intestinal obstruction is slightly higher after a negative appendicectomy compared to a positive one.

Literature studies have shown that the risk of death for patients undergoing an emergency appendicectomy is approximately seven times that of the general population of the same age and gender (17). The mortality rate for patients undergoing emergency appendicectomy for non-perforated and perforated appendicitis is 0.07 to 0.7% and 0.5-2.4% respectively (6). The operative morbidity rates for non-perforated and perforated appendicitis are 20% and 30% respectively. (ref 2..8,27) The operative mortality rises with increased age as follows: <0.1% in patients less than 40 years of age, 2.6% in patients more than 60 years of age, 6.8% for octogenerians and 16.6% for nonagenarians (17).

Hansson et al (3) found that the major complications were not significantly related to open or laparoscopic surgery. The common minor complications were wound infection in the appendicectomy group and diarrhoea in the conservative group. They concluded that conservative treatment with antibiotics was efficacious in 91% of cases with a relapse rate of 14% at 1 year follow-up.

A prospective study by Malik et al comparing antibiotic therapy to appendicectomy in acute appendicitis concluded that conservative treatment was both safe, efficacious and caused less patient pain than surgery, minimising the need for analgesia (p 0.001) (8). They found a relapse rate of 10% in the conservatively treated group within the first 12 months.

In children with perforated appendicitis who had an appendicectomy the morbidity is around 26-58% and for conservative management is 0–15% (23). There is evidence from retrospective studies showing that in patients with perforated appendicitis managed conservatively, the late recurrences showed a mild clinical course (24).

A recent metanalysis comparing conservative management and appendicectomy for complicated appendicitis concluded that conservative management was associated with a significant reduction in wound sepsis, pelvic or intra-abdominal abscesses, small bowel obstruction and need for reoperation (25). In a randomised controlled study by Styrud et al (4), the complication rate in the surgery group was 14% and was mainly due to infection and the time in hospital, sick leave and time lost from work were 2.6, 6 and 10 days respectively.

A study by Anderson reviewing small bowel obstruction after appendicectomy, (13) reported a cumulative risk of surgically treated small bowel obstruction after appendicectomy of 0.41% after 4 weeks, 0.63% after 1 year and 1.30% after 30 years of follow-up, compared with 0.003% at 1 year and 0.21% after 30 years of follow-up among a conservatively managed group. In another review of 1,777 patients who had an appendicectomy for acute appendicitis, the overall small bowel obstruction rate was 2.8% over an average 4.1-year follow-up (26).

Laparoscopic appendicectomy is associated with less postoperative pain and a reduced hospital stay, but it also carries risks as follows: intra-operative complications (0.7% to 3.1%), postoperative complications (1.9% to 6.1%) and re-operation rates ranging from 0.7 % to 3.4% (27).

A large population based study involving 32,683 patients documented the morbidity and mortality for both laparoscopic and open appendicectomy. (28). Their results for open versus laparoscopic appendicectomy were as follows, respectively: Overall morbidity (8.8%; 4.5%): serious morbidity (4 %; 2.6%); surgical site infection (6.6%;3.26%); mortality (0.13%; 0.07%); deep incisional SSI (0.99%; 0.24%): Organ space SSI (1.72%: 1.79%); wound disruption (0.45%; 0.06%): pneumonia (0.43%: 0.24%); pulmonary embolism (0.08%: 0.08%); sepsis and septic shock (2.16%; 1.15%); bleeding (0.01%; 0.04%) and UTIs (0.36%; 0.37%).

Non-operative management may be cost-effective compared to surgery in a larger number of patients without increasing the risk, and may reduce hospital stay and expenses in both developed and developing countries. However, delayed surgical treatment and a perforated appendix may increase morbidity, time off work and medical expenses. A study by Hansson et al concluded that patients who were managed conservatively had significantly fewer days of sick leave compared to the surgery group. The medical costs were also lower in the conservative group.

9. Hospital stay

The length of hospital stay in patients with acute appendicitis managed conservatively is shorter mainly because parenteral administration of antibiotics is necessary probably for only 24 hours. Thereafter, patients can be discharged on oral antibiotics for at least 10 days and follow-up examination scheduled. Studies have shown that antibiotic therapy alone is associated with a significant reduction in the intensity and duration of abdominal pain. (4) Hansson et al. concluded that the number of days with abdominal pain after hospital discharge was significantly lower in patients treated conservatively than those who underwent appendicectomy. (3)

Appendicectomy is associated with a significant financial burden both in terms of the operation, hospital charges and days lost from work. Figures from the USA (1997) estimated the overall costs of appendicectomy as one million hospital days and $ 3 billion in hospital charges, of which postoperative complications accounted for half of the hospital charges (29). With the recent increased popularity in laparoscopy, the financial burden is expected to rise even further. In one study, the costs of conservative treatment were 25-50% less compared to those who underwent surgery (3).

The feasibility of treating appendicitis on an outpatient bases has been facilitated by the increased availability of effective and improved oral antibiotics. The future management of uncomplicated appendicitis could be similar to the current management of uncomplicated diverticulitis, on an outpatient bases. Further cost reductions are expected as a result of elimination of the morbidity and mortality associated with surgery, which is the major contributor of the financial burden.

10. Negative appendicectomy

The negative appendicectomy rate recorded in the literature is 15 to 25% and is associated with significant morbidity such as wound sepsis, small bowel obstruction, pneumonia and incisional hernias. Interestingly, some investigators have found out that the risk of getting small bowel adhesive obstruction is higher in patients who undergo a negative appendicectomy compared to a positive appendicectomy. This underscores the importance of good diagnostic skills in order to reduce the negative appendicectomy rate and the associated morbidity.

The conservative management of acute appendicitis could be more beneficial in peripheral health centres especially in developing countries were resources and facilities might be scarce. This approach can also be useful in busy emergency facilities where it can be used to avoid unnecessary surgery and workload there by diverting resources to real emergency cases and reducing financial burden.

11. Missing other diagnoses

The carcinoid tumour is the most common tumour in the appendix with an incidence of 3-7 in every 1000 appendicectomies (30). Carcinoid tumour is commoner in man than women. This tumour can present as acute appendicitis following obstruction of the appendix lumen. Because of their small size they can be missed by imaging. More worrying is the possibility of missing colonic cancer in elderly patients masquerading as an acute appendicitis. Lai et al has shown that the incidence of appendicitis associated with colon cancer is 0.85% and the interval from appendicectomy to the diagnosis of the cancer was 5.8 months. From this study, the authors recommended that all patients above the age of 40 years presenting with symptoms of acute appendicitis should be investigated for possible underlying colonic cancer. They recommended a colonoscopy at least 6 weeks after surgery especially if the histology of the appendix was normal.

The routine imaging of patients with suspected appendicitis is not cost effective and is not recommended, however, several studies do support selective imaging with improved diagnostic criteria especially when cancer is included in the differential diagnosis (21, 31). A not uncommon typical scenario is an elderly patient who presents with recurrent right iliac fossa pain and anaemia; in these patients, a caecal tumour may cause obstruction of the appendix lumen resulting in appendicitis. Thus, a high index of colonic cancer should be maintained especially patients more than 40 years of age and those with risk factors for cancer. Conservative management of acute appendicitis can result in missing other diagnosis such as neuroimmune appendicitis (32) resulting in chronic right iliac fossa pains.

12. Allergy to antibiotics

The possibility of antibiotics allergic reactions should be borne in mind when a conservative approach is utilised. A good medical and drug history will identify most of these patients. Furthermore, there is a wide variety of types and combinations of antibiotics available which can be used to circumvent this problem. Acute appendicitis is one of the most common surgical conditions and if conservative antibiotic use becomes wide-spread, the possibility of increasing the risk of multidrug antibiotic resistance and susceptibility to resistant bacterial strains can become a major challenge especially if there is no strict adherence to guidelines and protocols. From this point of view, it may not be logical to recommend routine use of antibiotics to such a common surgical condition. This further underscores the importance of aiming for a high diagnostic accuracy for appendicitis before deciding on the use of antibiotics. Antibiotics treatment should be considered following the same high diagnostic accuracy similar to the one required before surgical intervention. This may include use of USS and CT scan of the abdomen. Other authorities in this area have suggested that no patients without an elevated C- reactive protein should be treated for suspected acute appendicitis.

13. Appendicitis and tubal infertility

The issue of the possibility of tubal infertility following conservative antibiotic treatment of suspected acute appendicitis has been raised by some investigators. They have reported the rate of tubal infertility to be between 3.2 and 4.8% (33). However, there is general agreement in the surgical community that a perforated appendix in childhood does not seem to have long-term effects on female fertility. This has important relevance in the management of females of childbearing age group presenting with suspected appendicitis where the practice of low threshold of surgical exploration for fear of increased risk of perforation following a perforation in no longer justifiable.

14. Patient selection for conservative management

The current surgical literature clearly supports the role of conservative antibiotic management for a selected group of patients with acute appendicitis. The prerequisites are to aim for a high diagnostic accuracy and to adhere to strict selection criteria in order to achieve the optimum outcome thereby avoiding the problem of negative appendicectomy. The criteria for selecting patients for conservative management of acute appendicitis should be a combination of clinical, laboratory and radiological investigations. Patients with mild clinical signs without complications could be considered for the conservative approach and in the presence of severe clinical features or signs of perforation / peritonitis, surgery should be contemplated unless the patient is unfit for surgery. Surgical intervention should also be considered in patients who are initially managed conservatively and then present with recurrent symptoms.

The value of white cell count in the diagnosis of acute appendicitis has been debated over the years and it has been found to be an unreliable marker of severe inflammation. Thus, a normal white cell count level cannot rule out severe acute appendicitis. This is particularly true in patients with immunosuppression, the elderly and paediatrics. . On the other hand CRP has been suggested as a more sensitive and specific marker of the severity of appendiceal inflammation compared to WCC. An elevated CRP is a marker of the degree of advanced pathology and serial CRP measurements has been shown to improve the diagnostic accuracy for acute appendicitis (6).

For conservative treatment to be successful, it is of utmost importance to make a correct diagnosis and assessment as possible so as to institute a correct treatment plan. Routine imaging is not recommended in cases of suspected acute appendicitis, except in atypical presentations. The specificity and sensitivity of CT scan and USS in diagnosing acute appendicitis has been reported as 100 and 97%, and 90 and 76% respectively (34). CT scan is especially useful in confirming acute appendicitis in paediatric patients and in looking for complications. Diagnostic laparoscopy has a role to play especially in patients with a recurrent history of right iliac fossa pain.

Studies have shown no statistical difference in the postoperative complication rates between primary and conversion cases. However, the duration of hospital stay was significantly higher and thus medical costs might be increased in the conversion cases (35). Thus, predictors for the negative outcome of conservative treatment are important in patient selection. A major concern is diagnostic uncertainty which may result in a negative appendicectomy or a delay in treatment. The presence of an appendiceal faecolith has been found to be associated with a complicated acute appendicitis and a higher recurrence rate after antibiotic therapy, often within the first year of the initial presentation. Thus appendicectomy is often recommended in patients with acute appendicitis associated with a faecolith so as to avoid the possible complications and the risk of recurrences.

An elevated CRP and signs and symptoms of small bowel obstruction have been suggested as possible predictors for a failure of conservative treatment (36, 37). Authorities still differ on the significance of a poorly marginated focal mesenteric infiltration as a marker of poor prognosis in the conservative management of appendicitis. Collection size, complexity or the presence of extra-luminal air has not been shown to be significant as predictors of clinical outcome (38). A sound clinical acumen is needed in the assessment of clinical progression of acute appendicitis and decides the need for surgery in the expected 5-10% subgroup of patients. The use of antibiotics has been shown to delay the need for an emergency operation for at least 24 hours without associated adverse consequences. Antibiotics can be used as a definite treatment of acute appendicitis or as a bridge to surgery, converting an emergency operation to a planned procedure. This applies mostly to paediatric patients who present late at night.

15. Choice of antibiotics

Currently there are no strict guidelines or recommendations for the optimal antibiotics treatment for acute appendicitis. Several different types and combinations of antibiotics exist and the choice is mainly affected by availability and surgeon preference. Recent advances in antibiotics therapy have made triple antibiotics regimens for the treatment of intra-abdominal infection almost obsolete. Furthermore, the improvements in antibiotics bioavailability has made it possible to treat severe intra-abdominal infections with enteral antibiotics on an outpatient bases. The current non-operative treatment for acute appendicitis involves intravenous antibiotics for a period of 24 to 48 hours followed by oral medication for 10- 12 days as an outpatient and follow-up thereafter.

16. Interval appendicectomy

Current opinion is that there is no need for an interval appendicectomy following successful conservative treatment for acute appendicitis even in complicated cases with an abscess or inflammatory mass (39). Recurrences can be managed by a repeat in conservative treatment or observation. Some authorities report that recurrences following conservative treatment tend to follow a milder course (40). It is recommended that appendicectomy should be reserved for multiple recurrences (more than 2) and for those who fail to improve. Interval appendicectomy may prevent recurrent appendicitis in about 7% of patients presenting with an appendiceal mass. This implies that 93% of patients may end up with an unnecessary appendicectomy (41).

17. Summary

A growing body of evidence supports the role of conservative management of acute appendicitis in carefully selected patients who can be followed-up with close monitoring of the clinical course. Emergency appendicectomy for acute appendicitis may not always be necessary. The success rates range from 68 to 95%. Other advantages include cost-effectiveness, shorter hospital stay, minimal sick leave and less pain. With a diagnostic accuracy rate for acute appendicitis greater than around 71% to 87% the conservative management of suspected or proven acute appendicitis seems justified. The recurrence rates are low and the complications are comparable to that after an appendicectomy.

In conclusion, acute uncomplicated appendicitis can be treated successfully with antibiotics with a short duration of hospital stay, minimal sick leave and limited degree and duration of pain. However, the risk of recurrence needs to be compared with the risks of appendicectomy.

18. References

[1] Fitz RH. Perforating inflammation of the vermiform appendix. *Am J Med Sci* 1886; 92: 321-346

[2] Coldrey E. Five years of conservative treatment of acute appendicitis. *J Int Coll Surg* 1959; 32:255-261

[3] Hansson J, Korner U, Khorram-Manesh A et al. Randomized clinical trial of antibiotic therapy versus appendicectomy as primary treatment of acute appendicitis in unselected patients. *Br J Surg* 2009; 96: 473-481.

[4] Styrud J, Eriksson S, Nilsson I et al. Appendicectomy versus antibiotic treatment in acute appendicitis. A prospective multicenter randomised controlled trial.*World J of Surg* 2006; 30:1033-1037.

[5] Eriksson S, Granstrom L. Randomised controlled trial of appendicectomy versus antibiotic therapy for acute appendicitis. *Br J Surg* 1995; 82: 166-169.

[6] Luckmann R. Incidence and case fatality rates for acute appendicitis in California: a population-based study of the effects of age. *Am J Epidemiol* 1989; 129: 905-209.

[7] Migraine S, Atri M, Bret PM et al. Spontaneously resolving acute appendicitis: Clinical and sonographic documentation. *Radiology* 1997; 205: 205-209.

[8] Malik AA, Bari SU. Conservative management of acute appendicitis. *J Gastrointest Surg* 2009; 13:966-970.

[9] McPherson A, Kinmonth J. Acute appendicitis and the appendix mass.*Br J Surg* 1945; 32: 365-370.

[10] Anonymous. Combined traditional Chinese and Western medicine in acute appendicitis. *Chin Med J* 1977; 3: 266-269.

[11] Adams ML. The medical management of acute appendicitis in a non-surgical environment: a retrospective case review. *Milit Med* 1990; 155:345-347.

[12] Tingstedt B, Johansson J, Nehez L et al. Late abdominal complaints after appendicectomy –readmissions during long-term follow-up. *Dig Surg* 2004; 21:23-27.

[13] Anderson RE. Small bowel obstruction after appendicectomy. *Br J Surg* 2001; 88: 1387-1391.

[14] Anderson RE. The natural history and traditional management of appendicitis revisited: spontaneous resolution and predominance of prehospital perforations imply that a correct diagnosis is more important than an early diagnosis. *World J Surg* 2007; 31:86-92.

[15] Mui LM, Ng CS, Wong SK et al Optimum duration of prophylactic antibiotics in acute non-perforated appendicitis. *Aust N Z J Surg* 2005; 75: 425-428.

[16] Winslow RE, Dean RE, Harley JW. Acute non-perforating appendicitis. *Arch Surg* 1983; 118: 651- 655.

[17] Blomqvist P, Ljung H, Nyren O et al. Appendectomy in Sweden 1989-1993 assessed by the Inpatient Registry. *J Clin Epidemiol* 1998; 51: 859-865.

[18] Hale DA, Molloy M, Pearl RH et al. Appendicdctomy: A contemporary appraisal. Ann Surg 1997; 225: 252-261.

[19] Bijnen CL, van den Broek WT, Bijnen AB et al. Implications of removing a normal appendix. *Dig Surg* 2003; 20:215-221.

[20] Heller MB, Skolnick ML. Utrasound documentation of spontaneously resolving appnedcitis. *Am J Emerg Med* 1993; 11:51-53.

[21] Varadhan KK, Jumes DJ, Neal KR et al. Antibiotic therapy versus appendectomy for acute appendicitis: a meta-analysis. *World J Surg* 2010; 34: 199-209.

[22] Wiegering VA, Kellenberger CJ, Bodmer N et al. Conservative management of acute appendicitis in children with haematologic malignancies during chemotherapy-induced neutropaenia. *J pediatr Hematol Oncol* 2008; 30: 464-467

[23] Abes M, Etik B, Kazil S. Non-operative treatment of acute appendicitis in children.*J Pediat Surg* 2007;42:1439-1442.

[24] Anderson RE, Petzold MG. Nonsurgical treatment of appendiceal abscesses or phlegmon: a systematic review and meta-analysis. *Ann Surg* 2007; 246:741-748

[25] Simillis C, Symeondes P, Shorthouse AJ et al. A meta-analysis comparing conservative treatment versus acute appendicicectomy for complicated appendicitis (abscess or phlegmon). *Surgery* 2010; 147: 818-829.

[26] Leung TT, Dixon E, Gill M et al. Bowel obstruction following appendicectomy: what is the true incidence? *Ann Surg* 2009; 250:51-52

[27] Brugger L, Rosella L, Candinas D et al. Improving outcomes after laparoscopic appendectomy: a population-based 12-year trend analysis of 7446 patients. Ann Surg. Published online first: 17 December 2010. *Doi: 10.1097/SLA.0b013e3181fc9d53.*

[28] Ingraham AM, Cohen ME, Bilimoria KY et al. Comparison of outcomes after laparoscopic versus open appendectomy for acute appendicitis at 222 NSQIP hospitals. *Surgery* 2010; 148:625-635; discussion 635-637.

[29] Davis GM, Dasbach EJ, Teutsch S. The burden of appendicitis-related hospitalisations in the United States in 1997. *Surg Infect (Larchmt)* 2004; 5:190:950-954

[30] Roggo A, Wood WC, Ottinger LW. Carcinoid tumours of the appendix. *Ann Surg* 1993; 217:385-390.

[31] Augustin T, Bhende S, Chavda K et al. CT scans and acute appendicitis: a five-year analysis from a rural teaching hospital. *J Gastrointest Surg* 2009; 13: 1306-1312.

[32] Franke C, Gerharz CD, Bohner H et al. Neurogenic appendicopathy: a clinical disease entity? *Int J Colorectal Dis* 2002; 17:185-191

[33] Mueller BA, Daling JR, Moore DE et al. Appendectomy and the risk of tubal infertility. *N Engl J Med* 1986; 315:1506-1508.

[34] Horton MD, Counter SF, Florence MG et al. A prospective trial of computed tomography and ultrasonography for diagnosing appendicitis in the atypical patient. *Am J Surg* 2001; 182:305-306

[35] Shindoh J, Hiwa H, Kawai K et al. Predictive factors for negative outcomes in initial non-operative management of suspected appendicitis. *J Gastrointest Surg* 2010; 14: 309-314

[36] Nadler EP, Reblock KK, Vaughan KG et al. Predictors of outcome for children with perforated appendicitis initially treated with nonoperative management. *Surg Infect* 2004; 5: 349-356.

[37] Kogut KA, Blakely ML, Schropp KP et al. The associationof elevated percent bands on admission with failure and complications of interval appendectomy. *J Pediatr Surg* 2001; 36:165-168

[38] Levi T, Whyte C, Borzykowsi R et al. Nonoperative management of perforated appendicitis in children: can CT predict outcome? *Pediatr Radiol* 2007; 37: 251-255.

[39] Eriksson S, Styrud J. Interval appendicectomy: a retrospective study. *Eur J Surg* 1998; 164: 771-775.

[40] Dixon MR, Haukoos JS, Park IU et al. An assessment of the severity of recurrent appendicitis. *Am J Surg* 2003; 186: 718-722

[41] Tekin A, Kurtoglu HC, CanI et al. Routine interval appendectomy is unnecessary after conservative treatment of appendiceal mass. *Colorectal Dis* 2008; 10:465-468

7

Appendicitis in the Elderly

Stephen Garba and Adamu Ahmed
Ahmadu Bello University, Zaria,
Nigeria

1. Introduction

Appendicitis in the elderly is a pathological process. It is common in many locales, populations and cultures. It is a potentially life threatening pathology. Lifetime incidence is 1 in every 15 persons (7%) with a prevalence rate of ten in one hundred thousand people (10/100,000) (Condon RE, 1986). Appendicitis usually affects people who are previously healthy. The rate of appendicitis among the elderly varies from 5% to 10% of appendicitis cases. Appendicitis is often thought of as a disease of the young but it has now become a disease of the elderly because of increasing life expectancy of the modern day man resulting from improved medical attention. It is the most common cause of acute surgical condition of the abdomen (Hardin D, 1999, Storm-Dickerson T.L. & Horattas, M.C., 2003). Appendicitis requires immediate surgical excision in most cases as soon as the condition is diagnosed unless contraindicated. If appendicectomy is carried out early, the end result is low morbidity and mortality. The cure rate is high if managed early without any long term sequelae (Birnbaum BA & Wilson SR, 2000; Ellis H, 1989). This write up will focus on appendicitis in the elderly. The elderly as defined in this discussion are people who are sixty years of age and above. The high occurrence of appendicitis has made the pathology a very important entity that should not be under estimated. The usual peak incidence of appendicitis in the general population is in the range 15 to 24years age group. This accounts for 5% of all acute abdominal conditions in the aged 65years and above (Sheu, B F. et al, 2007; Storm-Dickerson T.L. & Horattas M.C., 2003).
The elderly patients have a lowered physiological reserve. Inflammatory effect is much increased in the elderly. Hence appendicitis has a more fulminant outcome in this group of patients. The mortality can be as high as 16 times as what is obtainable in the young adult with appendicitis (Hui TT, et al, 2002; Semm K, 1983). There has been increased use of computed tomography (CT) in the last two decades. This investigative tool has improved the diagnosis of appendicitis (Horattas M, 1990). In the area of care, laparoscopy has revolutionized the care of appendicitis since the introduction of the first laparoscopy appendicectomy performed in 1983 by Semm (Tehrani H, 1999). A high rate of misdiagnosis of appendicitis in the elderly has been documented (Hale D, 1997). This is because this disease simulates much other pathology in the elderly. The elderly people have deteriorating functions of their organs system which in that state may mimic the pathology of appendicitis. Some of these pathologies shall be discussed latter in this write up. The presentation of appendicitis can be traditional or non classical. There is high rate of atypical or non classical presentation among the elderly patients than in the general setting. In contrast to this, the majority of young adults present classically. This atypical presentation in the elderly patients leads to delay diagnosis with resulting high

complications among them. This peculiarity has made many to say appendicitis in the elderly is a separate entity (Carr NJ, 2000; Blomqvist P, 2001).
The young adult with appendicitis presents mainly with classical features and this made it easy to make correct diagnosis, early and appropriate treatments can then be easily instituted. The elderly presents with a higher degree of non classical features, has delay attention because of delay correct diagnosis. In general the non classical features made diagnosis difficult hence higher morbidity and mortality. Appendicitis has a perforation rate of 17-20% in general. Bear in mind that in the elderly however, appendicitis appearance is usually not apparent, presenting as if it is not present. Hence delay in diagnosis and treatment is common with poorer outcome. There is need for expedient diagnosis of appendicitis in the elderly today. This is because the elderly proportion in the society has increased due to improved medical attention (Lee JF, 2000). Better Medicare has resulted in increased proportion of the elderly in the population. Physicians must always have in mind that appendicitis is a regular pathology in the elderly with irregular presentations. A high index of suspicion is a good practice principle. Every physician must familiarize himself with appendicitis unusual presentations. Apart from the elderly patients, other group of patients with a high degree of non classical presentations include the children, the pregnant and the acquired immune deficiency syndrome (AIDS) patients (Krisher S, 2001). They all have peculiar pathologic appendices.
Treatment outcome for young adult and the elderly with appendicitis are similar if correct diagnosis is made and patients are treated promptly. That is to say the result of treatment of appendicitis in the elderly can be as excellent as in the young adult (Rao P, et al 1999; Schumpelick V, et al 2000). Despite the profound improvements in the diagnosis and treatments of appendicitis in general and in the elderly in particular, the morbidity and mortality is still high (Gupta H & Dupuy D, 1997; Temple C, et al, 1995, Yamini D, 1998). Some have even reported a perforation rate as high as 70% at presentation because of this peculiar problem (Paranjape, et al 2007). Can we then say appendicitis is a separate entity in the elderly? There is no doubt that the outcome in this group of patients is poorer because of delay diagnosis and delay treatment all on the account of non-classical mode of presentation. Very few young adult patients present with 'out of character' manifestations of appendicitis (Nguyen D, et al 1999). When Reginald Fitz first described the condition of appendicitis in 1886, the mortality from acute appendicitis was 40 %.(Lin CJ, et al, 2005). Now with the introduction of general anaesthesia, antiseptic techniques and the availability of powerful antibiotics, the reported mortality rate has dropped significantly. However these improved medical practices have not completely eradicated the issue of delay diagnosis and late administration of appropriate treatments (Hardin D, 1999). This chapter will further address the characteristics of appendicitis in the elderly and where necessary compares it with appendicitis in the young adults. It will discuss the factors that are contributory to its high morbidity and mortality and how to regulate these morbidity and mortality modifiers of appendicitis in this category of patients. The modern imaging systems that are helpful in speedy diagnosis shall be highlighted in this discussion. Treatments and ways to improve the treatments shall be fully discussed with special regards to the elderly.

2. Pathology

This discussion on the pathogenesis of appendicitis will center more on the classical form of obstructing lesion leading to appendicitis. Only where necessary will the non obstructive form of appendicitis be mentioned. This vestigial organ can be involved in inflammation like other organs of the body. There are many factors that may lead to its inflammation but in general the inflammation starts in the mucosa and progresses into the deeper tissues of the appendix wall (Yamini D, et al, 1998). In no doubt there are many factors exacerbating the process of appendicitis in the elderly. These factors may be anatomic or physiologic in origin. What are the anatomical and physiological changes that enhance a different inflammatory response of appendix to inflammation in the elderly as compared to the young adults? The inflammatory process occuring in appendix following some initiators is greatly modified by many factors in this group of patients. Most of these factors are due to anatomical and physiological changes in the elderly. It is therefore very important for all attending physicians to know the peculiarity of inflammatory changes affecting the appendix in the elderly. It is this peculiarity that makes more of the appendicitis in the elderly to present atypically hence has worse prognosis as compared to the young adults with similar pathology (Hardin D, 1999;Yamini D, et al, 1998).

2.1 Anatomy

This section describes the changes in the appendix with age that make it respond to inflammations differently from the young adults. With aging the serosa of appendix becomes relatively less elastic compare to the elasticity quality of the mucosa of the appendix. In the young the elasticity of both is good and comparable. Because of significant differences in the elasticity of the serosa and the submucosa, the response to intraluminal pressure is different. The adaptation of them to stretch from luminal accumulation of secretions is different leading to relative ischaemia and early gangrene of the wall of appendix. This is a great factor in the pathogenesis of early perforation of appendicitis in the elderly. There is however other anatomical changes that enhances worse inflammatory response in the pathogenesis of appendicitis in the elderly which are associated with aging. Another important factor is that with age, the blood supply to the appendix is affected by atherosclerosis. It reduces the pliability of arterial and venous supply to the appendix. The wall of the appendix is weakened by fibrosis and fatty infiltration. There is progressive atrophy of lymphoid tissue with concomitant fibrosis of the wall of the appendix. This causes partial or total obliteration of the lumen. One of the overall effects is narrowed or occluded appendix. These make appendix more prone to ischaemia in any problem that involves a reduction of blood flow to the appendix as found in luminal blockade. The elderly has weakened peristalsis. This weakened peristalsis encourages food residue to form in the appendix. The food residue forms bezoar allowing secretions to accumulate in the appendix lumen (Maxwell JM & Ragland JJ, 1991). At old age the openings of appendix will atrophy which aids regurgitation of stool, undigested food, parasites, making it easy to enter the appendix lumen causing obstruction, local tissue ischaemia and necrosis of the appendix (Peltokallio P & Jauhianinen K, 1970). The weakened wall of appendix also encourages the accumulations of these materials. Appendix in the elderly therefore has tendency for secretions to accumulate and prone to ischaemia on the platform of anatomic changes enumerated above.

2.2 Physiologic changes

Physiologically, the elderly patients with deteriorating organs have lower physiological reserve than the young adults. They also have higher pain threshold response. They have poor reflexes in general and poor localisation of pain. The initial symptoms in the elderly patients with appendicitis are usually attributed to indigestion or constipation, thus ignoring the initial symptoms until they worsened. These declining physiologic functions exacerbate morbidity and mortality in the elderly. Another important factor contributing to increased pathological changes in the appendix is reduced local immunity in the appendix. There is poor inflammatory response from inflammatory cells. All these will also cause decrease ability to eliminate bacteria invasion hence faster bacterial multiplication without much interference. Local tissue factor in bacterial control is poor. The overall effects of these changes in the anatomy and the physiology of appendix is narrowing of the appendix lumen, decreased local tissue defence capability, and loss of mucosal integrity paving way for bacterial invasion of appendix (Horattas MC & Haught R, 1992). Bacterial invasion leads to rapid pus formation and gangrene with perforation and generalised inflammation of the peritoneum.

2.3 Aetiology

The process of inflammation in appendix starts most times from the mucosa with luminal obstruction of the appendix. As in other forms of intestinal obstruction, the obstructing lesion may be extrinsic, intramural or intraluminal. Appendix inflammation can however occur without any form of obstruction. In appendicitis, obstruction is more commonly of intraluminal variety than other forms of initiators. Obstructive appendicitis is commoner than catarrhal appendicitis even among the elderly. In catarrhal appendicitis, inflammation occurs without any form of obstruction. In cases of obstructive appendicitis, obstruction is usually due to matters such as faecolith which starts the process of inflammation from the mucosa of the appendix. The opening of appendix into the large bowel is prone to blockade from the content of the large intestine hence encouraging stasis in the lumen of the appendix. Inflammation resulting from non obstructive changes in the mucosa of the appendix is purely bacterial in origin (Carr NJ, 2000; Maxwell JM & Ragland JJ, 1991). The other obstructive lesions are response to a generalized lymphoid tissue from systemic infectious diseases by bacterial enterocolitis or by fecalith from foreign body or blockade from intestinal parasites. The bacterial that are usually involved in the inflammation are usually coliform organisms. Most of the obstructions are followed by infection with streptococcus pneumoniae.

2.4 Pathogenesis

In the majority of cases, the initiating factors of obstruction above leads to luminal stasis and obstruction causing impediments to the flow of the content of appendix. The obstruction distends the wall starting from the mucosa. As stated earlier there is relative unequal elasticity of the mucosa and the submucosal area of the appendix. Therefore there is unequal stretch effect on the mucosal distinct from that of submucosal area leading to early necrosis of the mucosa. A continued secretion within the lumen further increases the pressure in the lumen of the appendix (Lee, J. F. Y., et al 2000). This leads to an initial stage of lymphatic obstruction being the first culprit. This initial impairment of the lymphatic system causes edema, diapedesis of bacteria and mucosa ulceration. Bacterial begins to multiply and there is impairment of integrity of the wall of the appendix. These will therefore cause migration of cells of inflammation through the walls of blood capillaries into the tissue spaces. This leads to organ infection. Mucus further accumulates within the lumen of the appendix. The intraluminal pressure increases steadily as accumulation increases in volume within the appendix (Gupta H & Dupuy D, 1997; Temple C, et al, 1995). The rapidly proliferating intraluminal bacteria convert the accumulated mucus within the appendix into pus. This is an important reaction of appendix to insult of obstruction and infection. This proximal obstruction of the lumen of the appendix by fibrosis or otherwise has long been considered to be the major cause of appendicitis.

If the obstruction is not relieved, there is a further rise in luminal pressure from additional luminal secretion which causes venous obstruction subsequent to the initial lymphatic obstruction. The additional venous obstruction increases the edema, and cause further ischemia of the appendix. The end result of all these changes is suppurative appendicitis (Freund HR, Rubinstein E, 1984). The progression of this pathologic process results in lymphatic, venous and arterial thromboses in the wall of the appendix. As the pressure increases without a relive, the arterial component of the appendiceal vascular supply is jeopardized. A patch or a total gangrenous appendicitis may result from the ischaemia. The final stage in the progression of acute appendicitis is perforation through a gangrenous infarct and spilling of accumulated pus into the peritoneal cavity. This spillage will lead to a localized or generalized peritonitis depending on how fast the body can wall off the offending agents and the degree of perforation. Throughout the stages of inflammation, the body tries to cope with the pathological process with attempts to overcome the insult. The body can fight the offending agent and there can be a complete resolution of the inflammation. However these coping strategies may result in partial restriction of the inflammation leading to formation of appendiceal mass or appendiceal abscess formation (Paajanen H, et al 1994; chapter 83). The classical end result of this inflammation follows a natural course in which there may be a complete resolution of the inflammation, healing with fibrosis, chronic inflammation and/or abscess formation. The common result is however a form of complete resolution, formation of appendiceal mass, development of abscess formation and peritonitis which may be localized or generalized.

An increase in intraluminal pressure in the area distal to the obstruction from increased mucus secretion is followed by an increase in bacteria and, finally, the formation of frank pus. The appendix becomes swollen and the appendiceal wall becomes edematous from obstruction of lymphatic and venous drainage. Ulceration of the mucosa allows invasion of the wall by bacteria. Further progression causes venous thrombosis and obstruction of blood flow through the appendiceal artery. Because this is an end-artery, no collateral circulation is available to prevent ischemic necrosis and gangrene with eventual rupture of the wall. Escape of bacteria through the perforation causes peritonitis. Unless necrosis of the base of the appendix occurs, continued fecal contamination of the peritoneal cavity is prevented by the initial blockage of the appendiceal lumen. The infection in the right lower quadrant can be walled off efficiently in young, healthy patients. In females, this abscess usually involves the right adnexal organs to some extent. The end result is how well the body is able to cope with the inflammatory insult. In appendiceal mass, the inflammatory mass is composed of the inflamed appendix at the core, surrounded with the caecum, the terminal part of the ileum and omentum wrapped all together (Maxwell JM & Ragland JJ, 1991). The course of the appendiceal mass also may be in the form a complete resolution with the involved organs freed or it may take the form of abscess formation. In appendiceal abscess formation, the previous mass becomes softer, increase in size and patient also will have swing temperature

Generalized peritonitis may ensue in advanced age or in the presence of reduced host resistance from other illnesses or immunosuppression. Perforation is more likely with retrocaecal appendix unnoticed. This is so because in the retrocaecal position, the diagnosis of appendicitis is difficult. The difficult diagnosis causes delay in presentation and in the treatment of the pathology hence a high possibility of perforation among the patients (Maxwell JM & Ragland JJ, 1991). Even with a mild increase in luminal pressure during the early phase of appendicitis, these anatomical and physiological changes may enhance the appendix to early perforation. These changes are exaggerated in the elderly because of the anatomic and physiologic peculiarity. The elderly are not sensitive to pain, symptoms are not typical and therefore there is a rapid progression to perforation without patients' awareness of an ominous disease (Barcia JJ & Reissenweber N, 2002). Perforation with peritonitis in the elderly appendix is a serious complication. The anatomical and physiological changes rapidly boost perforation of appendix. In the general population, perforation rates range from 20 to 30%, but increase to 50–70% in the elderly. When is appendicitis considered perforated? The appendix is considered perforated if there is free rupture of intraluminal contents (Fitz HR, 1886). The rupture leads to spillage of intestinal juice into the peritoneum. The peritoneum becomes inflamed as a result of the bacterial contamination of the peritoneal cavity. The characteristics of perforation of appendix in the elderly are suggested by a very sick patient with fever, left shift leucocyte count (increased WBC) and anorexia in addition to abdominal pain. when these features are present, suspect perforation of appendix.

2.5 Microbiology

Talking about the biology of the microorganisms involved in inflammatory appendicitis; the flora of the lumen of the appendix is that of the flora of the lumen of the colon. There is a mixture of aerobic and anaerobic organisms involved in appendicitis (Vorhes CE, 1987). The various organisms involved in the inflammatory conditions of appendicitis include anaerobes and aerobes. The common organisms include Escherichia coli, Klebsiella-Enterobacter, Enterococcus faecalis group, Streptococci Clostridia. Fungal infection has also been documented. Any of these organisms can be found in the culture of appendiceal abscess. In an article published by Bernard and Owen in 1978 the organisms cultured in cases of appendicitis include the following: E. coli in 68% of the patients, the remaining 32% included organisms such as B *fragilis*, streptococci, Staph aureus and Klebsiella. In more than 60% of the cases they were monomicrobial and the remaining polymicrobial (Bernard and Owen, 1978). They were all sensitive to various antibiotics. There is poor response to inflammation from invasion of pathogenic microorganisms and the elderly mount inappropriate response to fever. The total white cell counts are not proportionally increased in inflammation of appendix in the elderly (Barcia JJ & Reissenweber N, 2002). These peculiarities lead to rapid progression of inflammation, early perforation, and abscess formation in the elderly. Those who develop perforations among the elderly patients with appendicitis usually have higher morbidity and mortality. They are very sick and present more with high and swinging fever, left shift leucocyte count and anorexia.

2.6 Implications of anatomical and physiological changes

Is the inflammatory process the same as in the young adults with appendicitis? No, the delay in seeking medical attention and delay in making diagnosis make this inflammatory process in the elderly more serious than in other categories of patients. The anatomical and physiological changes that are noted in the elderly also contribute to a more aggressive inflammatory change in the elderly appendicitis. The outcome of treatments in them is critical because of this delay in presenting to the hospital and also on the account of a more aggressive inflammatory response (Lau WY, et al, 1985). There are serious implications for changes in the anatomy and physiology of the appendix of the elderly patients. The consequences of these changes are a different inflammatory response in appendicitis. This different response causes delay and misdiagnosis of this entity in the elderly patient presenting with appendicitis. These changes are the causes of high incidence of atypical presentation in the adult. It can lead to a faster progression of the disease with early perforation of appendix (Smithy WB, 1986). In essence the hardened blood vessels, degradations of appendix, reduced local lymph nodes, poor ability to eliminate inflammation; all encourage aggressive inflammatory response in the elderly appendicitis. Appendix easily perforates and cause localised or diffused peritonitis. Awareness of possibility of appendicitis in the elderly is the master key to successful management of this pathology in the aged people. This group of patients have poor response, their symptoms and pathological changes are often inconsistent with the chief complaint of abdominal pain. The chief symptom in appendicitis is lower abdominal pain and this is most often less severe. Sometimes abdominal pain is not typical, only abdominal distension, nausea and other symptoms are noted. These inconsistent symptoms resulting from differences in the anatomic and physiologic changes are responsible for a high rate of non classical presentation of appendicitis in the elderly. One must bear in mind that many other pathologies mimic appendicitis of this age group. The differential diagnoses therefore are wide and difficult due to their atypical presentations and their aging state. One must consider appendicitis in every elderly patient with lower abdominal pain. This is important because appendicitis takes a more rapid and virulent course in the elderly with weaning organs if treatment is delayed (Horattas MC, et la 1990). On the basis of the pathologic process the following types of appendicitis can be noted: simple, complicated, acute, recurrent and chronic appendicitis.

3. Clinical features

The features of appendicitis in the elderly are similar to what is obtainable in the young adults though its presentation is more varied and subtle. Appendicitis can present classically (typically) or nonclassically (atypically). The cardinal symptoms of appendicitis are usually classical and it occurs also in elderly appendicitis (Burns RP, et al 1985). One of the classical symptoms of appendicitis as reported by Burns et al is right lower abdominal pain. In classical cases the pain of appendicitis follows a known classical course. The pain usually starts with sudden periumbilical pain, which becomes localised in the right iliac fossa. Typically the pain is initially diffused, central and minimally severe presenting as visceral pain. In a period of about six to eight hours after the onset of the pain, the pain migrates to the right lower quadrant of the abdomen. This time around the pain is somatic, more severe and usually localized. This is described as visceral - somatic sequence of presentation of pain of appendicitis, This visceral- somatic sequence occur less in the elderly appendicitis as compared to other categories of patients. Atypical form of presentation is common among the elderly patients. Many elderly patients with pain of appendicitis have out of character type of pain. This non classical type of pain stem from the anatomical and physiological changes in the elderly and the anatomic variations in the location of the appendix. These age related and non age related changes account for the non classical sequence of the pain. In the elderly patient with the pain of appendicitis, the pain may be localised in the right lower quadrant from the beginning. This pain also in some patients may be diffused and may never become localized

(Paajanen H, et al 1994). An elderly patient with retrocecal appendix may have diffuse pain only in the right flank of the abdomen. If the appendix is wholly in the pelvis, there may not be any manifestation of somatic pain but patient may present with tenesmus and lower abdominal discomfort. It is difficult to give a dogmatic sequence of pain presentation in the appendicitis of the elderly. High index of suspicion is needed in every elderly patient with abdominal pain. Every physician must be aware of these forms of pain presentations in appendicitis of the elderly. The next common symptoms after lower abdominal pain are anorexia and nausea. They are present in all cases of appendicitis. Vomiting is present in some cases but not as constant as pain and nausea. Vomiting comes only after the onset of pain and usually once or twice in most cases. If vomiting is persistent, the diagnosis of simple appendicitis should be questioned (Carr NJ, 2000).

Other patients may just have symptoms of irritation of the nearby organs from inflamed appendix. Depending on the location of appendix, if the bladder is being irritate in pelvic appendix, patient may only present with frequent urination and in some cases with haematuria. In some other cases it may be loose stool as a result of irritated bowel. When vomiting is present and profuse it may indicate generalized peritonitis associated with perforation or the diagnosis of appendicitis may be wrong. There is what is called Murphy description of features of appendicitis. The classical presentation as described by Murphy is present in only 50% of patients of appendicitis. This description starts with colicky central abdominal pain, progressing to pain intensification within 24hours. Pain becomes constant and sharp with loss of appetite, nausea, vomiting and constipation in the elderly. Atypical presentation is usually common with anatomic variations in location of appendix. There will be pain in the right loin in retrocecal appendix, suprapubic pain with urinary frequency or diarrhoea in subcaecal appendix. Remember that left sided appendix occur in 0.25% of the population resulting from situs inversus or intestinal malrotation. Elderly patients with appendicitis may present only with confusion. From this discussion, it is obvious that appendicitis takes many forms of presentations. In any abdominal pain in the elderly, consider appendicitis.

Anaemia is a common finding associated with appendicitis in the elderly. Patient may be dehydrated, pale, febrile and with foetor oris. Swinging temperature may be noted especially if there is appendiceal abscess from perforation of appendicitis. On further examination of the patients, they may present with other classical signs of appendicitis which include localised tenderness, muscle guarding, and rebound tenderness. There is usually an area of maximal tenderness in the McBurney point (Langenscheidt P, et al 1999). The most important sign is tenderness or rebound tenderness over McBurney point where the bases of majority of all appendixes are located. Charles McBurney (1845-1914) was an American surgeon who, in 1889, described the classic location of sharp pain on a spot exactly between an inch and a half and two inches from the anterior superior process of the ilium on a straight line drawn from the bony prominence to the umbilicus. It is interesting to remember the positions of other parts of the appendix may vary but the bases are constant. Whether the appendix is located in the pelvis, retroileal or in other positions, the point of maximum tenderness of the base is in the McBurney's point. In cases where the appendix is located in the retrocaecal region, tenderness may cover a large area diffusely. Because of the changes in the anatomy and physiological alterations in the aged, these classic signs may be absent. One may be able to elicit the presence of Psoas and obturator signs in these patients. Furred tongue and some levels of dehydration may be noticeable. A rectal examination may reveal right sided pelvic tenderness on rectal examination.

Basically there are two categories of patients when it comes to presentations of appendicitis in the elderly. There are patients with simple (uncomplicated) appendicitis and patients with complicated appendicitis. Therefore the presentation of patients with perforated appendicitis is quite different from uncomplicated cases in the elderly. Presentation therefore varies depending on the type of appendicitis one is dealing with. For these reasons, the diagnosis of acute appendicitis in the elderly bears many pitfalls due to a broad range of differential diagnoses and uncommon clinical presentation that one may confuse this pathology with. The elderly patients have deteriorating organs, at this age symptoms of which may also imitate appendicitis. Other examination findings include tachycardia, skin flushing, dry mouth, abdominal tenderness, with rebound tenderness and point of maximum tenderness at McBurney point which clinically is at two third along a line from umbilicus to anterior superior iliac spine. There may be muscular rigidity, pain in the right iliac fossa which is intensified with coughing. The pain is usually worse on movement. Patient who presents with atypical features may come with no evidence of muscular rigidity but with tenderness on deep palpation if the appendix is retrocaecal. In subcaecal or pelvic appendix Psoas stretch sign may be present. There may be positive *k* sign which is tenderness on posterior abdominal wall in patients with retrocaecal or paracolic appendicitis. We must always remember that there are signs we can elicit to exacerbate or localise appendix pain. These signs include Rovsing sign, obturator sign, and psoas sign. In complicated appendicitis where for example there is perforation of appendix and spillage of the content, the physical findings change. Additional findings depend on the nature of the complications the patient had developed. If the infection is contained, the patient often develops a soft, tender mass in the right lower quadrant, and the area of tenderness now encompasses the entire right lower quadrant.

A point for practice is that when patients develop perforated or gangrenous appendicitis with peritonitis, the fever may be high grade and the fever may be swinging. Note that patients with perforation have high temperature as high as 38.3^{oc}. There is slight elevation of temperature (37.80oc) in patient with no perforation. Perforated cases have pronounced left shift leucocyte count and anorexia. People with early appendicitis do not look very ill most times except complicated. Remember the elderly mount poor response to inflammatory changes so in some cases there may not be fever. Absent fever is not an indication that the patient has no appendicitis. The factors that have been found to increase the chance of perforation include: increased age, male sex, presence of fever or anorexia, retrocaecal anatomical position of appendix, peritoneal signs, left-shift leucocytes, a higher C-reactive protein level, and delay in presentation and surgical intervention (Carr NJ, 2000). When these factors are present, possibility of perforation is very high. Several studies have shown that elderly patients have a tendency to present late after the initial onset of symptoms (Barcia JJ & Reissenweber N). Many authors believe that the delay in presentation is multifactorial. Some of these elderly patients live alone and have difficulty in accessing medical care early while others, with a higher pain threshold, would attribute the symptoms to indigestion or constipation, thus ignoring the initial symptoms until they worsened (Carr NJ, 2000). Another major factor in the delay presentation is the morbid fear of hospitalization among our elderly patients because they equate hospital admission with certain death. Symptoms and pathological changes are often inconsistent with the chief complaint of abdominal pain and less severe (Smithy WB, et al, 1986). Hence patients and attending physician do not take these patients serious until complications develop. Although elevated leukocyte count and CRP value cannot effectively establish the diagnosis of acute appendicitis in the elderly, unelevated values exclude it. Accordingly, appendectomy is not recommended to be performed in an elderly patient with unelevated leukocyte count and CRP value, even though clinical symptoms and signs indicate acute appendicitis (Horattas MC, et al, 1990). Awareness is the watch word in elderly appendicitis as several studies have shown that elderly patients have a tendency to present late after the initial onset of symptoms (Carr NJ, 2000; Franz MG, et al, 1995; Smithy WB, et al, 1986). Again, remember to consider appendicitis in all cases of abdominal pains in the elderly.

4. Diagnosis

Making the diagnosis of appendicitis is largely clinical and it is based on history, physical examination, and imaging studies. Appendicitis in the elderly has inconsistent manifestations. There are high percentages of patients with atypical presentations in the elderly. Appendicitis is less common in the elderly than in the young, but symptoms are more likely to be ignored by the elderly patient, and the mortality is higher in this aged group, up to 10%. Similarly appendicitis in the elderly often has a delay in diagnosis owing to often vague symptoms, blunted tenderness, and diminished leukocytic responses. Thus, a higher index of suspicion is again required. Diagnosis is difficult as many of the symptoms mimic those associated with aging. Atypical appendicitis is common in the elderly and the diagnosis can elude even the most experienced surgeon. How do we make an early diagnosis of appendicitis in the elderly with a reduced rate of complications? High index of suspicion is the practice principle. The classical sequence of symptoms is uncommon. In a nutshell however, the presentation of appendicitis in the elderly still follows the classical form of presentation, though more of the elderly patients manifest atypically. It must be restated that awareness is the main thing when it comes to making diagnosis of appendicitis in the elderly. The corner stone of diagnosis is localised tenderness over McBurney's point (Carr NJ, 2000; Horattas MC, et al, 1990)..

The classical presentation is an elderly patient with a sequential progression of acute central abdominal pain migrating to the right lower quadrant of the abdomen. Majority of the patients have nausea. It may be associated with vomiting and low grade fever. There is slight temperature elevation (1°C), tachycardia, constipation and diarrhoea. If vomiting is more than twice in a patient with suspected appendicitis it indicates a complicated appendicitis or a wrong diagnosis (Carr NJ, 2000; Horattas MC, et al, 1990). What is the cornerstone of diagnosis for acute appendicitis? The basis of diagnosis is classic history of anorexia with periumbilical pain localizing to right iliac quadrant. In an article published earlier pain was found to be the most common complaints followed by anorexia and vomiting in 100, 67 and 59% respectively (Schumpelick V, et al, 2000). The usual complaint in appendicitis is abdominal pain. This was found in the article reviewed to vary from 92 to 100% of patients. The pain may be in the right iliac fossa, periumbilical, vague or diffuse. According to this publication the next common symptom was found to be anorexia nausea which was found in 52% of their patients. Patient may present with a mass in the right iliac fossa, which may come as appendiceal mass or an abscess. Other symptoms include vomiting, fever and diarrhoea. In the same article, tenderness in the right iliac fossa was found in 80 to 99% of patients. Other signs were abdominal mass, rectal tenderness, and high temperature. Leukocytosis was a very common laboratory finding. This was found in at least 71 to 94% of patients (Krisher S, et al, 2005). . Palpatory pressure in left iliac fossa may cause pain in the right iliac fossa (Rovsing sign). Other signs that may be elicited include, psoas (pain with right thigh extension), pain with internal rotation of flexed thigh, (obturator sign). In retrocaecal appendix, there may be flank tenderness in the right iliac fossa. The diagnosis of appendicitis is difficult in the elderly for many reasons that have been highlighted earlier. Diagnosis of this condition should be expedited in the elderly for good outcome of treatment. Clinical features and definitive investigations are indispensable in making the correct diagnosis of appendicitis in the elderly.

If vomiting occurs first the diagnosis of appendicitis is doubtful. The common sequence of presentation is the sequence of anorexia, then abdominal pain, then vomiting which occur in 95% of cases. Summarising their findings, the classical diagnostic features of appendicitis are fever, elevated WBC, anorexia, and right lower quadrant (RLQ) pain. In an attempt to improve diagnostic accuracy clinical scoring systems have been developed. In a meta-analysis of diagnostic studies, Anderson concluded that, although individual variables had weak discriminatory power, when combined they have strong predictive power. Diagnostic variable are better combined to improve the diagnosis of appendicitis. The most powerful variables were laboratory tests of inflammation - high WBC, the percentage of neutrophils and C reactive protein levels and clinical indicators such as history of migration of pain and evidence of peritoneal irritation - rigidity and rebound tenderness (Jaffe B, 2005; Naaeder SB, Archampong EQ, 1999). This method has been found to tremendously improve diagnostic accuracy. A prompt diagnosis is invaluable in the management of appendicitis in the elderly. A combination of delay in presentation and misdiagnosis with subsequent delay in surgical intervention contributes to perforation. The slight differences in pathophysiology of appendicitis also contribute to this complication as reported by Carr (Carr NJ, 2000). Remember not to place appendicitis lower than second in the differential diagnosis of acute abdomen in the elderly.

5. Investigation

What are the routine preoperative tests we should carry out? While symptoms can guide the selection of ancillary tests in persons under age 40, the prevalence of acute illness with a nonspecific presentation in the elderly dictates a lower threshold for screening. Elderly persons undergoing surgery should have the following routine tests: a fasting glucose level to screen for hidden or ongoing diabetes; a complete blood count to indicate any infection or anaemia and the blood pictures; electrolytes; blood urea nitrogen; creatinine to determine risk of cardiac arrhythmias and postoperative renal failure; chest radiograph to screen for pulmonary disease; and an electrocardiogram (ECG) to detect any ischemia or arrhythmia. All these tests are valuable in the general assessment of the patients for proper outcome of surgery. If patients are not adequately evaluated and all the defects or derangements are corrected before surgery, incorrect management can worsen the morbidity and mortality of the patient. Studies have shown that if these tests have been performed within 3 months prior to admission in persons without new symptoms, they need not be repeated. Nevertheless, most practicing physicians and surgeons repeat the tests within a few days of surgery as a matter of habit (Graber MA, et al, 1999; Wolfe JM, 2000). It is advisable that all these tests be repeated in the elderly each time they are being taken for any operative procedure as the organ systems at that age group are declining in function with low reserve as compared to the young candidates who are being taken for surgery. The elderly must be adequately resuscitated before undergoing any form of surgical procedure.

These investigations must not be seen in isolation but must be combined with clinical findings for proper assessment and management of patients. Carrying out these investigations astutely is important as many diseases present the same ways appendicitis manifest in the elderly. No time is wasted in taking our time to screen the elderly for other problems in order to reduce the incidence of unnecessary surgeries. Hence there is need for proper assessment by way of investigations. Appendix various locations in the abdomen has anatomical basis. Its intraabdominal location depends on the way it is attached by the mesoappendix. The presenting symptoms therefore vary according to the location of the inflamed portion and the affected contiguous structures. Adequate investigation is indispensable in knowing the exact cause of abdominal pain in the elderly. Appendix is variously located in order of frequency in the low cecal position, the pelvis and the retrocaecal position (Cordon RE, 1986; Paulson EK, 2003). The focus of the investigations should be directed against those conditions that can imitate appendicitis in the elderly. In this age group, the differential diagnosis of acute appendicitis includes the following: diverticulitis perforated peptic ulcer, acute cholecystitis, acute pancreatitis, intestinal obstruction, perforated caecal carcinoma, mesenteric vascular occlusion, and rupturing aortic aneurysm. Although rare, amoebic infection of the caecum with caecal dilation can mimic appendicitis especially in the tropical countries. Infection with salmonella species can also mimic appendicitis. The presence of a cecal malignancy must be seriously considered in the differential diagnosis of appendicitis in the elderly. Many cases of colonic cancers have been diagnosed as appendicitis and had also been treated as such. Risk of perforation is greater, and because of advanced age, mortality and morbidity are elevated in the elderly. In all patients with gastroenteritis, appendicitis must be considered (Freund HR & Rubinstein E, 1984). The main bearing is that in all cases of abdominal pain in the aged; please consider investigating for appendicitis strongly. All efforts should be made to rule out these pathologies as delay and wrong diagnosis worsen the outcome of appendicitis treatment among the old patients.

What are the values of white blood cell count in this group of patients? The white blood cell count must be noted and urine analysis should be included especially in the elderly patients with acute abdomen. Remember subcaecal or pelvic appendicitis may be associated with microscopic haematuria and leukocytes. The important of the Haemogram is the differential of the white blood cell count. There is a high level of leucocytes count in most of the patients. This is a normal reaction to bacterial infections in the body. In appendicitis of the elderly, this laboratory index is a strong parameter. This parameter is highly rated as it is stated that elevated WBC count and right lower quadrant pain appear to be the most sensitive clinical indicators of appendicitis but are highly nonspecific. Remember no single laboratory parameter is diagnostic. The urea and electrolyte only indicate the function of the kidney. If the patient will need to undergo surgery, the kidney must be function well in order to clear the system of anaesthetic drugs (Oliak D, 2000 et al. Saidi HS&Adwok JA, 2000). Many of these patients are already having a decline function of their kidneys. The incidence of diabetes is high in this category of patients hence the blood sugar estimation is necessary before anaesthesia.

Imaging studies are important among the many investigations to consider in the assessments of the patients for the purpose of proper management of the aged. These imaging investigations should not exclude the non specific tests such as complete blood count, C - reactive protein (CRP), and urinalysis as stated. The definitive diagnosis is easily enhanced with imaging studies such as computed tomography with or without contrast addition of intravenous or oral medium. The addition of contrast enhances its sensitivity. Two other

imaging studies that are important in the assessment are ultrasound and magnet resonance imaging. The first advocated imaging study is a non ionising study test, the ultrasonography scanning. In most cases if the diagnosis is not certain after ultrasound, computed tomography should be used to confirm or rule out appendicitis. Some surgeons maintain that the clinical diagnosis of appendicitis by a surgeon is sufficient without any radiologic study before surgery. The occasional discovery of normal appendix at the time of surgery may be considered an acceptable false positive clinical diagnosis in order to minimize the occasional error of false negative diagnosis that would result in delayed operation, ruptured appendicitis, and associated complications (Mahadevan M & Graff L, 2000).
As studies have shown, ultrasonography (US) and computed tomography (CT) scans have demonstrated high efficacy. US has a sensitivity of 75% to 90%, a specificity of 86% to 100%, a positive predictive value of 89% to 93%, and an overall accuracy of 90% to 94%. CT scanning is even more accurate, with a sensitivity of 90% to 100%, a specificity of 91% to 99%, and a positive predictive value of 95% to 97%. Ultrasound we should know cannot rule out appendicitis but very useful in its confirmation. For the vast majority of patients who present with typical appendicitis, however, obtaining a CT scan may only delay the time of operation and may prove to be unnecessary in the end. It also adds to the cost of care. A reasonable approach for that reason is to reserve the use of radiologic studies for patients with an atypical presentation or in patient populations in whom the possibility of a misdiagnosis is greater. Such patients in which the risk is greater include the young sexually active females with high likelihood of PID, pregnant women (US), and elderly patients with confounding factors. For patients with a classic presentation of appendicitis, radiologic studies are unnecessary (Naoum JJ, et al, 2002. Patrick DA, et al, 2003)

5.1 Plain abdominal X ray

One is not always able to diagnose appendicitis from plain abdominal x ray, but it is helpful. There may be localized air fluid levels, with increased soft tissue density in the lower quadrant of the abdomen. There may be presence of stones, altered right psoas shadow or an abnormal right flank stripe. In general the findings on plain films are non specific and rarely of help in diagnosis of appendicitis (Lawrence Way, 2006).

5.2 Ultrasonography

The sensitivity of ultrasound in the diagnosis of appendicitis from several centres has been reported to be as high as 80%, with specificity as high as 90%. Standard abdominal radiography may show a calcified faecolith in the right lower quadrant along with a paucity of gas in the right lower quadrant of the abdomen. A loss of the right psoas shadow may be noted and represents late appendicitis with retroperitoneal inflammation. A perforated or gangrenous appendix may exhibit extra abdominal gas on radiographs, but this occurs in only 1% of cases. A sentinel loop ileus or a soft-tissue mass with or without gas bubbles also be may seen in advanced cases. Ultrasound may diagnose acute appendicitis, but negative ultrasound does not appear to rule out appendicitis (Naoum JJ, et al, 2002; Patrick DA, et al, 2003). Ultrasound though useful has its own short coming in the diagnosis of appendicitis.

5.3 Barium contrast

Barium contrast studies remain a simple, safe, and readily available test that may be helpful. However, ultrasound and CT examinations now are preferred. A barium study assures luminal patency of the appendix, colonic wall for mass effects or secondary effects of appendicitis, and right colonic or terminal ileal mucosal disease that may simulate appendicitis. When the barium contrast fills the appendix, a diagnosis of acute appendicitis is very unlikely but not impossible. Up to 10% to 20% of normal appendices do not fill during a barium study. These inconsistencies should be noted in the use of barium contrast studies in the diagnosis of appendicitis.

5.4 Laparoscopy

Laparoscopy can be both diagnostic and therapeutic for acute appendicitis. Laparoscopy may be indicated in problem patients. In almost all circumstances, a laparoscopy with negative findings is preferred to expectantly watching the appendix rupture. No harm if negative laparoscopy is carried out. When the classical features are present, diagnosis of appendicitis by laparoscopy are not difficult. However in whatever form of presentation, diseases that will mimic appendicitis that do not require operative therapy and can be made worse by operation must be rule out. Such diseases include pneumonia of the bases of the lung, myocardial infarction and pancreatitis among others (Franz MG, et al, 1995). Laparoscopy is very useful in ruling out other intraabdominal problems that may mimic appendicitis in the elderly.

5.5 Computed tomography

CT is the diagnostic test of choice for appendicitis and to rule out abscess formation. It should be employed in cases of elderly appendicitis to avoid delay in diagnosis. The use of CT to delineate abdominal pain in a select population is an excellent tool that the surgeon should not hesitate to use early in patient for evaluation (Saidi HS & Adwok JA, 2000). CT scan accurately detected appendicitis in 90% of the cases according to an article published by Storm Dickerson and Horratas. According to Storm and Horratas, CT should be reserved for cases in which suspicion warrants confirmation prior to surgery. Radiologic evaluation should be based on the radiologist interpretation of acute abdominal series (AAS) or computer tomography (CT) or both. CT can be utilized selectively to confirm the diagnosis in equivocal cases. CT in their series was considered positive only if it was diagnostic for or suggestive of appendicitis. Their CT criteria for a positive appendicitis included pericaecal inflammation or visualization of the appendix with inflammation. While the use of CT has opened new avenues in medicine and may be the most significant advance made in the treatment of appendicitis in the elderly over the last 20 years, history and physical examination remains the hallmark of patient evaluation. Note according some authors, appendicitis need to be considered in the differential diagnosis for all acute abdominal pain in the elderly (Horattas MC & Haught R, 1992). CT scanning may decrease the incidence of appendiceal rupture and also the frequency of exploratory laparotomy for what turns out to be a normal appendix. However, removal of a normal appendix in a symptomatic patient who is thought to have appendicitis, a potentially lethal disease, should not be considered an unnecessary operation. The number of elderly patients and children who die of appendicitis because of failure to operate early enough when the diagnosis is in doubt is much higher than the number of patients who die from a complication following removal of a normal appendix. The morbidity of negative laparotomy is minimal and is much more acceptable than the significantly higher morbidity of a perforated appendix. Unfortunately, after 60 years of age, about 50% of patients are found to have a ruptured appendix when the operation is finally done. A normal appendix may be difficult to locate on CT examination and may require extra scans at finer intervals. Appendicoliths are seen in one fourth of all people as a ring-like or homogenous calcified density on CT. CT imaging has 90% sensitivity for detecting intraabdominal inflammation. CT findings suggestive of appendicitis include a pericaecal phlegmon or abscess, and small amounts of right lower quadrant intraabdominal free air that signals perforation.

6. Treatment

In 1989, Harold Ellis wrote that "the treatment of acute appendicitis is appendectomy - and the sooner it is done, the better" (McCallion J,et al, 1987). This statement is true today as it was many years back in the history of treatment of appendicitis. Controversies now exist in the treatment of appendicitis in the present day. Some now question the rational for removing all inflamed appendices without selective excision of appendix. There is general agreement that the treatment of acute appendicitis is appendicectomy. However, in the elderly it is advisable that if the diagnosis is certain, and surgery is indicated a patient who is fit for surgery; appendicectomy should be carried out for cases of appendicitis in the elderly (Sherlock DJ, 1985). Like any other patients with appendicitis, basic investigations for patients going for surgery must be performed in the elderly. Proper preoperative assessment is very important. The high probability that older patients will require surgery and the increased risk of morbidity and mortality in the elderly necessitate a thorough preoperative assessment in older adults than any other group of patients. Typical postoperative mortality rates of older patients undergoing major intra-abdominal surgery range from 3 to 5%, about twice that of persons under age 65 (Sherlock DJ, 1985).. What we need to do is to identify any significant risk factors of adverse outcomes and to provide recommendations for the evaluation and management of these risk factors. The high prevalence of multiple comorbidities in the elderly necessitates a comprehensive history and physical examination. The treatment of appendicitis in the elderly should be individualised. These patients have varied pathologies above sixty years of age. Treat appendicitis as indicated individually in the elderly. No single modus operandi can be followed but surgical principles should be observed. The type of procedure as well as the presence of several risk factors can be identified by a review of the patient's medical history. In general, a comprehensive physical examination should be conducted. A proper evaluation of clinical presentation allows the index of suspicion to be set at the proper level so that a threshold for intervention can be reached before the appendix ruptures. If after proper assessment of patient, appendix is still removed with the idea of what constitute unnecessary surgery, no harm is done. According to Condon, the removal of a normal appendix in appropriate clinical circumstances never constitutes an unnecessary appendectomy (Condon RE, 1986).

6.1 Preoperative assessment

All derangements found in the assessment of the patients should be corrected before surgery. Anaemia should be corrected. Dehydration and renal functions should be corrected. High blood sugar if present should be controlled. All other deranged parameters involving other organs apart from gastrointestinal system should not be disregarded. Proper and appropriate preoperative treatment depends most time on the type of presentation of appendicitis. Are we dealing with simple appendicitis, appendiceal mass or perforated appendicitis with peritonitis? In other word is it an elective patient or an emergency patient? Where the cases are patients for elective appendicectomy, cessation of smoking prior to surgery is helpful and should be undertaken at least 2 weeks prior to surgery. Training in coughing and deep breathing exercise should be undertaken prior to surgery. If chronic obstructive pulmonary disease (COPD) is present, aggressive use of bronchodilators should be implemented both before and after the operation. Prophylaxis of thromboembolic events is based on the type of procedure and level of risk of the patient. In high-risk general surgical patients, e.g., those with previous history of thromboembolic phenomenon who is to undergo surgery especially major one, a low dose heparin should be administered before and continued after surgery. Heparin 5000 to 7500 U every 12 hours begun on the day of surgery is effective. Low-molecular-weight heparin twice a day with or without intermittent pneumatic compression is also effective.

6.2 Preoperative analgesia

Should we or should we not give pain killer before surgery in order not to mask the diagnosis of appendicitis where we are not yet certain? There has been a growing concern of IV analgesia masking an ongoing intraabdominal catastrophe, leading the surgeon to miss the diagnosis and potentially endanger the patient. This code of belief has been challenged in recent times, however. In fact, it has been established that IV analgesia results in a significant pain reduction without concurrent normalizing effects on the abdominal examination. There is strong evidence suggesting that contrary to traditional teaching, it is, in fact, safe to administer opioid analgesics and other forms of analgesia in the setting of surgical evaluation of acute abdomen without increasing the chance of misdiagnosis. One can still be able to elicit all the necessary signs of the abdomen even after analgesia. It is also humane and since it will completely mask the signs, patients with pain should be relieved with pain killer before surgery. Patient should be properly assessed by the anaesthesiologist to ascertain the fitness and grade of fitness of patient for surgery. No patient should be rushed for surgery without appropriate consideration and duly signed informed consent obtained. Patient or patient relation must fully understand the procedure to be carried out and the possible outcome of the surgery. Delay treatment and misdiagnosis have been found to correlate with perforation of appendicitis. In cases of suspected appendicitis where the index of suspicion is too low to mandate immediate operation, active observation, comprising in patient admission with serial clinical and laboratory examinations, is an acceptable and valuable tool, both in reducing unnecessary appendectomies and preventing missed diagnoses (Watters JM, et al, 1996). Even though delayed surgical management is associated with increased risk for Appendiceal rupture in the elderly undue operation should be reduced. We should remember that extreme of ages are associated with high risk of surgical procedures. Delay in the elderly should be avoided.

6.3 Intraoperative management

Appropriate form of anaesthesia should be administered to the patient. Considerations should be given to individual patient. General or regional anaesthesia can be prescribed depending on the patient and the nature of operation to be carried out. Is patient going for simple appendicectomy or to undergo exploratory laparotomy? Treatment is seen in two major categories, simple appendicitis and complicated appendicitis. The complicated cases include appendiceal mass, appendiceal abscess and ruptured appendicitis with peritonitis among others. The peritonitis may be localised or generalised depending on how the body is able to wall off the offending agent (Paranjape, C., et al, 2007)

6.4 Simple appendicectomy

In cases of certainty of diagnosis of uncomplicated acute appendicitis, appendectomy should be performed as an emergency procedure. If we need to lay further emphasis on the type of incisions suitable for this surgery, the recommended incision for a routine appendectomy (uncomplicated cases) is a transverse incision (Brown CV, et al, 2003). Both midline and grid iron incision can be used equally. The midline has an added advantage for easy extension of the incision if the diagnosis is found to be something else that may require a complete laparotomy. Exposure of the appendix through this incision is much better than that obtained through the classic McBurney incision, particularly in patients who have a retrocaecal appendix or are obese. The gridiron, or muscle-splitting, incision (McBurney incision) is the one most widely used for uncomplicated appendicitis, largely because of surgical tradition rather than its particular utility. The exposure through a McBurney incision can be awkward, especially for a retrocaecal appendix, unless the appendix lies immediately below the incision. If necessary, the incision can be extended medially, partially transecting the rectus sheath, but this manoeuvre is usually helpful only for a pelvic appendix (Kaminski A, et al, 2005). If the diagnosis of acute appendicitis is in doubt and exploratory laparotomy is indicated, a vertical midline incision is appropriate. If an appendiceal mass is encountered, the midline incision can be closed and a more direct approach to the lesion made through a right lower quadrant incision.

6.5 Open technique

The benchmark incision for the management of appendicitis has been through a small right lower quadrant incision. Patient abdomen should be palpated under anaesthesia. McBurney's point marks the bearing of appendicectomy incision. It does not generally indicate the tip of the appendix but locates the base. In general, an inferior incision below the area of maximal tenderness helps in rotating the caecum into the wound. The McBurney incision is the classical oblique appendectomy incision through McBurney's point to the lateral edge of the rectus sheath; it can be extended into the lateral rectus sheath, if necessary. It is quite cosmetically acceptable when healed. On the other hand, a skin line or transverse incision placed 1 to 2 cm medial to the anterosuperior iliac spine can be used. These incisions are performed with a muscle-splitting technique through all layers lateral to the rectus abdominis muscle. The incision is continued through the superficial fascia until the external oblique muscle aponeurosis is exposed. The fibres of the aponeurosis are opened, and the muscle fibres are bluntly separated, as are the fibres of the internal oblique and transverse abdominis muscles. The peritoneum is opened and intraperitoneal cultures can be obtained. The caecum is mobilized into the wound, and the appendix is mobilized as adhesions are bluntly and/or sharply dissected. The taeniae of the colon converge at the base of the appendix, an arrangement that helps in locating this structure at operation. The base of the appendix always lies at the confluence of the taeniae. In mobile appendices, the mesoappendix can be grasped near the tip of the appendix with a clamp. The appendix can be grasped with a Babcock at its base. The mesoappendix can be ligated en masse with no. 3-0 absorbable suture if the pedicle is not too large or edematous (Brown CV, 2003; Condon RE, 1986).

Ligation of the mesoappendix usually is performed from the distal tip to the base of the appendix (antegrade appendicectomy), but sometimes reversing the sequence can facilitate appendectomy (retrograde appendicectomy). The accessory branch of the posterior cecal artery securely should be ligated. The appendix is double clamped with straight hemostats across the base, leaving sufficient space between clamps to permit passage of the cautery or scalpel. The space between clamps can be crushed or milked prior to clamping to minimize contamination into the peritoneal cavity. The appendix is amputated with the scalpel or with cautery, and the appendix and the attached clamp are dropped into a small basin to avoid contamination. The appendiceal stump is then doubly ligated with 2-0 absorbable or delayed absorbable suture. The appendiceal stump may be cauterized to prevent mucocele formation or inverted with a purse string suture or Z-stitch in the caecum. If this is done, a purse-string suture of medium silk is placed around the base of the appendix. The circumference of the purse-string suture should be large enough to permit easy inversion of the stump. A half-knot is placed in the silk; after the appendix is amputated, the stump is inverted and the purse-string is drawn tight. The site of the inversion should be covered with mesoappendix or any convenient flap of fat (Brown CV, 2003; Condon RE, 1986, Ellis H, 1989). However, inversion of the stump is no longer considered necessary by many authors. It is not recommended when the appendix is inflamed. Copious irrigation with saline or antibiotic solution should be performed in cases of perforated appendicitis to reduce the risk of a pelvic. The peritoneum and muscular fasciae are usually closed with a running absorbable suture. The skin can be closed in nonperforated cases of appendicitis, but delayed primary closure is routine in cases of ruptured appendicitis.

6.6 Laparoscopy appendectomy

This procedure has revolutionized the removal of appendix with minimal morbidity and mortality. Since it was first described by Semm in 1983, laparoscopic appendectomy has gained acceptance as both a diagnostic and treatment method for acute appendicitis. It is safe and effective. There is less surgical tissue trauma, a better postoperative course, the ability to explore the entire abdominal cavity, assessment for the existence of associated pathologies, better cosmetic results, and a rapid return to normal activity. The ability to completely evaluate the pelvis and the entire peritoneal cavity when a healthy appendix is found is extremely important for the surgeons as many conditions in the elderly that mimic appendicitis can be rule out immediately (Fitz HR, 1986). Removing a normal appendix during laparoscopic evaluation for suspected acute appendicitis can be performed with no added morbidity or increased length of hospitalization as compared to diagnostic laparoscopy. The laparoscopic approach offers the advantage of shorter hospitalization and less morbidity, with a lower rate of abdominal wall infection. There is no significant difference in the rate of abscess formation in patients with perforated appendicitis. The interval until the patient may return to work is shortened and postoperative pain is decreased with the laparoscopic approach, and the quality of life appears to improve faster than when the traditional open approach is used. Obese patients may benefit substantially from the laparoscopic approach as it obviates the problems of a large incision, strong retraction, prolonged surgery, and wound infection that are associated with open surgery in the obese (Fitz HR, 1986; Hui TT et al, 2002).The disadvantages of the laparoscopic approach have been longer duration of surgery and higher costs. However, the length of surgery has been significantly reduced with improved surgical skills and experience. Also, the immediate cost difference appears to be diminished with the use of reusable laparoscopic equipment, and when the more rapid return to work and other activities is included, the laparoscopic approach turns out to be extremely cost effective. It is increasingly recommended as the procedure of choice for the diagnosis and treatment of suspected acute appendicitis.

The detail procedure is beyond the scope of this write up. See other references for details of the procedure. How does the laparoscopic approach to appendectomy compare with that of the open approach? Laparoscopic appendectomy is superior to the open approach in terms of decreased postoperative wound infections and recovery time. In a large review, patients who underwent laparoscopic appendectomy were found to be as follows when compared with patients who underwent open appendectomy: Are about half as likely to develop postoperative wound infections (odds ratio 0.47, 95% confidence interval between 0.36 and 0.62) Have decreased pain on postoperative day 1 by the visual analog score of 8 mm on a scale of 100 mm (95% confidence interval between 3 and 13 mm) Have reduced length of hospital stay by 0.7 days (95% confidence interval between 0.4 and 1.0) Have reduced time of recovery in terms of earlier return to normal activity, work, and sport by 6 days (95% confidence interval between 4 and 8 days), 3 days (95% confidence interval between 1 day and 5 days), and 7 days (95% confidence interval between 3 days and 12 days), respectively Have increased cost of the operation, but decreased cost outside the hospital Have reduced rates of negative appendectomies or unestablished final diagnosis. But the laparoscopic appendectomy was inferior to the open appendectomy in the following ways: Nearly three times as likely to develop postoperative intraabdominal abscesses (odds ratio 2.77, 95% confidence interval between 1.61 and 4.77) Increased duration of surgery by 14 minutes (95% confidence interval between 10 minutes and 19 minutes) The reviewers concluded that the laparoscopic appendectomy would be advantageous over the open appendectomy in most cases of suspected appendicitis, except in patients in whom laparoscopy is contraindicated or unfeasible, in patients with gangrene, and patients with perforated appendicitis. In these patients, the laparoscopic approach carries a higher risk of intraabdominal infections (Sauerland S et al, 2004, van Sonnenberg E et al, 1987; Vargas HI, et al. 1994)

What would have been done if a tumour had been discovered in appendix? How often are tumours found in the appendix? What is the most common tumour of the appendix? What is the usual presentation of appendiceal tumour? The most common type of appendiceal tumour is carcinoid, usually on the tip of the appendix. Carcinoid, comprising 77% of appendiceal tumours, was discovered in only 1.4% of 1,000 consecutive appendectomies (Dymock RB, 1977). If the carcinoid tumour is small, a simple appendectomy is adequate; if the tumour is large, a more extensive resection is indicated. A retrospective literature review noted that tumours larger than 2 cm had a much higher incidence of regional metastasis than smaller ones. For this reason, simple appendectomy for tumours smaller than 2 cm and right hemicolectomy for tumours larger than 2 cm is recommended. Primary adenocarcinoma of the appendix is exceedingly rare (0.1%). The usual presentation of an appendiceal tumour is similar to that of appendicitis.

6.7 Incidental appendicectomy

What are the arguments for and against performing an incidental appendectomy during this patient's laparoscopic examination? What evidence supports incidental appendectomy in this patient? Removing the appendix during a negative exploration is controversial. The argument for incidental appendectomy is that the absence of the organ obviates any future question of appendicitis should the patient develop recurrent abdominal pain. The argument against incidental appendectomy is largely the risk of peritoneal or wound infection, especially during clean procedures in which resection through the appendiceal stump may spill the contents of the caecum. In a prospective randomized study of 139 trauma patients, there was no significant difference in intraperitoneal or wound infections between the patients who received incidental appendectomy and the control group who did not. The factors that would sway the surgeons to perform incidental appendectomy include easy access to the appendix and technical feasibility, contaminated peritoneum (i.e., concomitant bowel content spillage), young age, and the likelihood of future abdominal pains (e.g., history of PID, family history of Crohn's disease). In this young patient with a strong history of recurrent RLQ abdominal pain, an incidental appendectomy is justified. Vargas HI et al, 1994)

6.8 Peritoneal fluid culture

When the peritoneum is opened, cloudy intraperitoneal fluid is noted. A culture and sensitivity sample of the fluid is sent to the microbiology laboratory. Further dissection reveals a gangrenous appendix with distal perforation in the pelvic brim. How valuable is the practice of sending a sample of the intraperitoneal fluid for bacterial culture and sensitivity? Not valuable. In a retrospective study of 308 pediatric patients, the results of routine culture and sensitivity did not lead to improvement in patient management. Only 16% of the patients had their antibody management changed as a result of the culture and sensitivity. However, specific antibiotic treatment based on culture result was associated with increased infectious complications. The use of empiric antibiotics without modification to culture results was associated with a lower incidence of infectious complications, fever duration, and length of hospitalization. The practice of routine culture is not helpful in most cases of acute appendicitis, and empiric broad-spectrum antibiotic coverage should be adequate (Van Sonnernberg, et al, 1987)

6.9 Complicated appendicitis

We shall briefly consider the management of the complicated cases of appendicitis. The three complications that shall be considered include appendiceal mass, appendiceal abscess, and perforated appendicitis with peritonitis. These are various stages in the pathological processes of appendicitis. The development of each depends on how well the body can wall off the offending agents. If these complications are well tackled in the Elderly patients, the morbidity and mortality increase sharply.

6.10 Appendiceal mass treatment

Appendiceal mass are managed expectantly. The diagnosis can be made preoperatively or at induction of anesthesia when the patient is well relaxed and the abdomen can easily be re assessed. If appendiceal mass is detected at any state, the operation should be abandoned in favor of conservative management. Some of the patients may be having malignancy masquerading as appendicitis. If the decision has been made to manage the patient expectantly, patient should be admitted into the hospital. Intravenous fluid should be instituted, patient should inititialy be placed on nil per os. Intravenous antibiotics should be administered covering aerobic and anaerobic organism as indicated under pathology above. The patient should be kept under close observation with the pulse closely followed because tachycardia is one of the first signs of sepsis. Other clinical parameters to follow include change in pain quality, white blood cell counts, differential counts, and serial radiologic evaluations including ultrasound and/or CT. Failure to respond to therapy after 24 to 48 hours indicates that operative intervention should be reconsidered. Patients with well-formed periappendiceal abscesses can undergo CT-guided placement of pigtail drainage catheters to help resolve the abscess more rapidly, rather than depending on the abscess to drain internally into the cecum.

Naturally appendiceal mass can resolve completely or develop into an abscess. The vital signs monitoring and serial ultrasound and other possible imaging examinations will settle the outcome of the mass. If the mass forms an abscess, the abscess should be drained. If the mass resolves completely patient should have interval appendicectomy. If a distinct mass in the right iliac fossa is palpated and the patient has no systemic manifestations, the patient is kept nil per os (NPO) while intravenous fluids and broad-spectrum antibiotics are given to cover enteric organisms. There are growing schools of thoughts regarding the management of appendiceal mass. Apart from the usual method adopt by the majority of surgeons as described above, many have proposed a more aggressive methods of treatments of appendiceal mass. Another group of surgeons believe that patient should have immediate appendicectomy following appendiceal mass resolution before patient is discharged from the hospital (Terasawa T, et al, 2004). A school of thought has also proposed a more aggressive approach of immediate right hemicolectomy following a diagnosis of appendiceal mass. Each has its own advantages and disadvantages. The more aggressive method sorts out the cases at once even though it may turn out to be an overtreatment for the patients. Many of the patients may end up not requiring right hemicolectomy.

6.11 Appendiceal abscess treatment

Patient may present from the onset into the hospital as a case of appendiceal abscess especially among the elderly people. Some other patients may develop appendiceal abscess during expectant management for cases of appendiceal masses. The treatment however is the same in most patients. The abscess should be drained. The drainage of the abscess should be done extra peritoneally avoiding contamination of the general peritoneal cavity. The usual grid iron incision can be used and the peritoneum is not opened. The abscess is drained extra peritoneally with a drain inserted and directed out into the cavity of the abscess. If the peritoneum is breached and pus spills into the cavity, generalize peritonitis may ensue which will worsen the outcome of the abscess drainage. The conventional treatment of this patient further involves an interval appendicectomy which should probably be carried out 6-10 weeks after the initial sickness (Terasawa T, et al, 2004). Age passé is not a contraindication to surgery of interval appendicectomy in the elderly. Complications of appendiceal abscess include pelvic, subphrenic and intraabdominal abscess, faecal fistula, peritonitis, pyelonephritis, venous thrombosis, and intestinal obstruction. Septicaemia, pneumonia, septic shock, renal failure, and pulmonary embolus can lead to death in the most advanced or neglected cases. It is relatively safe to remove the appendix in virtually any patient. However, if there are significant medical contraindications to surgery in a nontoxic patient with a clear diagnosis of an appendiceal abscess, a nonoperative approach can be considered (Fitz HR, 1986).

In patients with perforated appendicitis, is there an alternative to immediate appendectomy? Yes, percutaneous drainage and interval appendectomy may be an alternative. If the appendiceal abscess is known to be well loculated and walled off on CT and the patient is not septic, one may percutaneously drain the abscess cavity in lieu of immediate appendectomy, laparoscopic or open, and treat with antibiotics for a few weeks. The patient returns later to have the appendix resected when the inflammation has decreased. Reports indicate a success rate of 70% to 90%. The benefits of percutaneous drainage under radiologic guidance include precise anatomic identification of complex, multiloculated abscess; avoidance of operation for drainage without appendectomy; temporization of high-risk patients; and temporization of emergency appendectomy for an elective appendectomy. Interval appendectomy reportedly has been performed with the laparoscopic approach safely and effectively. Not all surgeons support this approach, however, and they continue to prefer open appendectomy and drainage (Van Sonnernberg, et al, 1987).

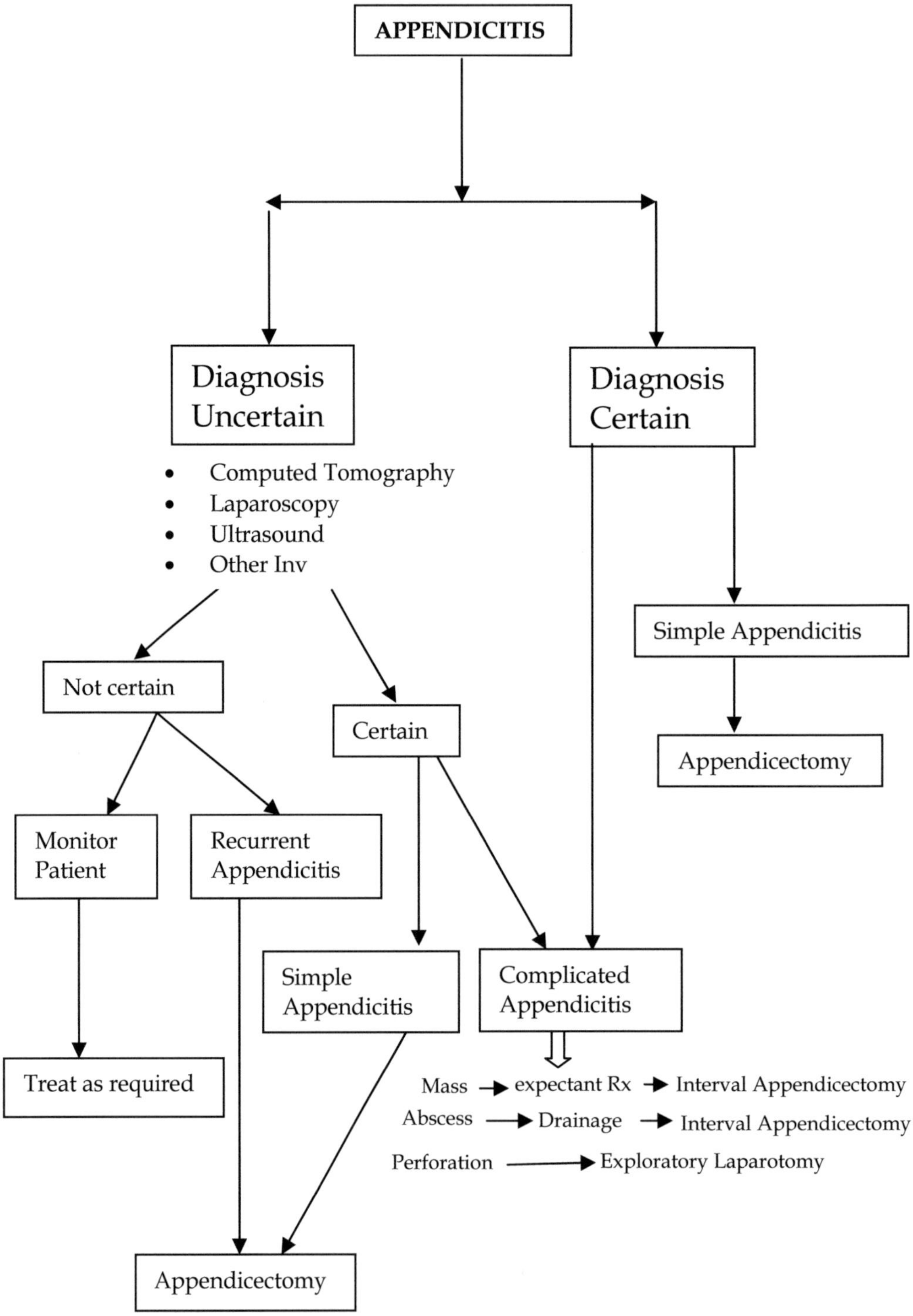

Fig. 1. Simple Management Pedigree of Appendicitis in the Elderly

6.12 Perforated appendicitis with peritonitis

Delay in seeking for medical care appears to be the principal reason for perforations in appendicitis of the elderly. The disease is allowed to progress through its natural course with alteration and this result in perforation at presentation. The appendicitis has progressed to perforation by the time of appendicectomy in people over 60 years of age. Most mortalities of appendicitis occur in this group of patients. Localised peritonitis results from microscopic perforation of gangrenous appendix, while spreading or generalised peritonitis implies gross perforation into the free peritoneal cavity. Patients with perforated appendicitis with generalised peritonitis should be well resuscitated before embarking on any surgical intervention. This category of patient requires exploratory laparotomy, appendicectomy and copious peritoneal larvage (Blomqvist P, et al, 2001). The mortality among these patients is high therefore patient must be adequately resuscitated before embarking on surgery (Lawrence Way, 2006). Management of appendicitis in the elderly is summarised in figure 1.

7. Conclusion

These initial investigations should include WBC, CRP (if available) and urinalysis. A higher index of suspicion with liberal early utilization of CT in uncertain cases may result in more appropriate management of these cases (Storm-Dickerson T.L. & Horattas M.C, 2003). A high index of suspicion is necessary to guard against misdiagnosis, especially in the elderly. We should exercise caution as delay in presentation and diagnosis are associated with higher rates of appendiceal perforations and hence higher morbidity and mortality. Appendicitis needs to be considered in all cases of acute abdomen in the elderly. A high degree of index of suspicion should be maintained always. Equivocal cases should undergo early computed tomography scan. This will facilitate appropriate and timely surgical interventions. The complications that may follow Appendicectomy commonly are wound infection, intraabdominal abscess, faecal fistula, pylephlebitis, and intestinal obstruction. The common organisms include anaerobic Bacteroides species and the aerobes Klebsiella and Enterobacter species and E coli. Successful management of acute appendicitis depends on early diagnosis and early surgical intervention. Elderly patients, who present to emergency departments with abdominal pain suspicious of appendicitis, should have an early surgical consultation and laboratory investigations to rule out appendicitis.

In dealing with wound infections following Appendicectomy in the elderly patients, the skin and subcutaneous tissue should be opened. The wound should be packed with saline-soaked gauze and reclosed with Steri-Strips in 4 to 5 days. Intraabdominal abscesses are common in patients with a perforated or gangrenous appendix. Intraabdominal abscesses are suspected when a patient with appendicectomy presents with recurrent fever, malaise, and anorexia. Computed tomography can be done to make the diagnosis of intraabdominal abscesses. Intraabdominal abscesses should be drained either operatively or percutaneously under CT or ultrasound guidance. Faecal fistula is a possible complication following appendicectomy. Many fistulas will close spontaneously if there is no anatomic basis. Those that do not close spontaneously and has anatomic reasons should be operated (Hardin D, 1999). The strong association between delay in presentation and appendiceal perforation supported the proposition that appendiceal perforation is the advanced stage of acute appendicitis; however, previous epidemiological studies also have suggested alternatively that non-perforated and perforated appendicitis may be different diseases (BOR-FUH SHEU, TE-FA, 2007). In caring for the elderly patient, a high index of suspicion and an awareness of the insidious symptoms of acute abdominal disease are mandatory. All aged patients with sudden lower abdominal pains should be screened for possibility of appendicitis. Appendicitis in the elderly is a difficult problem with a high incidence of atypical presentation resulting in incorrect diagnosis and consequent delay in medical care. This lead to relatively high rates of perforation often with associated postoperative complications and a high mortality (Hardin D, 1999).

8. References

Alvarado A. (1986). A practical score for the early diagnosis of acute appendicitis. *Ann. Emerg. Med.* 15: 557–64.

Paranjape C., Dalia S., Pan J., Horattas M. (2007) Appendicitis in the elderly: a change in the laparoscopic era *Surg Endosc* 21: 777–781 DOI: 10.1007/s00464-006-9097-4

Barcia JJ, Reissenweber N. (2002)Neutrophil count in the normal appendix and early appendicitis: diagnostic index of real acute inflammation. *Annals of Diagnostic Pathology;* 6(6):352-356.

Birnbaum BA, Wilson SR. (2000). Appendicitis at the millennium. *Radiology;* 215(2):337-348.

Blomqvist P, Andersson R, Granath F. (2001) Mortality after appendectomy in Sweden, 1987-1996. *Ann Surg;* 233:455–60.

Brown CV, Abrishami M, Muller M, Velmahos GC. (2003). Appendiceal abscess: immediate operation or percutaneous drainage? *American Surgeon;* 69(10):829-832

Burns RP, Cochran JL, Russell WL, Bard RM. (1985) Appendicitis in mature patients. *Ann. Surg.;* 201: 695–704.

Carr NJ. (2000). The pathology of acute appendicitis. *Annals of Diagnostic Pathology;* 4(1):46-58.

Condon RE. Acute appendicitis. (1986) In: Sabiston DC. Davis Christopher *Textbook of Surgery.* Vol. 13. Philadelphia, PA: WB Saunders;:967-982.

Ellis H. Appendix. (1989) In: Schwartz & Ellis, editor. Maingot's Abdominal Operations. Norwalk, Conneticut: Appleton & Lange,: 953-977.

Fitz HR. (1886) Perforating inflammation of the vermiform appendix; with special reference to its early diagnosis and treatment. *Trans. Assoc. Am. Physicians;* 1: 107–44.

Franz MG, Norman J, Fabri PJ. (1995) Increased morbidity of appendicitis with advancing age. *Am. Surg.;* 61: 40–4.

Freund HR, Rubinstein E. (1984) Appendicitis in the aged. Is it really different? *Am. Surg.;* 50: 573–6.

Friedell ML, Perez-Izquierdo M. (2000) Is there a role for interval appendectomy in the management of acute appendicitis? *American Surgeon;* 66(12):1158-1162

Graber MA, Ely JW, Clarke S,. (1999) Informed consent and general surgeons' attitudes toward the use of pain medication in the acute abdomen. *Am J Emerg Med.;* 17:113-116.

Gupta H, Dupuy D. (1997) Abdominal emergencies: has anything changed? *Surg Clin North Am;* 77:1245–64.

Hale D, Molloy M, Pearl R, et al. Appendectomy: (1997) A contemporary apprasial. *Ann Surg;* 225:252–61.

Hardin D (1999) Acute appendicitis: review and update. *Ann Fam Phys;* 60: 2027-36

Hogan MJ. (2003) Appendiceal abscess drainage. *Techniques in Vascular & Interventional Radiology;* 6(4):205-214.

Horattas MC, Guyton DP, Wu D. (1990) A reappraisal of appendicitis in the elderly. *Am. J. Surg.;* 160: 282–5.

Horattas MC, Haught R. (1992) Managing appendicitis in the elderly patient. *AORN J.*; 55: 1282–54.
Hui TT, Major KM, Avital I, Hiatt JR, Margulies DR (2002) Outcome of elderly patients with appendicitis: effect of computed tomography and laparoscopy. *Arch Surg* 137: 995–998;
Kaminski A, Liu IL, Applebaum H, Lee SL, Haigh PI. (2005) Routine interval appendectomy is not justified after initial nonoperative treatment of acute appendicitis. *Archives of Surgery*; 140 (9):897-901
Kraemer M, Franke C, Ohmann C, Yang Q, (2000) Acute Abdominal Pain Study Group. Acute appendicitis in late adulthood: incidence, presentation, and outcome. Results of a prospective multicenter acute abdominal pain study and a review of the literature. *Langenbecks Archives of Surgery*; 385(7):470-481.
Krisher S, Browne A, Dibbins A, Tkacz N. (2001) Intra-abdominal abscess after laparoscopic appendectomy for perforated appendicitis. *Arch Surg*; 136:438–41.
Langenscheidt P, Lang C, Puschel W, Feifel G. (1999); High rates of appendicectomy in a developing country: an attempt to contribute to a more rational use of surgical resources. *European Journal of Surgery* 165(3):248-252.
Lau WY, Fan ST, Yiu TF, Chu KW, Lee JM. (1985) Acute appendicitis in the elderly. *Surg. Gynecol. Obstet.*; 161: 157–60.
Lawrence W.W. 2006. Appendix. In:, *Current surgical diagnosis and treatment*. Gerard Doherty 648-653Lange Medical Books. ISBN 0-07-142315-X.
Lee J. F. Y., Leow C. K., Lau W. Y. Appendicitis In The Elderly. *aust. N.Z. J. Surg.* (2000) 70, 593–596
Lin CJ, Chen JD, Tiu CM. (2005) Can ruptured appendicitis be detected preoperatively in the ED? *Am. J. Emerg. Med.*; 23: 60–66
Mahadevan M, Graff L. (2000) Prospective randomized study of analgesic use for ED patients with right lower quadrant abdominal pain. *Am J Emerg Med.*;18:753-756.
Maxwell JM, Ragland JJ. (1991) Appendicitis, improvements in diagnosis and treatment. *Am. Surg.*; 57: 282–5.
McCallion J, Canning GP, Knight PV, McCallion JS. (1987) Acute appendicitis in the elderly: A 5-year retrospective study. *Age Ageing*; 16: 256–60.
McHale PM, Lo Vecchio F. (2001) Narcotic analgesia in the acute abdomen-a review of prospective trials. *Eur J Emerg Med.*; 8:131-136.
Naaeder SB, Archampong EQ. (1999) Clinical spectrum of acute abdominal pain in Accra, Ghana. West African Journal of Medicine; 18(1):13-16.
Naoum JJ, Mileski WJ, Daller JA,. (2002). The use of abdominal computed tomography scan decreases the frequency of misdiagnosis in cases of suspected appendicitis. *Am J Surg.*, 184.587-589
Okafor PI, Orakwe JC, Chianakwana GU. (2003) Management of appendiceal masses in a peripheral hospital in Nigeria: review of thirty cases. *World Journal of Surgery*; 27(7):800-803.
Oliak D, Yamini D, Udani VM (2000). Can perforated appendicitis be diagnosed preoperatively based on admission factors? *J. Gastrointest. Surg.*, 4. 470–74.
Omundsen M, Dennett E. (2006) Delay to appendicectomy and associated morbidity: a retrospective review. *ANZ J. Surg.*; 76: 153–5.
Paajanen H, Kettunen J, Kostiainen S. (1994) Emergency appendectomies in patients over 80 years. *Am. Surg.*; 60: 950–3.
Patrick DA, Janik JE, Janik JS, (2003). Increased CT scan utilization does not improve the diagnostic accuracy of appendicitis in children. *J Pediatr Surg.*; 38:659-662.

Paulson EK, Kalady MF, Pappas TN. (2003) Suspected appendicitis. *N Engl J Med.*; 48:236-242.

Peltokallio P, Jauhianinen K. (1970) Acute appendicitis in the aged patient. *Arch. Surg.*; 100: 140–3.

Rao P, Rhea J, Rao J. (July 1999) Plain abdominal radiographs in clinically suspected appendicitis: diagnostic yield, resource use, and comparison with CT. *Am J Emerg Med.*; 17:325–9.

Saidi HS, Adwok JA. (2000) Acute appendicitis: an overview. *East African Medical Journal*; 77(3):152-156.Sauerland S, Lefering R, Neugebauer EAM. Laparoscopic versus open surgery for suspected appendicitis (Cochrane Review). In: The *Cochrane Library. Chichester*, UK: John Wiley and Sons; 2004:2.

Schumpelick V, Dreuw B, Ophoff K, Prescher A. (Feb 2000) Appendix and cecum, embryology, anatomy, and surgical applications. *Surg Clin North Am*; 80:295–318.

Semm K. (1985) Endoscopic appendectomy. Endoscopy(1983) 15: 59– 64

Sherlock DJ. Acute appendicitis in the over-sixty age group. *Br. J. Surg.*; 72: 245–6.

Sheu B.-F.; Chiu T.-F.; Chen J.-C; Tung M.-S.; Chang M.-W.; Young Y.-R. (2007) *ANZ J. Surg.*; 77: 662–666 doi: 10.1111/j.1445-2197.2007.04182.x

Sivanesaratnam V. (2000) The acute abdomen and the obstetrician. *Best Practice & Research in Clinical Obstetrics & Gynaecology*; 14(1):89-102.

Smithy WB, Wexner SD, Dailey TH. (1986) The diagnosis and treatment of acute appendicitis in the aged. *Dis. Colon Rectum*; 29: 170–3.

Storm-Dickerson T L, Horattas MC, (2003) What have we learned over the past 20 years about appendicitis in the elderly? *American journal of surgery*; 185 198-201.

Tehrani H, Petros J, Petros J, . (1999) Markers of severe appendicitis. *Am Surg*; 65:453–5.

Temple C, Huchcroft S, Temple W. (1995) The natural history of appendicitis in adults, a prospective study. *Ann Surg*; 221:279–82.

Terasawa T, Blackmore CC, Bent S, Kohlwes RJ. (2004) Systematic review: computed tomography and ultrasonography to detect acute appendicitis in adults and adolescents. *Annals of Internal Medicine*; 141(7):537-546.

Van Sonnenberg E, Wittich GR, Casola G, (1987). Periappendiceal abscesses: percutaneous drainage. Radiology. 163:23-26.

Vargas HI, Averbook A, Stamos MJ. Appendiceal mass: conservative therapy followed by interval laparoscopic appendectomy. Am Surg. 1994;60:753-758

Vorhes CE. (1987) Appendicitis in the elderly: The case for better diagnosis. *Geriatrics*; 42: 89–92

Watters JM, Blakslee JM, March RJ, Redmond ML. (1996) The influence of age on the severity of peritonitis. *Can J. Surg.*; 39: 142–6.

Wolfe JM, Lein DY, Lenkoski K, (2000). Analgesic administration to patients with an acute abdomen: a survey of emergency medicine physicians. *Am J Emerg Med.*; 18:250-253.

Yamini D, Hernan V, Bongard F, (1998). Perforated appendicitis: is it truly a surgical urgency? *Am Surg*; 64:970–5.

Yang HR, Want YC, Chung PK. (2005) Role of leukocyte count, neutrophil percentage, and C-reactive protein in the diagnosis of acute appendicitis in the elderly. *Am. Surg.*; 71: 344–7.

8

Appendicitis in Children

Ngozi Joy Nwokoma
Addenbrooke's Hospital, Cambridge University Hospitals, Cambridge
United Kingdom

1. Introduction

Abdominal pain is a common clinical problem in children. The challenge is to determine which could be secondary to serious pathology. For the paediatric surgeon, the evaluation of a child with abdominal pain is often to ascertain if there is a surgically amenable pathology. The first clinical report of appendicitis in 1711 is credited to a German surgeon called Lorenz Heister (Ramsted et al., 1993). Appendicitis is the commonest acute childhood surgical abdominal emergency in developed countries. The peak incidence of acute appendicitis in children is in the second decade of life, at about 12years of age (Pearl et al., 1995; Tsze et al., 2011). It is uncommon in children less than 5years old, rare in infants and neonates, slightly more frequent in males than females with an incidence ratio of 1:1.5. The overall lifetime risk of appendicitis is 7%, slightly higher in females.

2. Embryology

The appendix develops as a true diverticulum of the caecum and becomes visible at the eighth week of gestation. It becomes more distinct as the inferior border of the caecum fails to enlarge as rapidly as the rest of it (Swain, 2005). As the proximal colon enlarges the caecum undergoes a downwards displacement into the right iliac fossa region of the abdomen. In certain congenital anomalies the final position of the appendix is outside the right lower quadrant. In situs inversus, the orientation of the intra-abdominal organs is reversed so that left sided organs are on the right and vice versa. The thoracic organs may also be involved in situs inversus totalis. In this condition, the appendix ends up in the left lower quadrant. In developmental arrest of the normal rotation of the midgut, the appendix may lie in the subhepatic region or towards the left side of the abdomen.

3. Anatomy

3.1 Position

The base of the appendix is located in the posteromedial aspect of the caecum; below and within 3cm of the ileocaecal junction. Though the base of the appendix assumes a relatively fixed position the final position of the appendix body and tip is variable (Figure 1). It commonly lies behind the caecum (retrocaecal: 64%) or crossing the pelvic brim into the pelvic cavity (pelvic: 32%). It could also lie posterior to the proximal colon (retrocolic), posterior to the terminal ileum (retroileal), anterior to the terminal ileum (preileal), just below the caecum (subcolic), along the lateral border of the caecum and colon (paracolic/precaecal) or it may be an obturator appendix crossing over the obturator internus muscle (Moore & Dalley, 2006; Standring et al., 2005). Rarely, the appendix may lie on the right kidney or duodenum with a retroperitoneal tip and has been reported to ulcerate into the duodenum (Ellis & Mahadevan, 2010).

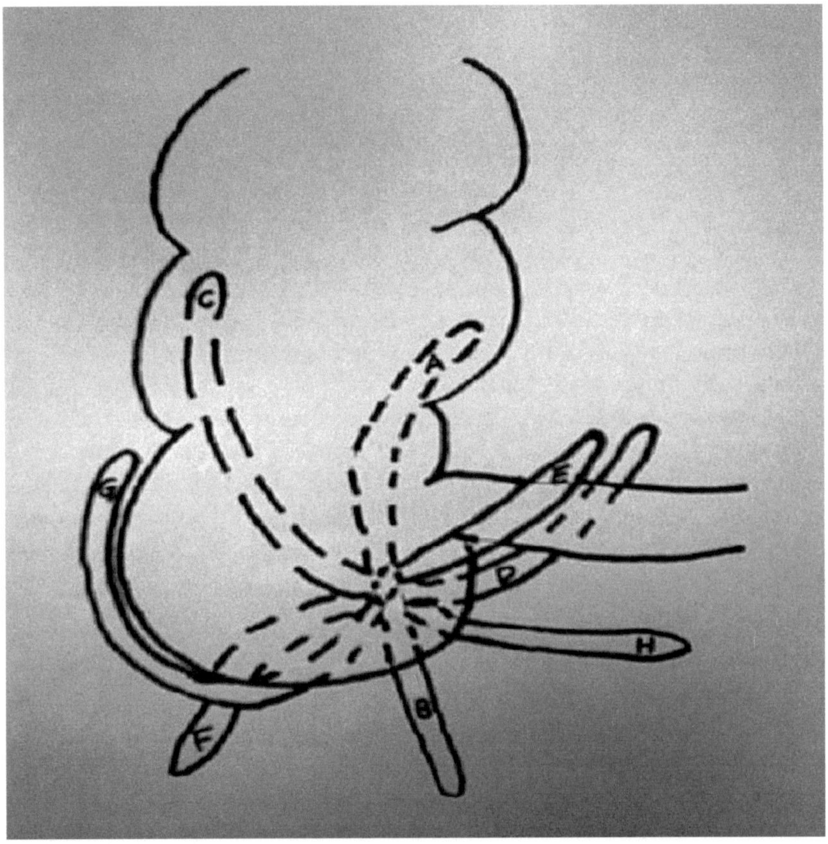

Fig. 1. Positional variation of appendicular body and tip: A. retrocaecal; B. Pelvic; C. retrocolic; D. retroileal; E. preileal; F. subcolic; G. paracolic/precaecal; H. obturator.

The superficial landmark of the base of the appendix corresponds to the level of the first segment of the sacral vertebrae (S1) at the McBurney's point. The McBurney's point is the junction of the outer and middle thirds of an imaginary line running from the right anterior superior iliac spine to the centre of the umbilicus. However, the appendix is located within 5cm of the McBurney's point less than 50% of the time (Karim et al., 1990).

3.2 Innervation

The midline development of the intra-abdominal viscera and associated innervation results in visceral pain being perceived in the midline. The level of pain may also be different from the level of the organ from which the pain stimulus arises due to the cranial migration of the nervous system. In line with the foregoing, epigastric pain is typically associated with pathology or irritation of the organs that originate from the foregut, periumbilical pain relates to midgut organs while infraumbilical or suprapubic pain relates to disease in the hindgut. The midgut stretches from the second part of the duodenum to the midpoint of the transverse colon. Being a midgut-originated structure, the initial pain sensation from the appendix is felt in the periumbilical region. Perception of abdominal pain occurs when the nociceptors in the respective organ or region of the abdomen have been stimulated by appropriate agents. Appendicitis represents inflammation of a magnitude great enough to stimulate these nociceptors.

The nerve supply to the appendix is derived from the autonomic nervous system and has fibres that respond to stretch rather than pain which explains the poorly localised symptoms until the parietal peritoneum becomes involved. The sympathetic nerve supply is from the superior mesenteric plexus while the parasympathetic nerve supply is from the Vagus nerve.

3.3 Structure

The appendix is commonly referred to as the *vermiform appendix* because of its worm-like tubular structure. The length of the appendix is variable ranging from 2 - 25cm but can be up to 31cm. It is longer in children, than in adults probably due to age-related atrophy. The external diameter could range from 3 - 8mm and the luminal diameter between 1 - 3mm (Williams & Myers, 1994; Petras & Goldblum, 1996). The maximum transverse diameter of the appendix is attained by the age of 4 years. It progressively narrows with age with increasing fibrosis after 40 years.

The three taeni coli of the proximal colon converge at the base of the appendix. The anterior taenia colon is commonly used as a landmark to identify the base of the appendix. In the neonate, the characteristic haustration of the large bowel are absent appearing within the first 6months and the taenia coli are thin (Standring et al., 2005).

The appendicular wall consists of four main layers: mucosa, sub-mucosa, muscularis propria and the serosa. The mucosa is similar to the colonic mucosa and consists of the epithelial lining, the lamina propria and the muscularis mucosa. The epithelial lining is a single layer of surface epithelial cells including columnar cells with basally located nuclei, goblet cells, apical mucin and absorptive cells as well as scattered paneth and endocrine cells. The lamina propria contains crypts of Lieberkühn. The muscularis mucosa of the appendix is poorly developed unlike the rest of the gastrointestinal tract. The sub-mucosa contains a rich network of arterioles, venules, capillaries and lymphatics in a connective tissue framework. It also contains a plexus of nerves, the Meissner's plexus. The neurosecretory cells in the submucosa are few till the age of 9years. The age-related increase in the number of these cells is thought to explain the increase in number of carcinoid tumours in older patients.

The muscularis propria contains muscles which are arranged in a similar pattern as those of the small intestine. The outer longitudinal muscle fibres aggregate into the taenia coli to become continuous with them at the base of the appendix. The inner circular muscles are thicker. Between these muscle layers is the myenteric or Auerbach's plexus of nerves which is morphologically similar to the Meissner's plexus in the submucosa, unlike the rest of the gastrointestinal tract where the Meissner's plexus is thinner.

3.4 Lymphatics

The appendix belongs to the group of lymphatic organs called the Mucosa Associated Lymphatic Tissue which also includes the intestinal Peyer's patches, the tonsils and the lymphoid follicles in the walls of the bronchi. They are thought to protect the gastrointestinal tract and the respiratory tract from recurrent infections from foreign matter and organisms entering these body cavities (Snell, 2004b). However, its role in immune protection in the gastrointestinal tract is unclear. The submucosa of the appendix contains prominent lymphoid tissue similar to that in the terminal ileum; this feature differentiates the appendix from the colon. These may become hypertrophic in the presence of inflammation and may obstruct the lumen in acute appendicitis. Lymphoid hyperplasia is at its peak during the second decade of life. This has been postulated to be the reason behind the high incidence of appendicitis in this age group. Lymphoid hyperplasia is thought to be responsible for 60% of acute appendicitis and occurs mainly in children.

The appendicular lymphatic vessels drain into the lymph nodes in the mesoappendix, the anterior ileocolic lymph nodes which often become enlarged during acute appendicitis and then into the right para-aortic lymph nodes.

3.5 Vasculature

The appendicular artery arises from the inferior branch of the ileocaecal artery and the vein drains through the ileocaecal vein into the portal venous system. The meso-appendix connects the appendix to the ileal mesentry. The artery enters the mesoappendix a short distance from the appendicular base where it gives off the recurrent branch which anastomosis with a branch of the posterior caecal artery. It is common to find accessory arteries associated with the appendix (Standring et al., 2005). These must be handled carefully to limit blood loss during appendicectomy. The appendicular artery runs through the meso-appendix along its free edge and lies on the appendix wall in its distal aspect. The anastomosis at the base gives rise to a good blood supply but it is an end artery from the midpoint to distal appendix where its close proximity to the appendix makes it susceptible to thrombosis as the appendix enlarges during acute inflammation.

4. Aetiology of appendicitis

The aetiology is multi-factorial and may involve interplay of factors including obstruction, infections, ischaemia and hereditary factors. Obstruction from lymphoid hyperplasia is a common causal factor and this has been addressed in detail elsewhere in this chapter. A faecolith is a small stone-like mass of stool. Its formation starts with entrapment of vegetable fibre. Like the colonic mucosa, the appendix mucosa is well equipped for water absorption resulting in concentration of its contents with mucous entrapment. Several layers of deposits eventually result in increase in diameter and a faecolith diameter of 1cm leads to appendicular obstruction. Faecoliths are less common in children than in adults; 7.7% versus 42% (Gillick et al., 2001). A primary neoplasm of the appendix is found in 0.5-1.0% of specimens removed for appendicitis. The neoplasm could be mucinous adenoma, mucinous adenocarcinoma, colonic type adenocarcinoma, non-Hodgkins lymphoma, classical carcinoid tumour, or goblet cell carcinoid tumour. 30-50% of patients with carcinoid present with acute appendicitis, being associated with obstruction of the appendix in 25% of cases. An appendicular diameter greater than 15mm should raise suspicion as to the presence of an appendicular tumour (Pickhardt et al., 2002). Carcinoid tumours mostly are located in the distal tip of the appendix, taking the form of a bulbous solid tumour of about 2-3cm diameter. In children it is usually of a diameter of less than 2cm. 75% is at the tip; 20% mid-appendix and 5% at the base. The incidence of carcinoid tumours in surgical specimens is about 0.08-0.7%; 0.2-0.5% in children. It is the most frequent tumour of the gastrointestinal tract in childhood and adolescence. It occurs more in white females. A mucocele is a dilated appendix filled with mucinous substance. It may present as an obstructed appendix containing insipissated mucin or be a consequence of mucinous cystadenoma or mucinous cystadenocarcinoma.

Bacterial and fungal infections can also lead to appendicitis. The bacteria involved are usually of a mixed aerobic and anaerobic population; most commonly Bacteroides fragilis and Escherichia coli. Others include Streptococcus milleri (associated with a seven-fold increased risk of abscess formation) and Campylobacter jejuni (Feneglio-Preser et al., 2008). Infections may further lead to fibrin thrombi which can block the small appendicular vessels leading to secondary ischaemia. The appendix is particularly prone to ischaemic insult because the appendicular artery is an end artery beyond the base of the appendix. Torsion of the appendix may occur resulting in ischaemic appendicitis; but, this condition is rare (Fenoglio-Preiser et al., 2008). Familial aggregation of appendicitis suggests polygenic inheritance and the appendicitis usually manifests before the age of 10years. The hypothesis of appendicitis being associated with low fibre diet is weakened by the finding in Africa that populations on high fibre diet did not have a lower appendicitis rate (Naaeder & Archampong, 1998).

5. Pathophysiology

The human appendix secretes up to 2ml of clear fluid containing mucin, amylase and proteolytic enzymes, which may be produced by bacteria each day. The appendicular aperture is guarded by semilunar mucosal folds which give it a valve effect. The basal intraluminal caecal pressure is approximately 5cm of water while the appendicular intraluminal pressure ranges from 15 - 25cm of water creating a pressure gradient of about 10cm of water. This is believed to keep gut contents from entering the appendicular lumen.

Experimental studies have shown that the obstruction of exteriorised human appendices can raise the intra-luminal pressures to an extent that exceeds the perfusion pressure in the vascular plexus within the wall of the appendix. The distal end of the appendix is most vulnerable to this reduction in blood flow. Electrical stimulation of the appendix has been demonstrated to cause closure of the ileocaecal valve (Williams and Myers, 1994). This may be a contributing factor to the nausea and vomiting associated with acute appendicitis.

The peritoneum consists of a continuous visceral and parietal layer. Both layers are of mesodermal origin, but develop separately with independent nerve supplies. The visceral layer covers the intra-abdominal organs and is supplied by autonomic nerves. The parietal peritoneum lines the under surface of the abdominal wall and is supplied by somatic nerves. Pathways for pain differ in each layer and so also the quality of pain. Visceral pain has a dull aching character, often crampy and may be associated with nausea and sweating. Parietal pain on the other hand is mostly sharp, severe and persistent in nature. Visceral organs have limited response to pain stimulus but the stretching of the mesentry and irritation of the parietal peritoneum produces severe pain.

Visceral afferent fibres carrying sensation of distension and pressure are responsible for the initial pain of appendicitis, poorly localised initially and referred to the periumbilical region. Afferent nerve fibres from viscera enter the dorsal horn of the spinal cord along with afferent nerve fibres from cutaneous structures of the corresponding dermatome. These two groups of nerve fibres overlap at the synaptic junctions in the dorsal horn leading to the phenomenon of referred pain whereby pain is perceived by the brain as arising from the corresponding cutaneous structures. Nerve fibres decussate and travel up to the thalamus along the lateral spinothalamic tract and then onwards to the cerebral cortex. Increased intravisceral pressure by stretch, distension or contraction of the viscus especially against an obstruction leads to visceral pain. The dermatomal distribution associated with the midgut relates to the umbilical region, with nerves entering the spinal column at the tenth thoracic spinal segment (T10). The midgut extends from the second part of the duodenum to the midpoint of the transverse colon. Therefore, pain arising from the midgut is felt initially in the umbilicus before the parietal peritoneum becomes involved (Klish, 2006).

In 1886, the American pathologist - Reginald Fitz became the first person to describe the pattern of the pathophysiological basis of appendicitis in literature. He noted that the condition started with onset of inflammation, followed by perforation, abscess formation and peritonitis (Morrow & Newman, 2005). Appendicitis is commonly secondary to luminal obstruction which is demonstrable in 50-80% of cases (Turner, 2010). As stated previously, the commonest cause of luminal obstruction in children is lymphoid hyperplasia or hypertrophy which mostly results from dehydration and viral infection. Faecoliths take several years to form. They are commoner in older children and may cause direct focal or diffuse mucosal ulceration. The stasis that results creates an environment which favours bacterial proliferation and also causes ischaemic injury.

The fore-going results in inflammatory changes including oedema, neutrophilic infiltration of the lumen, muscular wall and periappendicular soft tissue. In early appendicitis, subserosal vessels become congested and perivascular neutrophilic infiltrate develops within all the layers of the wall leading to loss of lustre which gives the appendix a dull granular erythematous appearance. Therefore, the histological diagnosis of acute appendicitis must demonstrate neutrophilic infiltration of the muscularis propria not just within the lumen (Turner, 2010). Figure 2 illustrates the sequence of events that follow appendicular obstruction.

Luminal obstruction → Increased mucous production
and bacterial overgrowth

↓

Dilatation/swelling of the appendix

↓

Impaired venous drainage ⇆ worsening congestion and oedema
Impaired lymphatic drainage
Increasing oedema and turgidity
Loss of the appendicular lustre

↓

Further appendicular swelling
Reduction in arterial blood flow
Thrombosis of appendicular vessels
Necrosis of the appendicular wall.

Fig. 2. Sequence of events that follow appendicular obstruction

More severe inflammation results in prominent neutrophilic exudate which generates serosal fibrino-purulent reaction that gives the appendix the creamy yellow appearance associated with this stage of the inflammatory process. If the inflammatory process is not curbed at this stage, it progresses to formation of focal abscesses within the appendicular wall; this is acute suppurative appendicitis. Progressive increase in the intraluminal pressure leads to venous flow compromise. Laplace law suggests that the wall tension of a tubular structure is directly proportionate to the thickness of the wall divided by the square of the radius. Further increase in the wall tension culminates in necrosis of the appendix. Further inflammation leads to the formation of large areas of haemorrhagic ulceration with gangrenous necrosis that extends to the serosal layer; this is acute gangrenous appendicitis. Rupture of the appendix follows with suppurative peritonitis (Turner, 2010). The risk of perforation of the appendix rises with the duration of symptoms being about 30% for <24hours and greater than 70% in >48hours (Swain, 2005). The perforation rate also varies with the age of the child. The average rate is 30-45% which may be as high as 80% in those under 5years and nearly 100% in those under 2years (Morrow & Newman, 2005; Stevenson, 2003).

The normally glistening serosal and peritoneal surface becomes dull and lustreless; serous or slightly turbid fluid begins to accumulate within 2-4hours of the onset of inflammation. With progression of the inflammatory process creamy suppurative material with increasing viscosity accumulates. At this point, the process can take the form of localisation by the omentum and viscera to be controlled in a small area of the abdominal cavity, or become widespread filling the entire abdomen. The cellular response results in the formation of dense collections of neutrophils and fibrinopurulent debris that coat the viscera and abdominal wall at the site of the inflammation (Turner, 2010). The greater omentum is smaller in children and only at the level of the umbilicus in the neonate containing small amount of fat and therefore providing limited omental protection (Standring et al., 2005).

Inflammation of the peritoneum and surrounding intra-abdominal organs follows with peritonitis. Bowel obstruction may result from the adhesive inflammatory process. Irritation of the rectosigmoid may lead to enteritis manifesting with frequent loose stools. Irritation of the bladder by the inflammatory process may cause dysuria, increased frequency of micturition and urgency simulating urinary tract infection. Severe inflammation may lead to haemorrhagic cystitis.

The inflammatory process may also be accompanied by increased tissue porosity or permeability with bacterial translocation. Peritonitis from bacterial translocation across the porous inflamed wall of the appendix may still occur in the absence of obvious perforation or faecal contamination.

6. Histopathological features

In the acute phase, serosal injection leads to loss of the normal appendiceal lustre; if inflammation progresses purulent exudate forms on the surface of the appendix followed by perforation. There may be fecolith within the appendix lumen; or the lumen may be distended with pus or mucous. Enterobius vermicularis may be present in the lumen and sometimes within the mucosa where they may induce a granulomatous reaction. They can be identified on microscopy by their lateral spines evident on the cross section of the transected worms (Sebire et al, 2010).

Histological features of acute appendicitis include

- Acute transmural inflammatory aggregation of neutrophils and eosinophils
- Hyperplasia of mucosal lymphoid tissue
- Haemorrhagic changes in the mucosa
- Pus within the appendicular lumen
- Mucosal ulceration
- Acute serosal inflammation
- Haemorrhagic necrosis of the appendicular wall
- Adenovirus inclusions may be seen in the epithelial cell nuclei
- There may be vasculitic changes with or without thrombi within the vessels in the wall
- Following interval appendicectomy, there may be chronic inflammatory changes with fibrosis of the wall with or without occlusion of the appendicular lumen (Sebire et al, 2010).

Inflammation without mucosal ulceration is of uncertain significance. In acute intraluminal appendicitis, there is increased neutrophil presence in the appendicular lumen with no evidence of mucosal infiltration. Similar findings have been documented in incidentally removed appendix specimens (Feneglio-Preser et al., 2008).

The issue of sending normal appearing appendix for histological analysis is supported by the fact that certain conditions may present in the appendix with macroscopically normal appearance. These include polyarteritis nodosa, tuberculosis, amoebiasis, parasitic infestations including bilharzisis, schistosomiasis, trichuriasis, ascariasis and clonorchiasis, actinomycosis as well as epithelial tumours. 2 - 5% of macroscopically normal appendices may have significant unsuspected pathological condition (Williams & Myers, 1994). Furthermore, neurogenic appendicopathy may appear macroscopically normal and can only be diagnosed with certainty on histological analysis (Zaupa et al., 2011).

7. Microbiological perspective

Peri-appendicular abscesses may occur from bacteria usually present in the bowel including *Escherichia coli, Proteus* species, other enterobacteriaceae, *Bacteroides* species, anaerobic cocci and other anaerobes. Infections are therefore commonly polymicrobial. The resultant secondary peritonitis commonly yields *Escherichia coli* and other enterobacteriaceae and anaerobes from intra-operative peritoneal pus swabs. Some authors argue that the precise value of peritoneal swabs in many cases of secondary peritonitis is difficult to assess because the bacteriology seldom influences antibiotic treatment which is given empirically on clinical grounds for short duration, often ending within 2-3days before the full bacteriology results become available (Baker et al, 2004).

The gastrointestinal tract like other portals of entry into the human body, has a normal flora that helps protect it against pathogenic micro-organisms. The flow rate reduces from the small intestine to the large intestine giving the bacteria more time to colonise and reproduce leading to higher concentration of the organisms. The amount of flora increases in number and varies in type as the gastrointestinal tract progresses from the oral cavity to the anorectum. About one thousand species of micro-organisms are present in the large intestine. Approximately 20% of the volume of faecal matter in the healthy person consists of bacteria, most of which come from the colon. The terminal ileum flora is similar to colonic flora. More than 90% of these are anaerobes, mostly Bacteroides, Fusobacterium, Eubacterium and Clostridium. Others include E. coli, enterococci, yeasts and numerous others (VanMeter et al, 2010). Organisms commonly isolated from peritoneal microbiological tests in secondary peritonitis are mostly anaerobes which outnumber aerobes in the bowel by a thousand fold (Forbes et al, 2007).

Enterobius vermicularis is the most common nematode infection in humans and can be found in up to 3% of appendices in the USA. Schistosomiasis of the appendix is rare. Strongiloides stercoralis infection results in eosinophilic appendicitis. Viral appendicitis has been associated with measles in the prodromal phase. Other viruses that may cause appendicitis are adenovirus and gastrointestinal cytomegalovirus infection. Acute infectious mononucleosis and Epstein Barr virus infection rarely may give rise to abdominal pain (Petras & Goldblum, 1996).

8. Diagnosis

8.1 Clinical presentation

Making a diagnosis of acute appendicitis in children can be a difficult task even for the experienced paediatric surgeon. Negative appendicectomy rate was found to be higher among children operated upon in district general hospital than in a specialist paediatric centre, 20% versus 4% (Whisker et al., 2009). Chang et al., (2010) found that approximately 12-15% of paediatric appendicitis were missed at the first visit to the emergency department with the rate of perforation of 73.1% versus 49% in those diagnosed at first presentation. The duration of symptoms was longer in the former group and the rate of perforation higher the longer the duration of symptoms.

Generally, clinical symptoms are the patient's report of the manifestation(s) of dysfunction in the normal body physiology. Thus, the younger the child, the less accurate the report of symptoms can be expected to be. Neurodevelopmental immaturity precludes accurate understanding, interpretation and description of symptoms by children particularly those younger than eight years of age. Not surprisingly, this is the age group that commonly presents late with advanced appendicitis. Furthermore, parents of infants often ascribe febrile illness and vomiting to "teething" and do not seek medical evaluation early. The clinical symptoms of appendicitis are often secondary to luminal obstruction leading to colicky abdominal pain at onset which progresses to constant pain with progression of the inflammatory process. Nausea and vomiting are commonly present. Clinical signs are discussed in detail later in this chapter and often include tenderness in the right lower quadrant of the abdomen.

Advanced appendicitis is often associated with delayed presentation especially in children below the age of five years and also with retroileal, retrocolic or pelvic appendicitis. Irritation of pelvic structures may produce symptoms and signs suggestive of urinary tract infection or enteritis.

8.2 History

Rigorous pursuit of a detailed history is invaluable in the diagnosis of appendicitis. In children, patience is an indispensable virtue and a rushed history increases the risk of misdiagnosis. Possession of the clinical skills required for eliciting appropriately focused and chronologically accurate history from the child and parent is key to early diagnosis. The surgeon therefore has to make the most of open-ended and direct questioning at appropriate key moments of the history taking applying sensitivity to the emotional climate.

Background information of the child's usual status of health should be obtained. The onset of the current symptoms should be carefully ascertained. Site of onset of abdominal pain and its present location may suggest migration of pain which may be associated with acute appendicitis; usually starting in the peri-umbilical region, the pain later localises to the region of the right iliac fossa. In addition it is often preceded by nausea or vomiting. Characterising the abdominal pain is key to accurate diagnosis of its source. The onset of the pain associated with acute appendicitis is often gradual, progressively worsening. It may be intermittent initially then sharp and constant within a few hours. Children may not give this typical presentation; even the older ones may become very quiet and distracted by other issues including pain, fear, strange environment with unfamiliar people or even psychosocial circumstances in the family.

The usual duration of symptoms at presentation is 24 - 36hours. There may be a history of pain being made worse by road bumps on the way to the hospital. This suggests the presence of rebound tenderness. Enquiry into the presence of associated factors should be made. Nausea and vomiting may be present in up to 90% of patients. Diminished appetite may be absent in children with appendicitis. Diarrhoea may suggest irritation of the anorectum by inflamed tissue in the rectovesical pouch. The sigmoid colon is often redundant in children, with a tendency to loop into the pelvis. Consequently, it may come in contact with an inflamed appendix manifesting as diarrhoea. Care must be taken not to mistake this for gastroenteritis. Dysuria may be associated with appendicitis from irritation of the urinary bladder by an inflamed pelvic appendix.

The history should also explore other possible causes of abdominal pain. Symptoms of upper respiratory tract infection may suggest mesenteric adenitis. Cough may suggest pneumonia with referred abdominal pain as a diagnosis. Vulvovaginal irritation with or without vaginal discharge may suggest pelvic inflammatory disease. Abdominal pain may also be referred from an acute scrotal condition and older boys in particular do not offer this important information without direct questioning. Constipation may produce symptoms in children that may imply the presence of pathology and should be considered. In addition, enquiry should be made about any previous history of abdominal pain, previous abdominal surgery, recent foreign travel, current or recent medications as well as the presence of similar condition in other family members or pupils in the same school.

8.3 Differential diagnosis of acute abdominal pain in children

The cause of acute abdomen in children may vary according to sex and age. Possible causes are presented below. The list is by no means exhaustive and not in order of frequency. In addition, some conditions may co-exist.

8.3.1 Infants

Viral enteritis
Intussusception
Pyelonephritis/ other urinary tract infection (UTI)
Gastro-oesophageal reflux
Bacterial enterocolitis
Chest infection
Appendicitis
Pyloric stenosis

Strangulated hernia of the anterior abdominal wall
Testicular torsion
Mesenteric cysts
Ruptured abdominal tumour
Pancreatitis
Meckel's diverticulitis
Hirschsprung's disease with or without enterocolitis
Poisoning
Trauma
Non-accidental injury

8.3.2 Children aged between 2-10years old

Meckel's diverticulitis
Cystitis
Pyelonephritis
Viral enteritis
Bacterial enterocolitis
Appendicitis
Non-specific abdominal pain
Crohn's disease
Abdominal trauma, including non-accidental injury
Chest infection
Mesenteric adenitis
Neutropenic enterocolitis
Pancreatitis
Ruptured intra-abdominal tumours
Poisoning

8.3.3 Children above 11years old

Viral enteritis
Bacterial enterocolitis
Appendicitis
Non-specific abdominal pain
Mesenteric adenitis
Pelvic inflammatory disease
Tubo-ovarian cysts
Tubo-ovarian abscess with or without rupture
Torsion of an ovarian cyst
Haemorrhage in an ovarian cyst
Endometriosis
Mittleschmerz
Crohn's disease
Pancreatitis
Neutropenic enterocolitis
Chest infection
Haematocolpos

Peptic ulcer disease
Psychosomatic condition
Trauma
Ectopic pregnany
Dysmenorrhoea
Gall stone disease including cholecystitis, biliary colic, cholangitis
Urinary tract infections
Neuronal abdominal wall pain including shingles, spinal or nerve root problem, iatrogenic peripheral nerve injury
Spontaneous rectus sheath haematoma

8.4 Physical examination

A thorough physical examination would compliment the clinical suspicion formed from the reported symptoms. A general examination of the child with abdominal pain is imperative and requires experience in identifying the sick child. The child's appearance should be noted - body habitus, facial expression, position, willingness or reluctance to move, alertness, pallor and whether the child is flushed or sweaty. Assess the child's pulse for volume and rate. The temperature in early appendicitis may be normal or mildly raised. A temperature above 38°C should prompt further investigation or evaluation to exclude other causes. Ears, throat and lymph nodes should be evaluated. Tachypnoea, recessions, shallow breathing and flaring of the alar nasi may suggest a respiratory tract problem or be secondary to circulatory system contraction. An antalgic gait, leaning to right side, limping on the right leg and slow motion are all cues to the presence of abdominal pathology. Flexion at the hip suggests abdominal wall discomfort with or without peritoneal irritation.

Younger children typically poorly localise pain. Most of the under five-year-olds point to their umbilical region as the site of all pain; perhaps because the umbilicus is a central feature with a unique appearance that sets it out as a point of focus which captures the child's attention. The demonstration of certain clinical signs may further qualify the pain but atypical abdominal pain is seen in about 40 - 45% of patients. One should beware of the child who is on antibiotic therapy for other presumed infection who presents with attenuated features of appendicitis.

The child's anxiety should be taken into consideration and reducing the number of people in the room or creating a distraction may help. Distraction may be accomplished with the help of a paediatric play therapist. Building a rapport with the parents gains the child's trust and allays anxiety. A warm child-friendly environment is desirable and is common practice in many paediatric specialist centres. Focused examination of the abdomen should commence with inspection for distension, abdominal wall excursions with respiratory activity, hernia orifices, external signs of trauma, scars or visible peristalsis. Percussion of the abdomen may reveal the presence of rebound tenderness suggesting peritonism. Palpation of the abdomen should in the first instance be superficial and general, starting away from the site of pain. This gives the examiner the opportunity to explore all the quadrants of the abdomen and improves the chance of identifying non-appendicular pathology. This gentle approach reassures the child and allows him or her to trust the examiner, and also to relax the abdominal wall. Guarding may be present as well as tenderness. Depending on the child's level of development and co-operation, he or she may be encouraged to cough, laugh, distend the abdomen or retract the abdominal wall. Rebound tenderness may be present if these activities elicit pain. This is followed by deep palpation to explore the presence of an intra-abdominal mass. The character of any palpable mass should be evaluated - soft, firm, mobile or fixed to surrounding structures, regularity of its palpable surface and possible organ of origin. Due to the variability of position of the appendicular tip as previously discussed, the parietal pain may be related to the right upper quadrant, right loin or pelvis. The practice of gently rocking the pelvis from side to side is still practised by some surgeons and may elicit rebound tenderness.

Auscultation should evaluate bowel sounds but is generally not very useful. Bowel sounds may be absent or diminished in advanced inflammation. However, the presence of normal bowel sounds does not exclude advanced appendicitis. For the tense anxious child, using the stethoscope as a palpation tool can help with the evaluation of the abdomen. Also palpating over the child's hand can play the same role. An auscultation of the chest is part of the evaluation for probable appendicitis to rule out or confirm chest pathology. In the presence of positive chest signs, the abdomen should still be carefully evaluated for the presence of possible co-existing intra-abdominal pathology.

Children are not good at responding to the question - "Does this hurt?" The young child is very likely to respond in the affirmative when asked such questions. Conversely, beware of the older child who denies any pain for fear of being admitted into the hospital. The child with acute appendicitis would often be reluctant to move and may express discomfort by facial grimace or tears rather than verbally. Therefore careful observation of the child's facial expression and non-verbal responses is paramount to the interpretation of clinical signs.

Right lower quadrant pain, tenderness and rebound tenderness should be elicited. The traditional method of eliciting rebound tenderness by suddenly withdrawing the hand following a deep palpation, is not advisable in children. It results in sudden severe pain which may make the child loose confidence in the doctor. Rather, rebound tenderness is usually tested for by asking the child to increase the intra-abdominal pressure by coughing (Dunphy sign). This brings the inflamed appendix or surrounding tissues to the anterior abdominal wall manifesting as rebound tenderness. Similarly, the abdominal pain may also be exaggerated by attempting to move the abdominal wall outwards - "blowing out the abdomen" or moving the abdominal wall inwards - "sucking the abdomen inwards". McBurney's sign is the presence of maximum tenderness over the McBurney's point. This was first described by McBurney who was the first to recommend appendicectomy for treatment of appendicitis (Morrow, 2005).

Rovsing sign is positive if there is perception of pain in the right lower quadrant on palpation of the left lower quadrant. Obturator sign may be positive. To elicit this sign, the patient lies supine with the right knee and hip flexed to 90degrees. The examiner, holding the patient's right ankle in the right hand, places the left hand on the knee. Outward rotation of the flexed right knee causes internal rotation of the right hip which causes the obturator internus to become tense. The test is positive if pain in the right lower quadrant is elicited; usually in appendicitis in the pelvic or obturator positions where the appendicular tip lies over the obturator fascia covering the obturator internus muscle. The iliopsoas comprising of the powerful hip flexors - iliacus and psoas major, can become inflamed in appendicitis which is retrocaecal and therefore retroperitoneal giving a positive psoas or iliopsoas sign. This can be evaluated by two approaches. With the patient lying supine, the examiner's hand is placed just above the right knee and the patient asked to flex the right hip against resistance. Eliciting pain means positive psoas sign. An alternative method is to have the patient lie on the left side, if hyper-extension on

the right hip elicits pain, the sign is positive. A psoas abscess from a different cause would elicit similar pain (Liu & McFadden, 2003).
The introduction of the algometry for the diagnosis of acute abdominal pain in children has been welcomed by many paediatric surgeons (Vajcner et al., 2011). This device is used to predict acute appendicitis by observing the abdominal tenderness threshold which is the minimum pressure applied to the anterior abdominal wall to produce discomfort. With regards to diagnosing acute appendicitis, when combined with other clinical findings, it was found to have a sensitivity of 82% specificity of 73% and positive likelihood ratio of 3.03. This new innovation may become popular in the future but it needs evaluation through appropriately designed clinical trials.

9. Investigations

In cases where the clinical history or physical signs are atypical and inconclusive for the diagnosis of acute appendicitis, various investigations may be used to complement the clinical findings, strengthen the diagnosis and exclude the presence of alternative pathology. They may also aid the peri-operatively management of the patient. These may be bed-side, laboratory, radiological or laparoscopic investigations.
There is no one investigation that can accurately diagnose appendicitis every time. The clinical value and economic benefit of laboratory investigations for the diagnosis of appendicitis has been the cause of much debate (Liu and McFadden, 2003).
The general rule to the selection of an investigation is that it would:

- Complement the history and examination
- Determine what other clinical tests may be required
- Alter treatment approach.

An ideal diagnostic test should offer the following benefits:

- High level of accuracy: high sensitivity and specificity
- Capable of assessing the extent of disease
- Cost effective: cost of investigation should be less than the consequences of treatment without the benefit of the information derived from the examination
- Short length of study
- Quick and easy access to result or diagnostic information
- Non-invasive
- Suited to local needs, resources and available expertise (Hernanz-Schulman, 2010)

9.1 Bedside investigations

Bedside investigations can be done alongside the initial evaluation. Urinalysis with urine dipstix may suggest urinary tract irritation or infection, diabetes or pregnancy-related conditions. A bedside blood sugar test is a quick check for possible diabetic ketoacidosis.

9.2 Laboratory investigations

Laboratory tests commonly used to evaluate acute abdominal pain include full blood count, electrolyte studies, C-reactive protein (CRP), urine microscopy and culture, liver function tests and serum amylase level. Approximately two-thirds of the patients would have elevated white blood cell (WBC) count with neutrophilia but this is not specific to appendicitis. The relative neutrophil count may be above normal range even in the presence of a normal total white blood count. Serum levels of inflammatory markers may not be raised in early appendicitis. Repeating the investigations at least 6hours after the initial test may increase the diagnostic yield (Wu & Fu, 2010).

Laboratory urine microscopy would assess for presence of pyuria and micro-organisms. Urinalysis may be abnormal in up to 48% of patients with acute appendicitis. This may show microscopic haematuria, pyuria or proteinuria (Rothrock & Pagane, 2000). Pyuria may arise as a consequence of irritation of the urinary bladder or the ureter by the inflamed appendix or surrounding inflamed tissue. Serum or urine βhCG tests should be performed in young women of child-bearing age and if positive, an ectopic pregnancy should be excluded by further evaluation involving the gynaecologist. Moreover, pregnancy and appendicitis can co-exist.

Serum electrolytes and creatinine levels should be requested and any abnormalities corrected appropriately. Blood glucose should be obtained and any abnormality appropriately managed. It must be borne in mind that diabetic ketoacidosis may present as acute abdomen. The CRP is an acute phase reactant synthesized in the liver which is often raised within 12hours of an acute inflammatory process. It may be raised in 50-90% of patients with acute appendicitis but again it is non-specific. Serum levels of inflammatory markers including CRP and WBC count cannot be reliably used to distinguish between acute appendicitis and other causes of abdominal pain (Dalal et al., 2005). They are more effective in supporting a clinical diagnosis of appendicitis than excluding the diagnosis (Birchley, 2006).

9.3 Radiological investigations

Radiological investigations should be tailored to the specific presentation and possible differential diagnoses. A chest radiograph may be useful in the presence of clinical suspicion of lower respiratory tract infection or complications there from.

9.3.1 Plain abdominal radiograph

Plain abdominal radiographs are not commonly used in the evaluation of abdominal pain in children particularly when appendicitis is felt to be a likely cause. There are several reasons for this stance, one being that children present with abdominal pain commonly and obtaining an abdominal radiograph each time may lead to a significant amount of radiation. Extremes of age are more sensitive to radiation and it should be avoided as much as possible. The average plain abdominal radiograph exposes the patient to a typical effective radiation dose of 0.7millisieverts (mSv), equivalent to 4months of natural background radiation which is equal to 35 chest radiographs (Hampson and Shaw, 2010). It is of limited use in the evaluation of abdominal pain in children but it may be useful in atypical presentation where no obvious diagnosis can be made after adequate history, examination and laboratory investigations. It is noteworthy that only 10% of patients with an acute abdomen have abnormalities on plain radiographs. A study in the adult population demonstrated that the specificity of abdominal radiograph for acute appendicitis can be as low as 0% (Hampson & Shaw 2010).

An adequate abdominal radiograph should include the diaphragm and pelvis; antero-posterior and lateral shoot through views may be required if the patient is unable to sit up. The preperitoneal fat often gives rise to a fine line of fat on a plain abdominal radiograph. Inflammation of a retrocaecal appendix may be associated with infiltration of the preperitoneal fat and lead to a focal absence of this fine line of fat. In addition, a mass between the preperitoneal fat and ascending colon, gas in the appendix lumen, a faecolith above the anterior superior iliac spine combined with haustral irregularity of the ascending colon can raise the suspicion of appendicitis on plain abdominal radiograph. As stated earlier faecoliths are uncommon in children. Retrocaecal extraperitoneal gas suggests perforation. Extraluminal gas on radiograph from a perforated appendicitis may be demonstrable in 1% of perforated cases. Loss of shadow of the right psoas suggests advanced appendicitis with retroperitoneal inflammation.

An abdominal radiograph may also demonstrate dilated loops of bowel suggesting obstruction or extraluminal gas in perforation of abdominal viscus. Bowel obstruction in the absence of features of peritonism may be secondary to adhesive obstruction. It has a significant role in the evaluation of the neonate with suspected intra-abdominal pathology where it may demonstrate radiological features of necrotising enterocolitis as clinical signs would not conclusively demonstrate perforations. In addition, it may demonstrate the renal outline with a huge outline being suggestive of obstructive uropathy.

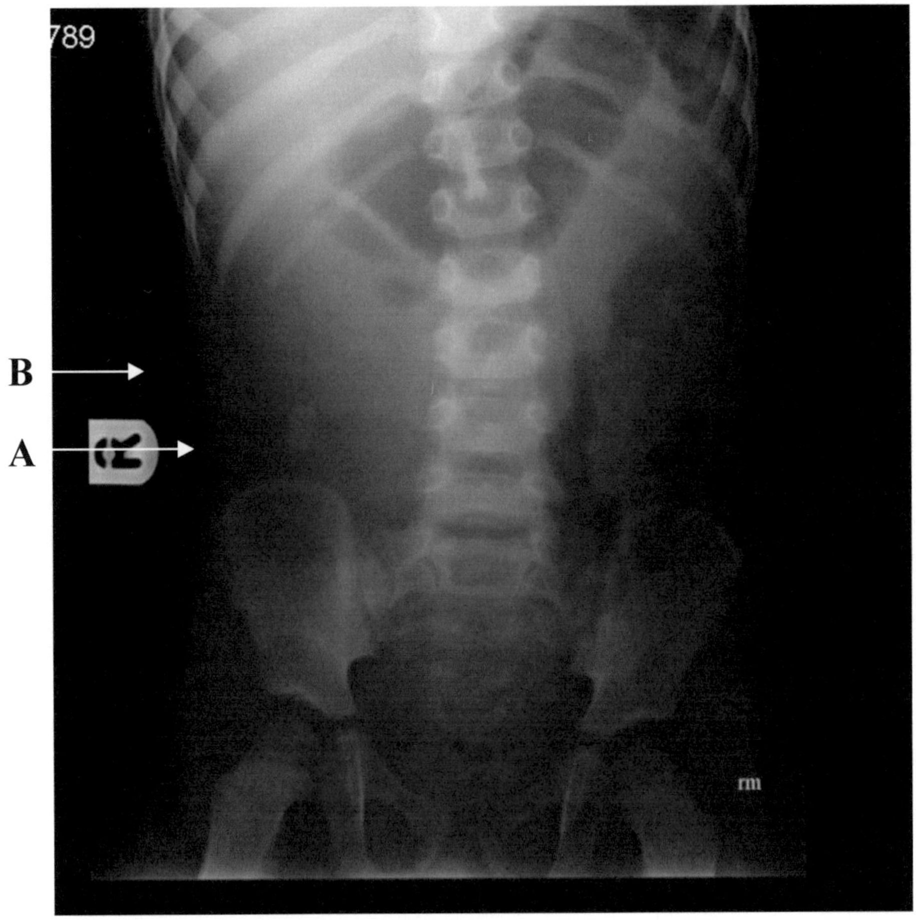

Fig. 3. Plain abdominal radiograph of a 2year old showing: A. Faecolith; B. Focal absence of fine line of preperitoneal fat (uninterrupted on the left side). Note also, the absence of bowel gas in the same region.

9.3.2 Ultrasonography

Where clinical observation by an experienced paediatric surgeon over a 48hr period still reveals equivocal diagnosis and suspicion of appendicitis persists, imaging is recommended, mainly by way of abdominal ultrasonography (Lander, 2007). Ultrasonography for the evaluation of appendicitis was introduced by Puylaert in 1986. It is a useful investigation in the further evaluation of abdominal pain with atypical and inconclusive findings. Some authors suggest that its specificity and sensitivity may be higher in children than in adults (Rothrock & Pagane, 2000). This is particularly relevant to peripubertal and older girls where ovarian pathology may mimick appendicitis. Even a left pedunculated ovarian cyst could present with right-sided symptoms if it assumes a right lower quadrant position. Abdominal ultrasonography can usually be performed without any sedation and the sonographer can communicate with the child and ask where the pain or tenderness is maximal. However, this may be distracting in children who localise pain poorly. The closeness is reassuring to the child and also allows the sonographer to observe the child's facial expression or reaction to contact with the examination probe. Appropriate application of the probe relies heavily on co-operation from the patient and the graded compression can be limited by the presence of guarding. In addition, ultrasound is operator dependent and has reduced efficacy in obese patients. It can achieve up to 98.5% sensitivity, 98.2% specificity, 98.0% positive predictive value and 98.7% negative predictive value in experienced hands (Strouse, 2010). A repeat ultrasound in case of persisting clinical borderline suspicion may increase diagnostic yield (Schuh et al., 2011).

Ultrasonographic features suggestive of appendicitis include:

1. Rigid non-compressible appendix
2. Tenderness on attempted compression
3. Non-peristalsing appendix
4. Appendicular wall thickness of > 6mm
5. Distension of the appendicular lumen
6. Presence of abscess in the peri-appendicular region
7. Increased amount of intraperitoneal fluid
8. Inflammatory changes in surrounding tissues
9. Discontinuity of the appendicular wall
10. Extruded faecolith
11. Thickening of ileum or caecum which may represent part of the inflammatory mass around the inflamed appendix but may also suggest a diagnosis of Crohn's disease.

9.3.3 Computed Tomography (CT)

CT has been demonstrated to be more effective than ultrasonography in the diagnosis of appendicitis and evaluation of abdominal pathology in general. The radiation load from an abdominal CT remains a hindrance to its widespread application in children. The typical effective radiation dose from a CT of abdomen/pelvis is 10 mSv (Hampson and Shaw, 2010). For a single abdominal CT study in a 5 year old child, the life time risk of radiation induced malignancy would be 26.1/100 000 in girls and 20.4/100 000 in boys.

Reported CT sensitivity is 79-98%, increased with intravenous contrast. Luminal contrast may further improve its sensitivity (Theoni and Thornton, 2007). Kaiser et al., (2002) demonstrated that compared to graded compression ultrasound in acute childhood appendicitis, CT sensitivity is 97%, with accuracy of 95%, negative predictive value of 92% while ultrasound sensitivity was found to be 80%, accuracy of 89% and negative predictive value of 88%. CT is also preferable in obese patients and those with significant ileus or bowel gas. It was found to lead to a reduction in negative appendicectomy rates in children. The negative appendicectomy rate without imaging was found to be 14%, 17% with ultrasound but reduced to 2% with CT. No difference was observed in perforation rate (Theoni and Thornton, 2007). Lower abdominal CT should be performed with intravenous contrast where possible. Features suggesting appendicitis include (Theoni and Thornton, 2007):

- Appendicular diameter of more than 6mm
- Presence of inflammatory changes in the peri-appendicular area combined with a dilated or thickened appendix
- Inflammatory changes extending to the psoas muscle
- A calcified faecolith may be seen
- There may be free fluid with or without an enhancing rim suggesting abscess
- Thickened caecum and terminal ileum with inflamed appendix
- Periappendicular fat stranding
- Air in the appendix wall, retroperitoneum or abdomen associated with inflammatory changes in the area around the appendix
- Advanced appendicitis may give CT findings of pericaecal phlegmon or abscess
- The right lower quadrant may demonstrate free air which suggests perforation.

Early appendicitis may not be distinguishable from normal appendix because the features mentioned above would be absent. Consequently, failure to visualise the appendix radiologically does not rule out acute appendicitis. It is noteworthy that air within the appendix lumen may be normal in the absence of other features of periappendicular inflammation and the appendix may not be demonstrable in the presence of focal inflammatory changes of the appendix. Thickening of the wall of the appendix observed on axial images as three concentric rings or as single thick ring of enhancement with or without periappendicular soft tissue stranding may be the only feature present. Disadvantages of CT include the following:

- Risk of radiation.
- CT costs more to perform
- Patients are at risk of allergic reaction to the contrast agent
- It takes longer to perform
- It may have a lower sensitivity in patients with low body fat (Rothrock & Pagane, 2000).

9.3.4 Radionuclide scanning

Radionuclide scanning using 99mTc-hexamethylpropyleneamine oxime (HMPAO) labelling of patient's leucocyte or technetium-99m-labelled antigranulocyte antibodies can be used to evaluate abdominal pain in children presenting with equivocal clinical and laboratory findings. Accumulation of the radionuclide material in the right lower quadrant of the abdomen indicates positivity for appendicitis. The sensitivity is between 91-94% and specificity is 82-94%. The disadvantages to its use include the issue that it is not universally available, takes long to perform and interpretation of the scan is operator dependent (Sarosi & Turnage, 2002).

9.3.5 Contrast studies

A contrast enema is not usually employed in children for the diagnosis of acute appendicitis because it is unpleasant to the child, may require sedation, involves contrast going through probably inflamed bowel and may not contribute much to the evaluation following the use of other radiological investigations. If it is done, it may show failure of the appendix to fill with contrast. However, 10-20% of normal appendixes do not fill during contrast study. False negative result may be caused by distal appendicitis at the tip without proximal obstruction or partial obstruction in early appendicitis. It may demonstrate right colonic or terminal ileal mucosal changes secondary to infective enterocolitis e.g from Yersinia enterocolitica, Salmonella spp. Shigella spp. Campylobacter spp. Bacteroides spp. Escherichia coli, as well as changes due to Crohn's disease or non-specific inflammatory bowel disease. It may compliment CT and US in equivocal cases, particularly in recurrent abdominal pain. An upper gastrointestinal contrast study may be used to evaluate the rotational status of the midgut in such cases.

Contrast studies offer advantages of being

1. Simple
2. Safe
3. Readily available where ultrasound and CT are not available

Disadvantages include:

- Up to 40% of barium studies may be equivocal where CT and US have been equivocal (Liu and McFadden, 2003)
- In the presence of perforation, contrast may extravasate into the peritoneal cavity
- It takes time to set up
- It may require sedation.

9.3.6 Laparoscopy

Up to 59% of patients with right lower quadrant pain may have appendicitis confirmed at laparoscopy for suspected appendicitis. 35% of the females with suspected appendicitis may be found to have gynaecological pathology at laparoscopy (Liu and McFadden, 2003). Laparoscopy also offers the advantages of direct inspection of all the intra-abdominal organs as well as the opportunity to treat the identified pathology where appropriate.

9.4 Clinical scoring systems

Several scoring systems have been put forward to facilitate the diagnosis of appendicitis. Unfortunately, paucity of validation studies limits their clinical application. It should be borne in mind however that achieving a maximum score in any of the scoring systems may still lead to a negative appendicectomy. Two of these are discussed.

The Paediatric Appendicitis Score (PAS) for the evaluation of children aged between 4-15years with probable appendicitis is based on scores assigned to the clinical history, presenting signs and laboratory results. A score of ≤5 implies the diagnosis is unlikely to be appendicitis; ≥ 6 is compatible and 7-10 indicates a high probability of appendicitis. PAS has been advocated and shown to reduce the rate of normal appendicectomy to less than 5% giving a mean score of 3.1 ± 1.1 in non-appendicitis cases and 9.1 ± 0.1 in appendicitis (Samuel, 2002). Samuel (2002) also demonstrated that the PAS had a sensitivity of 100%, specificity of 87%, positive predictive value of 90% and negative predictive value of 100%. Table 1 shows the details of the scoring system.

Diagnostic indicator	PAS (maximum 10)
Tenderness with cough or percussion or hopping	2
Anorexia	1
Pyrexia	1
Nausea/ vomiting	1
Tenderness in right lower quadrant	2
Leucocytosis ≥ 10,000 (10^9/L)	1
Neutrophilia	1
Migration of pain	1

Table 1. Paediatric Appendicitis Score

Similarly, the Alvarado score (Table 2) employs clinical and laboratory values in predicting the possibility that the cause of abdominal pain is acute appendicitis. Shreef et al., (2010) in their review of 350 children demonstrated that with an Alvarado score of ≥6, the sensitivity of the scoring system could be as high as 100%, specificity 84.4%, positive predictive value of 83% and accuracy of 91.1%.

Diagnostic indicator	Alvarado score(maximum 10)
Tenderness in right iliac fossa	2
Rebound tenderness in right iliac fossa	1
Anorexia	1
Pyrexia >37.3	1
Nausea/Vomiting	1
Leucocytosis	2
Neutrophilia (>75%)	1
Migration of pain	1

Table 2. Alvarado Score

10. Treatment

10.1 Suspected appendicitis

Where a definite diagnosis is not reached following history taking and examination in a child with significant symptoms, admission for observation should be undertaken. The child should be managed according to symptoms with analgesia and rehydration therapy where appropriate. The gastric emptying in children with inflammatory intestinal problems is delayed, therefore, these patients should be kept on clear liquid diet to avoid aggravating the condition and also to minimise the risk of aspiration during induction of anaesthesia should this subsequently becomes necessary. Surana et al., (1995) demonstrated that active observation of children with suspicion of appendicitis was not associated with a significant increase in complication rate; 5.5% vs. 4.2% in those diagnosed at presentation. Moreover, after the inflammation reaches the submucosa, it progresses quickly to involve the rest of the appendix (Fenglio-Preiser et al., 2008). Therefore, hospital admission and active observation is recommended with regular review of the patient at intervals of 4-6hours.

10.2 Immediate treatment

The immediate management of a child with presumed acute appendicitis should include resuscitation, analgesia +/- abdominal decompression with a nasogastric tube. The child's clinical status should be evaluated to determine the appropriate level of care most suitable for the individual child. Some children would require level 2 intensive care nursing, or higher, before and/or after surgical treatment. Fluid resuscitation should be commenced and the child should be well-hydrated to ensure safe surgery. Broad spectrum antibiotics should be administered once the diagnosis of acute appendicitis has been made and surgery planned. There is evidence that commencing antibiotics at least 4hours before surgery reduces the risk of post-operative wound infection particularly when the duration of symptoms is longer than 48hours (Krukowski et al., 1987; Lander et al., 1992). Using a protocol involving adequate fluid resuscitation and a minimum of two pre-operative doses of antibiotics (Coamoxiclav +/- Gentamicin), Cleeve et al., (2011) demonstrated a complication rate of 6% in children with advanced appendicitis. The choice of antibiotics should cover the micro-organisms expected at the site of infection as described in the microbiology section of this chapter. Commonly, a third or fourth generation cephalosporin is used with or without a penicillin. An aminoglycoside, often Gentamicin, should be added where there are features suggesting advanced appendicitis. In the supine position, the lowermost levels of the peritoneal cavity are the right subphrenic space and the pelvic cavity. In peritonitic patients the rate of absorption of toxins from the intraperitoneal infection can be reduced by keeping them in the 45° position to encourage gravitation into the pelvis where the rate of toxin absorption is slow (Snell, 2004).

10.3 Conservative treatment

Delayed diagnosis is associated with higher rate of perforation, pelvic abscess, longer duration of hospital stay, delayed return to normal activities and greater risk of adhesive bowel obstruction. Up to 30% of children under 3years of age present with appendix mass with a duration of symptoms usually longer than 4-5days (Stevenson, 2003). In cases with long duration of symptoms, ultrasound should be performed before planning surgery if the clinical status of the abdomen precludes adequate palpation, or if the presence of a mass cannot be excluded. In the presence of a clinically palpable or radiologically identified appendicular mass and absence of gross peritonitis, conservative management with broad spectrum intravenous antibiotics can be safely undertaken. Hoffman et al., (1984) demonstrated that up to 80% of patients successfully managed with antibiotics for an appendix mass required no further treatment, 14% of these presented with recurrent abdominal pain not related to appendicitis; 20% had recurrent appendicitis and 66% of these occurred within 2 years of initial treatment. Swain et al., (2005) also demonstrated that an appendix-related abscess of ≤ 2cm can be successfully treated conservatively. Larger abscesses should be drained whenever this can be safely undertaken either by radiology-guided approach or surgically using laparoscopy or into the rectum.

Careful monitoring of physical signs, both local and systemic should be undertaken at regular intervals. The temperature, heart rate, respiratory rate, abdominal tenderness and size of inflammatory mass should be observed. Laboratory investigations should be used to compliment clinical findings. Repeat radiological investigations may also be required. The resolution may take a few days to become evident though generally a definite improvement should be noticed after 48 hours. If the acute appendicitis settles, interval appendicectomy should be performed within 6 weeks to 3 months. For those who show persistent or worsening clinical signs, early appendicectomy should be undertaken to avoid more serious complications.

10.4 Definitive surgery

Complications of appendicitis include pyelophlebitis, portal venous thrombosis, cholangitis, liver abscesses and bacteraemia. Also, fistula formation may result from appendicitis including enteroenteric, enterovaginal, enterocutaneous and enterovesical fistulae. Therefore, in the presence of strong suspicion of appendicitis, it is less of a clinical risk to undertake the removal of a normal appendix than expose the patient to the significant morbidity associated with advanced appendicitis. A negative appendicectomy rate of 5-10% can be expected (Stevenson, 2003). Oyetunji et al., (2011) observed a reduction in the negative appendicectomy rate over the years from 8.1 % in 2000 to 5.2% in 2006, being higher in rural areas, younger children, and girls. Of patients with negative appendicectomy, 12% may have a different surgical condition, 18-20% may have non-surgical pathology and 60% may have no identifiable pathology. Complication rate for negative appendicectomy may range from 5-15% including wound related problems, pulmonary complications, urinary tract infection and small bowel obstruction (Sarosi & Turnage, 2002).

Following induction of anaesthesia, palpation of the abdomen should be undertaken. In the presence of a clearly defined mass which was not identified earlier, further management would involve two main secondary options: to continue with the planned surgery, or, to defer the operation and further evaluate the child with treatment using intravenous antibiotics. The latter view was strongly expressed by Surana and Puri (1995). Gillick et al., (2001) found that children who had a palpable mass under anaesthesia, which was not diagnosed clinically earlier, had a shorter duration of symptoms (mean 2days) than those with clinically palpable or ultrasound diagnosed mass (mean 4days). In their series, half of the children aged ≤ 2years and one-third of those ≤ 3years had an appendix mass present at the time of first evaluation. 15.8% of their patients failed to settle with conservative management, 41.5% of whom had abscess drainage followed by appendicectomy, while 26% required early appendicectomy; 50% of these had post-operative complications. 10% of those who settled with conservative management had recurrent appendicitis. Considering the short duration of symptoms associated with a mass that was not palpable before anaesthesia, the author recommends that surgical treatment should proceed in these cases; having commenced antibiotic therapy at least 4hours before surgery where the duration of symptoms was longer than 48hours as suggested above. This recommendation is also given by Stevenson, (2003) and adopted by many paediatric surgeons in the United Kingdom.

10.4.1 Anaesthetic considerations

Appendicitis is usually an acute illness in otherwise healthy persons. It is often associated with gastroparesis and a patient who is admitted for observation for a probable diagnosis of appendicitis should be given fluid diet if not nil per oral as the stomach may not empty as well as in other conditions. Intraoperative precautions should be observed as for patients with a full stomach with rapid sequence intravenous induction of anaesthesia (Oberhelman & Malott, 2004). Once anaesthetised, the stomach should be promptly emptied with a nasogastric tube. The presence of associated peritonitis and abdominal distension may lead to splinting of the diaphragm which in turn reduces the functional lung volume. Respiratory impairment may be present especially in very young children. Tachypnoea may be a manifestation of respiratory embarrassment, pain, dehydration or sepsis. The circulatory system may be affected by hypoperfusion from associated fever, vomiting, diarrhoea or nausea with resultant reduced oral intake. This may manifest as increased heart rate and end organ signs including increased capillary refill time, reduced peripheral temperature, dry mucous membranes and reduced urine output. Preoperative correction of any hypovolaemia is mandatory for safe anaesthesia. There may be coexistent electrolyte imbalance and this also needs to be appropriately corrected preoperatively (Oberhelman & Malott, 2004).

Muscle relaxation is required to facilitate surgery whether open approach where muscle splitting is applied or laparoscopy which requires adequate exposure by pneumoperitoneum using the lowest possible intra-abdominal pressure. The physiological challenges posed by the pneumoperitoneum required for laparoscopic surgery needs careful attention from the anaesthetists (Nwokoma & Tsang, 2011).

10.4.2 Laparoscopic approach

Since the description of laparoscopic appendicectomy by the German gynaecologist Kurt Semm in 1983 (Semm, 1983), this approach to appendicectomy has continued to gain wide acceptance. With the advances in laparoscopic surgery in recent years, it has become common practice in many centres to have laparoscopic approach to appendicectomy in the absence of contraindications (Table 3).

Patient unsuitable for open surgery
Uncontrolled bleeding or coagulation problems
Multiple previous abdominal surgery

Table 3. Contraindications to paediatric laparoscopy

Where the child presents with features of advanced appendicitis with bowel obstruction, this may constitute a relative contraindication to the use of laparoscopy due to increased risk of injury to the dilated bowel loops. Previous abdominal surgery predisposes the patient to intra-abdominal adhesions which increase the risk of bowel injury and bleeding but this risk is less if the previous surgery was performed laparoscopically (Nwokoma et al., 2009b).

Laparoscopic approach has been safely used to treat advanced appendicitis in children with results similar to that in open approach. We demonstrated that laparoscopic approach offered significant advantages with better outcomes than open approach in paediatric advanced appendicitis with less wound-related complications: 8.6% versus 17.6% (Nwokoma et al., 2009a), and a conversion rate of 0%. Brugger et al., (2011) and Garg et al., (2009) drew similar conclusions from their studies. Brügger et al., (2011) further demonstrated the rate of wound infections (0.50% vs. 6.98-7.97%), post-operative ileus (0.15% vs. 0.33%), urinary complications (0.13% vs. 0.66%) and pulmonary complications (0.18 vs. 1.19%) to be lower in their group of laparoscopically treated appendicitis than data from large studies using the open approach.

The age-long principles of safe surgery include quick and adequate access, adequate target organ visualisation and minimal tissue trauma. In children, access can be quite a challenge because of the smaller height/width ratio of the abdomen particularly observed in those under 8years of age. In many cases, however long the incision, gaining access to the target organ or indeed to the four quadrants of the abdomen and pelvis, can be very difficult. Laparoscopy offers the paediatric surgeon the advantage of been able to visualise these areas while reducing the trauma usually consequent upon use of large abdominal wall incisions (Nwokoma & Tsang, 2011).

There is growing evidence that laparoscopy has more advantages and benefits to offer children than was earlier presumed to be the case. These benefits have been widely reported (Table 4) and significantly outweigh any concerns regarding the technical difficulties (Table 5) which are largely overcome with increasing experience and further developments in the laparoscopic equipment.

Reduced wound size
Reduced wound trauma
Less wound infection
Less incisional hernia
Less wound dehiscence
Less wound pain
Early mobilisation
Less bleeding
Less heat loss from tissue
Wider field of vision
Less postoperative adhesions
Less postoperative ileus
Earlier return to usual activities
Earlier commencement of chemotherapy
Less respiratory complications
Less risk of thromboembolism
Reduction in nerve entrapment

Table 4. Advantages of laparoscopy

Loss of tactile sensation
Loss of spatial and depth orientation
Two-dimensional imaging
Difficulty with control of bleeding
Difficulty with extraction of resected tissue or organ

Table 5. Technical difficulties of laparoscopy

A 10mm primary port should be inserted using the Hasson's open technique either in the suprapubic region, half way between the symphysis pubis and the umbilicus making sure that the urinary bladder is not in the path of entry or in the umbilical region - centrally or

infraumbilically. Two secondary 5mm ports should be inserted under laparoscopic guidance in the left lower quadrant for instruments. Alternatively, with an umbilical primary port, each of the two secondary ports can be placed on either side in the left and right lower quadrants. Single port transumbilical laparoscopy-assisted appendicectomy is gaining popularity and has been demonstrated to give results comparable to standard laparoscopic appendicectomy for uncomplicated appendicitis (Guanà et al., 2010). It has been successfully used to treat uncomplicated appendicitis as day case procedures (Alkhoury et al., 2011). Local anaesthetic injection into the port sites is advisable. Safe pneumoperitoneum should be established with 5-8mmHg in the newborn, 10-12mmHg in infants and <15mmHg in older children (Nwokoma & Tsang, 2011). Pus can be obtained with the suction device for microbiological analysis. The appendix is dissected free, the appendicular vessels divided by diathermy cauterisation or between endoclips. Ligation of the appendix should be carried out with three endosurgical loops; two proximally and one distally, as close to the base as possible to avoid the complications of stump appendicitis and enterocutaneous fistula (Lintula et al., 2002). Stump appendicitis which can occur following open or laparoscopic appendicectomy may occur in residual appendix as small as 6mm (Waseem & Devas, 2008) and is associated with significant morbidity. Cauterisation of the appendicular stump may prevent later formation of a mucocele. All incisions ≥ 5mm should be closed with absorbable sutures to the deep fascia and subcutaneous tissue to avoid port site hernia.
Advanced appendicitis poses a significant challenge for the paediatric surgeon and many opt for the open approach if this is suspected preoperatively. This is because the abdomen in children is shorter in height and relatively wider than in adults, especially children younger than eight years of age which is the group that commonly present with advanced appendicitis. However, as we demonstrated above, advanced appendicitis can be safely managed laparoscopically in children with outcome comparable to those of open approach. An inflammatory mass may be present during surgery and this can be drained laparoscopically with good vision of all four quadrants of the abdomen. Following laparoscopic drainage of the abscess, liberal peritoneal lavage should be performed as appropriate and the inflammatory mass should be assessed with regards to safety of continuing with the operation. Where the tissues are very friable, it is preferable to postpone the appendicectomy and treat with intravenous antibiotics with a view of performing interval appendicectomy safely at a later date. It is preferable to place the patient in a reverse Trendelenburg position and drain the purulent material from the pelvic cavity before putting the patient in the Trendelenburg position required for good access for the appendicectomy. This practice should reduce the risk of post-operative subphrenic, subhepatic and parasplenic abscesses.
Following laparoscopic appendicectomy in 7446 cases (age range between 12 and 100years), Brügger et al. (2011) observed an overall complication rate of 8.63% with individual complications detailed in Table 6.

10.4.3 Open appendicectomy

The open approach to appendicectomy has been established for over a century. The first recorded appendicectomy was performed by Claudius Amyand in 1735 at St. George's Hospital in London (United Kingdom) where he removed an appendix containing a calcified mass around a pin in a patient presenting with inguinal hernia. Lawson Tait performed the first successful appendicectomy for appendicitis in 1880 (Williams and Myers 1994).

Complication	*% frequency*
Intraoperative complications	**1.88**
Haematoma/intra-abdominal bleeding	0.6
Haematoma/ abdominal wall bleeding	0.28
Injury to intra-abdominal organ	0.13
Injury to stomach/ bowel	0.08
Vascular injury	0.07
Inadvertent bowel puncture by trocar	0.07
Inadvertent puncture by Veress needle	0.01
Other intraoperative complications	0.63
Postoperative Complications	**6.75**
Surgical postoperative complications	**4.24**
Abscess	0.98
Peritonitis	0.59
Paralytic ileus	0.56
Haematoma/intra-abdominal bleeding	0.50
Haematoma/abdominal wall bleeding	0.34
Haematoma/bleeding requiring transfusion	0.13
Wound infection	0.50
Obstructive ileus	0.15
Intestinal perforation	0.04
Stricture	0.01
Other surgical complications	0.44
General postoperative complications	**2.51**
Cardiac complication	0.36
Pulmonary embolism	0.15
Urinary tract infection	0.13
Jaundice	0.05
Pneumonia	0.03
Deep vein thrombosis	0.01
Stroke	0.01
Nerve compression	0.01
Other general postoperative complications	1.75

Table 6. Complication rates following laparoscopic appendicectomy

The commonly applied incision in children is the Lanz incision. It is an almost transverse incision in the right lower quadrant, about 2cm above and medial to the anterior superior iliac spine with its centre in the McBurney's point. The Lanz incision is more popular in children than the gridiron incision which also has its centre as the McBurney's point but runs perpendicular to an imaginary line between the anterior superior iliac spine and the pubic tubercle. This is because the Lanz incision has better cosmesis and healing, being along the Langerhan's lines. It also offers the surgeon the qualities of a good incision including easy and quick access to the abdominal cavity, extendable if required and easy to close. It crosses less dermatomal regions making the post-operative pain less and easier to control. As mentioned earlier, the abdomen of young children is relatively wider than its height on the longitudinal axis. Therefore access to the abdominal organs during surgery is best achieved by an incision that can go across the abdomen; the Lanz incision offers this advantage. Some authors advocate palpating the abdomen just before induction of anaesthesia and placing the incision just below the point of maximum tenderness. The problem with this is that the point of maximum tenderness usually marks the appendicular tip and may be far from the base. This may result in a longer than necessary incision. For example a pelvic appendix tip may give maximum tenderness suprapubically and a retrocaecal appendix may give maximum tenderness in the right upper quadrant. An incision over the region of the base of the appendix works best with various positions of the appendix body and tip. In certain situations, lengthening of the incision is necessary to perform a four-quadrant examination and drainage of associated pus. The Lanz incision allows such an extension of the incision to be undertaken safely and effectively.

Muscle splitting is preferable to the muscle cutting approach because the reduced tissue trauma is associated with reduced risk of bleeding, infection and post-operative pain. The peritoneum should be entered between clips, avoiding damage to the underlying bowels by ensuring bowel clearance from the edges of the clips. A microbiological swab of the peritoneal fluid should be taken, preferably from the appendix itself to increase micro-organism yield. Pus is the creamy-yellow viscid fluid present in infected tissues which consists of bacteria - living and dead, dead polymorphonuclear leukocytes, extravasated plasma and damaged host cells or tissue debris (Eykyn, 1998). If purulent material is present, a sample of it should be sent for analysis as well as a swab sample. The caecum should be identified and the anterior taenia followed inferomedially to the appendix base. Any inflammatory adhesion should be carefully released by blunt digital dissection. The peritoneal folds along the lateral and inferior borders of the caecum may need to be divided to adequately mobilize the caecum and deliver the appendix into the wound, especially so when it lies retroperitoneally. The mesoappendix is narrowest at the tip and widest at the base with the appendicular vessels within its edge. Ligation of the vessels usually commences from the tip towards the base. This is the antegrade dissection. In some cases retrograde dissection from the base may be required for safe appendicectomy. The appendix base should be crushed with a straight clamp as close to the caecum as can be safely achieved. Reapplying the clamp just above the crushed portion, the appendix should be transfixed and ligated with strong absorbable suture material, then cut above this. Cauterisation of the appendicular stump reduces risk of formation of a mucocele. Inversion of the appendicular stump with a purse string suture or a Z- stitch anchored within the taenia coli on the caecum adjacent to the base is still common practice. Taking too much caecum into the purse string suture or Z-stitch may lead to the development of a mucocele or become a lead point for intussusception (Swain, 2005). With local purulent peritonitis, local irrigation is preferable to wide spread lavage in other to minimise any dissemination of infective agents. On the other hand, if free pus is present, liberal peritoneal lavage is recommended. The addition of Betadine (Povidone iodine) or antibiotic agent(s) to the lavage fluid is widely practiced. However, it is noteworthy that Schneider et al., (2005) reported no significant advantage from the use of adjuvant peritoneal Taurolidine lavage in children with appendicitis associated with localised peritonitis. Local anaesthetic injection into the wound at this point compliments immediate post-operative analgesia. The abdominal wall should be closed carefully with absorbable suture material in layers or as mass closure. Subcuticular absorbable sutures should be used to close the skin. Pauniaho et al., (2010) demonstrated a reduced incidence of wound-related complications in acute appendicitis using subcuticular absorbable sutures than with the use of non-absorbable sutures.

The complication rate following open appendicectomy in children varies with age and severity of the appendicitis. Intra-abdominal abscesses may complicate up to 20% of perforated appendicitis; wound abscess <5%; faecal fistula <1% and wound haematoma <0.5%. Other complications include intestinal obstruction, missed bowel injury and bleeding. Mortality for non-perforated appendicitis is <0.1% and for perforated appendicitis this rises to up to 2% (Oberhelman & Malott, 2004).

10.5 Post-operative management

Careful monitoring of the patient in the post-operative period should follow the principles of management of the critically ill surgical patient. As stated earlier, level 2 (or higher) nursing care may be required. Careful management of respiratory and cardiovascular system should be continued. In the very young patient a urinary catheter may be a useful adjunct to fluid management and opiate analgesia may make the child prone to urinary retention. A nasogastric tube may be required if features of bowel obstruction are present. A peripherally inserted central line may be inserted intra-operatively if prolonged antibiotics or significant delay to return of bowel function is anticipated.

Post-operative analgesia may initially be administered as a patient or nurse-controlled intravenous opiate analgesia. Where advanced appendicitis has necessitated a wide incision and laparotomy, an epidural analgesia may be preferable. If epidural analgesia is used, a urethral catheter should be placed. Oral analgesia should be introduced when gastrointestinal function returns.

The administration of antibiotics for any reason can potentially upset the balance of the normal gastrointestinal flora. This may create an environment that is favourable for the multiplication of exogenous pathogens as well as the overgrowth of select pathogenic strains. Antibiotic-related complications are common with use beyond 5 days (Mui et al., 2005).

Principles for the selection of antibiotic therapy (Raftery, 2002) are as follows;

- There should be clinical evidence of infection
- Best guess antibiotics to cover known likely infective micro-organism(s)
- Where possible, remove infected tissue or foreign body
- Appropriate specimen collection from the site of infection for microbiology examination
- Cheapest and most effective drug or drug combination with known effectiveness over known likely organisms
- Monitoring of clinical response to treatment
- Appropriate route to achieve therapeutic levels of drug at site of infection

- Duration of administration should cover acute infection period, avoiding prolonged antibiotic treatment
- Re-evaluate clinical response with microbiology result and change antibiotics if clinically indicated.

Appendicectomy creates a contaminated wound with an infection risk of 12%. In the presence of pus or a perforation, a dirty wound results, with infection risk of 25% (Raftery, 2002). Perioperative antibiotics administration should follow local sensitivities, usually - Amoxicillin/ Gentamicin/ Metronidazole or a cephalosporin given instead of Amoxicillin. The former combination is used in our institution. Antibiotics should be given at least one hour before the skin incision is made to ensure adequate therapeutic plasma levels. Further antibiotic therapy should be based on intraoperative findings. In the presence of normal looking appendix, no further antibiotic is required. Single dose combined antibiotic therapy has been demonstrated to be adequate surgical prophylaxis in non-perforated appendicitis (Mui et al., 2005). In addition, Lee et al., (2010) observed that single or double agent antibiotics were effective and of lower cost than triple therapy. The author's recommendation in the case of an inflamed non-perforated appendix with no pus present is that a 24hr antibiotic therapy of single or double agents be given. This is because inflamed bowel is known to be associated with some micro-organism translocation. If heart rate and temperature remain within normal limits at 24 hours, antibiotics can be discontinued. A perforation may not be evident on resected specimen due to the extensive inflammation (Fenoglio-Preiser et al., 2008). In a cutaneous abscess, it is possible to clear out the pus. In the abdominal cavity, this is not possible and one must assume that infective agents remain free in the peritoneal cavity even after extensive peritoneal lavage. Five days of intravenous antibiotics is recommended in the presence of pus or an obvious perforation, preferably a triple agent therapy. The results of the microbiology analysis of any pus sample should be ascertained before the end of the five-day antibiotic therapy There is evidence that intraperitoneal abscess formation is commoner with Streptococcus milleri (Feneglio-Preser et al., 2008) and a longer duration of antibiotics, about 7days, is recommended in these situations.

Thromboprophylaxis should be administered by mechanical and/or chemical means as appropriate to each patient. In particular, older children above average weight or on contraceptive medication or who smoke should have peri-operative thromboprophylaxis. Some children show signs of gastric irritation following appendicectomy more with advanced appendicitis. If features of gastric irritation are observed including new onset epigastric pain and coffee-ground appearance of the vomitus, H-2 antagonists or proton pump inhibitors should be given to cover the period of acute illness till symptoms resolve.

11. Special considerations

11.1 The normal appendix: Remove or not remove?

Since the introduction of the Antegrade Colonic Enema procedure to aid the management of functional problems of the large bowel, the need to preserve the normal appendix particularly in children has been the subject of much discussion. Children without functional bowel problem or spina bifida at the time of presentation are unlikely to require the ACE procedure in the future. The appendix is also used for urinary diversion or vesico-cutaneous channel in the Mitrofanoff procedure and for biliary drainage (Swain, 2005). Arguably, while this may not be required at the time of surgery, the child's condition might change in the future. The likelihood that a child would need an appendix-related reconstructive surgery in the absence of a previous health problem is less than the likelihood of having appendicitis (Morrow, 2005). On this premise, it would appear that incidental appendicectomy has more benefits to offer by avoiding a future appendicitis.

Contraindications of incidental appendicectomy include impaired immunity, presence of surgical implants, presence of Crohn's disease in the adjacent caecum, intra-operative instability, history of recent abdominal radiation and an inaccessible appendix (Stevenson, 2003).

As discussed earlier, a normal-appearing appendix may be pathological. It is arguable that the presence of a Lanz incision may imply that appendicectomy had previously been undertaken which could be misleading with needless delay to the diagnosis of appendicitis where the appendix had actually not been removed. On the other hand, removing a normal appendix converts a clean operation into a dirty operation with increased risk of complications. The author recommends appropriate pre-operative evaluation and the removal of the normal-appearing appendix discovered intra-operatively.

11.2 Neurogenic appendicopathy

This condition is caused by the proliferation of nerve fibres in the appendix and can only be diagnosed with certainty on histological analysis. It may be present in up to 4.2% of specimens removed for presumed appendicitis. It is commoner in girls and older children, with up to 80% of specimens showing no histological features of inflammation. The use of antiserotonin or antihistamine therapy is advocated in suspicious cases (Zaupa et al., 2011).

11.3 Inflammatory bowel disease in appendicitis

Crohns disease: The appendix is involved in 25% of Crohn's disease leading to surgical treatment. However, Crohn's disease manifesting as appendicitis at the time of diagnosis is rare with less than 100 cases reported in literature. 7-10% of these are thought to progress to Crohn's disease at other sites. Ulcerative colitis: The appendix is involved in up to 50% of resected ulcerative colitis specimens. Some of these manifest as skip lesions without caecal involvement or in continuity with caecal disease (Petras & Goldblum, 1996).

11.4 Acute appendicitis in the neonate

Neonatal acute appendicitis is rare but associated with high morbidity and mortality of about 50-80%. Diagnosis is often late or missed and found at post-mortem (Swain, 2005). It may result from the presence of necrotising enterocolitis, cystic fibrosis, Hirschsprung's disease or bacteraemia associated with maternal chorioamnionitis (Pressman et al., 2001).

The neonatal anatomy presents special challenge due to its difference from the rest of the paediatric population. The abdomen in these children is often protuberant due to the flat diaphragm, shallow pelvis and reduced sacral curvature. Consequently, the organs that would have been within the rib cage and pelvis are intra-abdominal (Standring et al., 2005).

11.5 Chronic appendicitis

An organising phase of acute appendicitis occurs with the finding of granulation tissue and a mixture of acute and chronic inflammatory changes as well as recently laid down connective tissue. However, true chronic appendicitis with lymphocyte and plasma cells present in the muscularis propria and serosa without significant acute inflammation is rare (Petras and Goldblum, 1996).

11.6 Tuberculosis of the appendix

Appendicular tuberculosis occurs in 0.1-3% of patients with tuberculosis but isolated tuberculosis of the appendix is rare. Appendicectomy followed by antituberculous chemotherapy is the treatment of choice. Abdominal tuberculosis in children affects the immunocompromised and those who have not received the BCG vaccine. It manifests with weight loss, malaise, abdominal distension, abdominal pain, anaemia raised white cell count and altered albumin: globulin ratio (Rangabashyam et al., 2000)

11.7 Neoplasm of the appendix

Neoplasm of the appendix is found in 1.08 to 1.3% of appendicectomy specimens. The carcinoid tumour is very rare but it is the most common neoplasm of the gastrointestinal tract in children. It may be found in 0.3% of paediatric appendicectomies. Mean peak age of incidence in children is 15years though children as young as 6years old may be affected (Stevenson, 2003). Carcinoid syndrome comprises of flushing, diarrhoea and cardiac disease. It is usually associated with liver or retroperitoneal metastasis; with increased urinary 5-hydroxyindoleacetic acid. Lymph node metastasis is seen in 4-5% of paediatric patients with carcinoid tumour but distant metastasis of appendicular carcinoid is very rare in children. It may also be associated with multiple endocrine neoplasia type 2. (Christianakis et al., 2008). Adenocarcinoma of the appendix is exceedingly rare. More a problem of older patients, it develops in the appendicular base with appendicitis from luminal occlusion being the commonest mode of presentation. 50% are metastasized at diagnosis. It commonly spreads to the peritoneum directly. Adenocarcinoids are also rare. The histological features are of combined carcinoid and adenocarcinomas. The treatment of neoplasm of the appendix is largely limited to appendicectomy. Extension beyond the appendix requires treatment by right hemicolectomy (Liu & McFadden, 2003). Cystadenocarcinomas are mucin-filled. Perforation results in mucin-secreting peritoneal deposits manifesting as pseudomyxoma peritonei which is treated by repeated debulking and eventually fatal. In advanced cases, the abdomen is filled with tenacious semisolid mucin.

11.8 Recurrent appendicitis

Recurrent appendicitis is becoming increasingly accepted as a diagnosis. Appendicitis like any other inflammation in the human body may become arrested and not progress to full-blown process. To lend support to this, approximately a quarter of patients with histologically proven acute appendicitis report a history of prior episodes of abdominal pain of similar character as that which culminated in appendicectomy. Furthermore, sometimes histopathological analysis of acute appendicitis specimen shows both acute and chronic inflammatory characteristics. Also, about 60% of patients who respond well to treatment of advanced appendicitis report abdominal pain suggestive of recurrent appendicitis prior to interval appendicectomy (Swain, 2005).

11.9 Antibiotic-associated Clostridium difficile infection

Clostridium difficile (C. diff.) is a spore-forming gram positive rod. It produces its pathogenic features by the production of toxins. Toxin A is an enterotoxin while toxin B is a cytotoxin. Diagnosis is by detecting these toxins in stool. C. diff. toxins can be detected in the stool of 2-5% of the general population and up to 50% of infants. Its clinical significance is anchored on being the causative agent of antibiotics associated diarrhoea included in this chapter as a likely complication of prolonged perioperative antibiotic administration. It has been found to be responsible for approximately 30% of cases of the simple uncomplicated diarrhoea that often follows antibiotic administration. It is associated with 90% of cases where pseudomembranous colitis is present. Alteration of colonic flora especially by Ampicillin or Cephalosporins and Clindamycin favours the proliferation and virulence of C. diff. The clinical manifestation of C diff. colitis depends on which toxin is predominant in the colon. In situation of toxin A predominance, watery diarrhoea manifests; with toxin B predominance pseudomembranous colitis results. C. diff. diarrhoea onset is usually 5-10 days after starting antibiotics but this could range from day 1 to weeks after cessation of the therapy. Clinical effects may be mild and watery or bloody with or without severe crampy abdominal pain, raised levels of white blood cells and raised temperature. Treatment of C. diff colitis consists of discontinuation of implicated antibiotics which would usually lead to complete resolution of symptoms. However, if there is no response to antibiotic withdrawal or the patient is severely ill, Metronidazole or Vancomycin given orally is recommended. The risk of relapse or re-infection requiring repeat treatment may be up to 20% (Ryan & Ray, 2010).

11.10 Appendicitis in cancer patients on chemotherapy

Appendicitis in the neutropaenic child on anticancer chemotherapy is a great challenge. As much as possible, surgery should be avoided and conservative management with antibiotics instituted with a plan to perform interval appendicectomy when the child is better. A CT scan is often required to differentiate this from typhlitis. Joint care should be undertaken with specialist paediatric oncology staff. Granulocyte Colony Stimulating agents are often used to improve the neutrophil count. Some authors recommend elective appendicectomy in patients diagnosed with malignancy who are about to commence chemotherapy if surgery for other reason was to be performed before chemotherapy with a view of preventing appendicitis that may occur in neutropenic patients while on chemotherapy. This practice was not found to be associated with increased complications rate but only 0.2% of patients who did not have incidental appendicectomy went on to have appendicitis during a median follow up period of 5years (Morrow, 2005).

12. References

Alkoury F.; Burnweit C.; Malvezzi L.; Knight C.; Diana J.; Pasaron R.; Mora J.; Nazarey P.; Aserlind A. & Stylianos S. (2011). A prospective study of ambulatory appendectomy for acute appendicitis: safety and satisfaction with same day discharge in 126 children. *Presented at the British Association of Paediatric Surgeons Conference.* Belfast, U.K. (July 2011).

Baker N.; Bushell A. & Hawkey P. M. (2004). Bacteriology of superficial and deep tissue infection. In: *Medical Bacteriology.* (2004) 157-160. Hawkey P. M. & Lewis D. (Eds.) Second edition. Oxford University Press Inc. New York, USA. ISBN: 019963778-4

Birchley D. (2006). Patients with clinical acute appendicitis should have pre-operative full blood count and CRP assays. *Annals of the Royal College of Surgeons of England.* Vol. 88, No. 1, (January 2006), pp. 27-32. ISSN: 0035-8843

Brügger L.; Rosella L.; Candinas D. & Güller U. (2011). Improving Outcome After Laparoscopic Appendectomy, A population-based, 12year Trend Analysis of 7446 Patients. *Annals of Surgery,* Vol.253, No.2, (February 2011), pp. 309-313, ISSN: 0003-4932

Chang Y.; Chao H. C.; Kong M. S.; Hsia S. H. & Yan D. C. (2010). Misdiagnosed acute appendicitis in children in the emergency department. *Chang Gung Medical Journal.* Vol. 33, No. 5, (September-October 2010), pp. 551-556, ISSN: 20720939

Cleeve S.; Jones N.; Joshi A.; Phelps S.; Misra D. & Ward H. (2011). Trends in childhood appendicitis. *Presented at the British Association of Paediatric Surgeons Conference.* Belfast, U.K. (July 2011).

Dalal I.; Somekh E.; Bilker-Reich A.; Boaz M.; Gorenstein A. & Serour F. (2005). Serum and Peritoneal inflammatory mediators in children with suspected acute appendicitis. *Archives of Surgery.* Vol. 140, No. 2, (February 2005), pp. 169-173 ISSN: 0004-0010

Doria A. S. (2009). Optimising the role of imaging in appendicitis. *Pediatric Radiology,* Vol. 39, Supplement 2, (April 2009), pp. S144-8, ISSN: 1432-1998

Ellis H. & Mahadevan V. (2010). *Clinical Anatomy.* Twelfth edition. Pp. 87-88. Wiley-Blackwell, West Sussex, United Kingdom. ISBN 978-1-4051-8617-9

Eykyn S. J. Surgical infections and the use of antibiotics. In: *The New Aird's Companion in Surgical Studies,* (1998). Second edition. K.G. Burnand and A.E. Young, (Eds.), 66, Churchill Livingstone, ISBN 0443 05326X, London, United Kingdom

Fenoglio Preiser C. M.; Noffsinger A. E.; Stemmermann G. N.; Lantz P. E. & Isaacson P. G. (2008). *Gastrointestinal Pathology: An Atlas and Text.* Third edition. 502-505. Wolters Kluwer/ Lippincott Williams & Wilkins, Philadelphia, USA. ISBN-13: 978-0-78-17-7146-7

Forbes B. A.; Sahm D. F. & Weissfeld A. S. (2007). *Bailey and Scott's Diagnostic Microbiology.* Twelfth edition. P. 905. Mosby Elsevier, St. Louis, Missouri, USA. ISBN: 139780323030656

Garg C. P.; Vaidya B. B. & Chengalath M. M. (2009) Efficacy of laparoscopy in complicated appendicitis. *International Journal of Surgery.* Vol. 7, No. 3, (May 2009), pp. 250-252, ISSN: 1743-9191

Gillick J.; Velayudham M. & Puri P. (2001). Conservative management of appendix mass in children. *British Journal of Surgery.* Vol. 88, No. 11, (November 2001), pp. 1539-1542, ISSN: 0007-1323

Hampson F. A. & Shaw A. S. Assessment of the acute abdomen: role of the plain abdominal radiograph. *Reports in Medical Imaging.* (2010), No. 3, 93-105. Dove Medical Press limited.

Hernanz-Schulman M. (2010). CT and US in the diagnosis of appendicitis: an argument for CT. *Radiology.* Vol 255, no. 1, (April 2010), pp. 3-7, ISSN: 0033-8419

Hoffman J.; Lindhard A. & Jensen H. (1984). Appendix mass: conservative management without interval appendicectomy. *The American Journal of Surgery.* Vol. 148, No. 3, (September 1984), pp. 379-382, ISSN: 0002-9610

Karim O. M.; Boothroyd A. E. & Wyllie J. H. (1990). McBurney's point – fact or fiction? *Annals of the Royal College of Surgeons of England.* Vol. 72, No. 5, (September 1990), 304, ISSN: 0035-8843

Krukowski Z. H.; Al-Sayer H. M.; Reid T. M. S. & Matheson N. A. (1987). Effect of topical and systemic antibiotics on bacterial growth kinesis in generalised peritonitis in man. *British Journal of Surgery.* Vol. 74, No. 1, (April 1987), pp. 303-306, ISSN: 0007-1323

Lander A. (2007). The role of imaging in children with suspected appendicitis: the UK perspective. *Pediatric Radiology.* Vol. 37, No. 1, (January 2007), pp. 5-9, ISSN: 0301-0449

Lander A. D.; Ward H. & Brereton R. J. (1992). Perforated appendicitis in children: progress towards non-urgent operative treatment. *Unpublished Report.* (January 1992).

Lee S. L.; Islam S.; Cassidy L. D.; Abdullah F. & Arca M. J. (2010). Antibiotics and appendicitis in the pediatric population; An American Pediatric Surgical association outcomes and Clinical Trials Committee Systematic review. *Journal of Pediatric Surgery.* Vol. 45, No. 11, (November 2010), pp. 2181-2185, ISSN 0022-3468

Lintula H.; Kokki H.; Vanamo K.; Antila P. & Eskelinene M. (2002). Laparoscopy in children with complicated appendicitis. *Journal of Pediatric Surgery.* Vol. 37, No. 9, (September 2002), pp. 1317-1320, ISSN 0022-3468

Liu C. D. & McFadden D. W. Acute abdomen and appendix. In: *Surgery – Scientific Principles and Practice,* (2003). Second edition. L. J. Greenfield, M. Mulholland, K.T. Oldham, G.B. Zelenock, K.D. Lillemoe, (Eds.), 1248-1260, Lippincott-raven-Publishers, ISBN 0-397-51481-6, Philadelphia, USA

Mui L. M.; Ng C. S. H.; Wong S. K. H.; Lam Y. -H.; Fung T. M. K.; Fok K. -L.; Chung S. S. C. & Ng E. K. W. (2005). Optimum duration of prophylactic antibiotics in acute non-perforated appendicitis. *The Australian and New Zealand Journal of Surgery.* Vol. 75, No. 6, (June 2005), pp. 425-428, ISSN 1445-2197

Naaeder S. B. & Archampong E. Q. (1998). Acute appendicitis and dietary fibre intake. *West African Journal of Medicine.* Vol. 17, No. 4, (October –December 1998), pp. 264-267, ISSN 0189-160X

Nwokoma N. J. & Tsang T. T. (2011). Laparoscopy in Children and Infants, Advanced Laparoscopy, Ali Shamsa (Ed.), ISBN: 978-953-307-674-4, In Tech, available from: http://www.intechopen.com/articles/show/title/laparoscopy-in-children-and-infants

Nwokoma N. J.; Hassett S. & Tsang TT. (2009). Trocar site adhesions after laparoscopic surgery in children. *Surgical Laparoscopic Endoscopic Percutaneous Techniques.* Vol. 19, No. 6, (December 2009), pp.511-513, ISSN 1530-4515

Nwokoma N. J.; Swindells M. G.; Pahl K.; Mathur A. B.; Minocha A.; Kulkarni M. & Tsang T. T. (2009). Pediatric advanced appendicitis: open versus laparoscopic approach. *Surgical Laparoscopic Endoscopic Percutaneous Techniques.* Vol. 19, No. 2, (April 2009), pp.110-113, ISSN 1530-4515

Oberhelman H. A. & Malott K. A. (2004). Intestinal Surgery. In: *Anethesiologists Manual of Surgical Procedures.* Third edition. Jaffe R. A., Samuels S. I. (Eds.), Pp. 407-410. Lippincott Williams & Wilkins. Philadelphia USA. ISBN: 0-7817-4332-X

Oyetunji T. A.; Ong'uti S. K.; Bolorundoro O. B.; Cornwell III E. E. & Nwomeh B. C. (2011). Pediatric Negative Appendectomy Rate: trend, predictors and Differentials. *Journal of Surgical Research.* (May 2011) 1-5. Epublication ahead of print. ISSN 0022-4804

Pauniaho S. L.; Vasama T.; Helminen M. T.; Iber T.; Mäkelä E. & Pajulo O. Non-absorbable interrupted versus absorbable continuous skin closure in pediatric appendectomies. *Scandinavian Journal of Surgery.* Vol. 99, No 3, (March 2010), pp. 142-146. ISSN 1457-4969

Petras R. E. & Goldblum J. R. (1996). Appendix. In: *Anderson's pathology.* Tenth edition. I. Damjanov and J. Linder. (Eds.) 1728-1732. Mosby-Year Book. St. Louis, Missouri, USA. ISBN 0801672368

Pickhardt P. J.; Levy A. D.; Rohrmann Jr. C. A. & Kende A. I. (2002). Primary neoplasms of the appendix manifesting as acute appendicitis: Ct findings with pathologic comparison. *Radiology.* Vol. 224, No. 3, (September 2002), pp. 775-781, ISSN: 0033-8419

Puri P.; McGuiness E. P. & Guiney E. J. (1989) Fertility following perforation appendicitis in girls. *Journal of Pediatric Surgery,* Vol. 24, No. 6, (June 1989), pp. 547-549, ISSN: 0022-3468

Raftery A.T. (2002). Basic Microbiology. In: *Applied Basic Science for Basic Surgical Training.* A.T. Raftery (Ed.) Pp. 139-157, Elsevier Science Limited. Philadelphia, USA. ISBN: 0443-061440

Ramsden W. H.; Mannion R. A.; Simpkins K. C. & deDombal F. T. (1993). Is the appendix where you think it is - and if not does it matter? *Clinical Radiology*. Vol 47, No. 2, (February 1993), p. 100, ISSN: 0009-9260

Rangabashyam N.; Anand B. S. & OmPrakash R. (2000). Abdominal tuberculosis. In: *Oxford Textbook of Surgery*. Second edition. P.J. Morris, W.C. Wood (Eds.) 3247-3249, Oxford University Press, New York, USA, ISBN: 0192628844.

Rothrock S. G. & Pagane J. (2000). Acute appendicitis in children: emergency department diagnosis and management. *Annals of Emergency Medicine*. Vol 36, No. 1, (July 2000), p. 39, ISSN: 0196-0644

Ryan K. J. & Ray C. G. (2010). Sherris Medical Microbiology. Fifth edition. Pp. 528-531. McGraw Hill Medical. USA. ISBN: 978-0-07-160402-4

Samuel M. (2002) Paediatric Appendicitis Score. *Journal of Pediatric Surgery*, Vol. 37, No. 6, (June 2002), pp. 877-881, ISSN: 0022-3468

Sarosi G. A. & Turnage R. H. (2002). Appendicitis. In: *Sleisenger and Fordtram's Gastrointestinal and Liver Disease*. Seventh edition. M. Feldman, L. S. Friedman, M.H. Sleisenger. (Eds.) Pp. 2089-2099. Saunders. Philadelphia, USA. ISBN: 0-7216-8973-6

Schneider A.; Sack U.; Rothe K. & Bennek J. (2005). Peritoneal taurolidine lavage in children with localised peritonitis due to appendicitis. *Pediartic Surgery International*. Vol. 21, No. 6, (June 2005), pp. 445-448, ISSN: 0179-0358

Schuch S.; Man C.; cheng A.; Murphy A.; Mohanta A.; Moineddin R.; Tomlinson G.; Langer J. C. & Doria A. S. (2011) Predictors of non-diagnostic ultrasound scanning in children with suspected appendicitis. *Journal of Pediatrics*. Vol. 158, No. 1, (January 2011), pp. 112-8, ISSN: 0022-3476

Sebire N. J.; Malone M.; Ashworth M. & Jacques T. S. (2010) *Diagnostic Pediatric Surgical Pathology*, p. 587. Churchill Livingstone Elsevier, Philadelphia. ISBN: 978-0-443-06808-9

Semm, K. (1983). Endoscopic appendectomy. *Endoscopy*,Vol.15, No.2, (March 1983), pp. 59-64, ISSN: 0013726X

Shreef K. S.; Waly A. H.; Abd-Elrahman S. & AbdElhafez M. A. (2010). Alvarado score as an admission criterion in children with pain in the right iliac fossa. *African Journal of Paeditaric Surgery*. (2010), Vo. 7. No. 3, pp. 163-165, ISSN: 0186-2391

Snell R. S. (2004). *Clinical Anatomy*. Seventh edition. P. 227. Lippincott Williams & Wilkins. Philadelphia, USA ISBN: 0-7817-4315-X

Snell R. S. (2004). *Clinical Anatomy*. Seventh edition. P. 782. Lippincott Williams & Wilkins. Philadelphia, USA ISBN: 0-7817-4315-X

Standring S.; Ellis H.; Healy J. C.; Johnson D. & Williams A. (2005). *Gray's Anatomy*. Thirty-ninth edition. 1188-1190. Elsevier Churchill Livingstone, Philadelphia, USA. ISBN: 0-443-06676-0

Stevenson R. J. (2003). Appendicitis. In: *Operative Pediatric Surgery*. Ziegler M. M., Azizkhan R. G., Weber T. R. (Eds.), pp. 671-689. McGraw-Hill Companies. New York, USA. ISBN: 0-07-121239-6

Strouse P. J. (2010) Paediatric appendicitis: an argument for US. *Radiology*. (Vol. 255, No. 1, (April 2010), pp. 8-13, ISSN: 0033-8419

Surana R. & Puri P. (1995a). Appendiceal mass in children. *Pediatric Surgery International*, (February 1995), Vol. 10, No. 2-3, pp. 79-81, ISSN: 0179-0358

Surana R.; O'Donnell B. & Puri P. (1995b). Appendicitis diagnosed following active observation does not increase morbidity in children. *Pediatric Surgery International*. Vol. 10, No. 2-3, (February 1995), pp. 76-78, ISSN: 0179-0358

Swain R. S. (2005). Appendix and Meckel's diverticulum. In: *Principles and Practice of Pediatric Surgery*. K.T. Oldham, P.M. Clobani, R. P. Foglia & M. A. Skinner. Vol.2, p. 1269, Lippincott Willaims & Wilkins, Philadelphia, USA. ISBN: 078174290-0

Thoeni R. F. & Thornton R. Radiology of the Colon. In: *Diseases of the Colon.* (2007). S. D. Wexner and N. Stollman (Eds.), 178-183, informa healthcare, ISBN: 0-8247-2999-4, New York, USA

Tsze D.S.; Asnis L. M.; Merchant R. C.; Amanullah S. & Linakis J. G. (2011). Increasing Computed Tomography Use for Patients With Appendicitis and Discrepancies in Pain management Between Adults and Children: Analysis of the NHAMCS. *Annals of Emergency medicine,* Vol. 58, No. 2, (August 2011), In press corrected proof) ISSN: 0003-4932

Turner J. R. (2010). The gastrointestinal tract. In: *Robbins and Cotran Pathologic Basis of Disease.* V. Kumar, A.K. Abbas, N. Fausto, J.C. Aster (Eds.), 825-828, Saunders Elsevier, Philadelphia, USA. ISBN: 978-1-4160-3121-5,

Vajcner G.; Postuma R. & Postuma R. (2011). Algometry: A novel tool in the diagnosis of children presenting with acute abdominal apin. *Presented at the 12th European Congress of Paediatric Surgeons.* Barcelona, Spain. (June 2011).

VanMeter K. C.; VanMeter W. G. & Hubert R. J. (2010). Microbiology for the Healthcare Professional. Pp. 237-240. Mobsy Elsevier. Missouri, USA. ISBN: 978-0-323-04594-0

Waseem M. & Devas G. (2008). A child with appendicitis after appendectomy. *Journal of Emergency Medicine.* Vol. 34, No. 1, (January 2008), pp. 59-61, ISSN: 0736-4679

Whisker L.; Luke D.; Hendrickse C.; Bowley D. M. & Lander A. (2009). Appendicitis in children: a comparative study between a specialist paediatric centre and a district general hospital. *Journal of Pediatric Surgery.* Vol. 44, No. 2, (February 2009), pp. 362-367, ISSN: 0022-3468

Williams R. A. & Myers P. (1994). *Pathology of the Appendix.* 1-11, Chapman & Hall medical, London, United Kingdom. ISBN: 0-412-54810-0

Wu H. P. & Fu Y. C. (2010). Application with repeated serum biomarkers in pediatric appendicitis in clinical surgery. *Pediatric Surgery International.* Vol. 26, No. 2, (February 2010), pp.161-166, ISSN: 0179-0358

Zaupa P.; Lange C.; Bäumel D.; Karpf E. & Höllwarth M. (2011). Neurogenic appendicopathy in children. *Presented at the 12th European Congress of Paediatric Surgery,* (June 2011).

9

Demographic and Epidemiologic Features of Acute Appendicitis

Barlas Sulu
Kafkas University Faculty of Medicine, Department of General Surgery, Kars, Turkey

1. Introduction

Acute Appendicitis (AA) is the most commonly encountered disease in emergency clinics, with about 250,000 cases of appendicitis reported in The United States and 40,000 in England each year (Deng et al., 2010; Simpson et al., 2008). The key form of treatment for the disease is surgery and the mortality, morbidity, and economic cost ratio rise the longer it remains untreated.

Despite the high prevalence of the disease, the uncertainty of just how many appendicitis patients will present to emergency clinics each day still remains an unpredictable situation for us surgeons, with some days bringing a large number of cases, and others relatively few. Ever since Amyand Claudius performed the first appendectomy in 1735 at St George's Hospital in London, this decrease and increase in cases has led researchers to conduct studies into both the etiology of AA and the disease's epidemiological and demographic characteristics.

The etiology of AA has, as of yet, not been clarified. Clarification of the etiology has been the main point of epidemiological studies and advancements in this area will influence the incidence of the disorder as well. There are various theories on the frequency and incidence of appendicitis at present and these are still debated, despite some having strong scientific backing.

2. Demographic features of appendicitis

Studies have demonstrated that AA is seen most commonly in western societies, particularly in youths and males (Addiss at al.,1990; Al-Omran et al., 2003; Noudeh et al., 2007; Sulu et al., 2010). Research carried out in our own region has also shown that AA is seen more commonly in young people aged 10-19 and in males **(Figure 1)**.

The appendix tissue possesses the features of a lymphoid organ and there is a larger amount of lymphoid tissue in young subjects. Lymphoid hyperplasia can be caused by any obstruction occurring in the lumen of the appendix and this can develop into appendicitis if the condition continues. Appendicitis is therefore seen more frequently in young people. Lymphoid tissue is vague. Lumen of the appendix enlarges after lymphoid tissue atrophies and probability of obstruction by decreases fall of in over aged people. For that reason, incidence of acute appendicitis decreases with age. Consequently only 5% to 10% of acute appendicitis cases are seen in the elderly (Jones et al., 1985). The more common involvement of young people and men is easier to discern in Western societies than other regions. The lower incidence of AA and the less pronounced gender gap in regions such as Africa and Asia is worth mentioning (Ajao, 1979; Arnbjörnsson, 1983; Oguntola et al., 2010; Walker & Segal, 1995). This may be because people living in these regions are less influenced by the western-type diet (fast-food diet) with the majority of foods consumed being high in carbohydrates and low in fiber. The height of males as a factor in the development of the disease is not clear (Addiss at al., 1990). However, the effect of sex hormones in females alongside the predisposition of males to consume 'fast-food' are considered to be important (Walker & Segal, 1979).

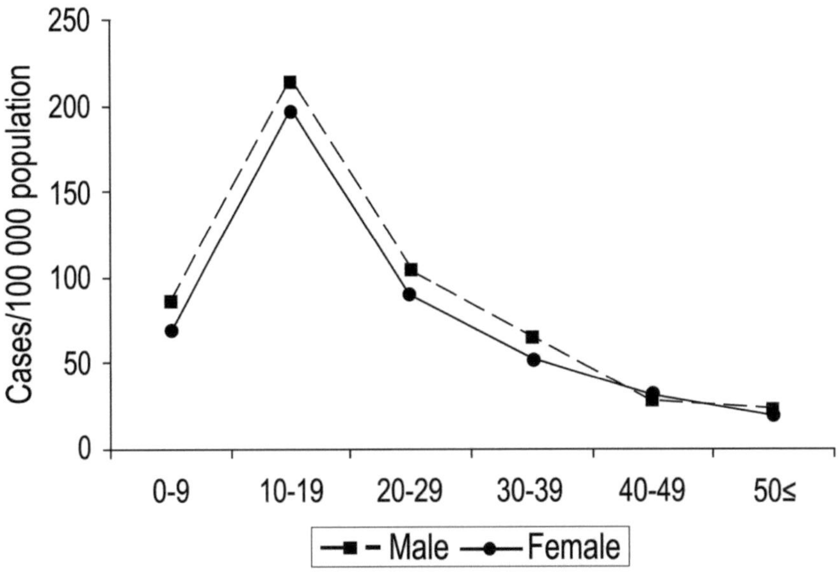

Fig. 1. The distribution of acute appendicitis according to age groups and sex (2004-2007).

3. Epidemiological theories for the development of appendicitis

The most widely accepted theories today are the diet and hygiene hypotheses (Walker & Segal, 1995). At the same time, these hypotheses have also formed the groundwork of AA's epidemiological features.

The dietary theory was first developed by Rendle Short in 1920. He stated that the AA incidence was higher with a lower ratio of cellulose in the diet and that this was the reason why Britain had been seeing an increase in the incidence of AA since the turn of the 20th century, as well as why the rate differed by country (Barker, 1985; Walker & Segal, 1995). This theory was further developed to reveal a positive correlation between AA and a diet poor in fiber but rich in such foods as meat, potatoes, and sugar, and a negative correlation between AA and a diet rich in fiber containing green vegetables, fruits, and tomatoes (Morris et al.,1987). In other words, a diet devoid of sufficient fiber triggers the formation of AA. A diet featuring low consumption of fiber reduces the colonic transit time by reducing the lumen of the appendix, and the resulting lymphoid hyperplasia causes obstruction, ultimately leading to infection and appendicitis.

The hygiene theory was promoted by Barker in articles in the 1980s (Barker, 1985; Barker et al., 1988). Barker felt that the diet did not explain the decrease in incidence of appendicitis in England in the 1930's. He found that the appendicitis incidence had decreased, together with that of many diseases, such as tuberculosis, in relation to the introduction of better housing and water supply following World War II. He felt that these improvements had decreased exposure of young children to enteric microorganisms and that the number of deaths due to diarrhea in childhood had been somewhat reduced. As a result, children and adults now avoided the effect of bacteria and viruses causing enteric and respiratory infections which pave the way for appendicitis and instead developed immunity against them. An insufficient number of bathrooms, toilets, hot water, and sewage systems in communal areas can promote the enteric bacterial, viral, and parasitic infectious agents that are responsible for the formation of appendicitis. These improvements will decrease the incidence of deaths due to enteric organisms in children and adults and also decrease the risk of appendicitis. This outcome is strongly related with the incidence of infectius disease and scocioeconomic status of the patients with appendicitis. For example, Schistosomiasis is a waterborne parasitic disease that can be prevented by following principles of good hygiene and preventing, by the management of sewage networks, the spread of parasite eggs in water that is used for consumption. As a result, the incidence of Schistosomal appendicitis is 0.2% in the USA, where sewage networks are well maintained, while it is 20 times this rate in Nigeria (Terada, 2009). Interestingly, the patients who suffered from this illness in the USA were African Americans.

4. Factors influencing appendicitis incidence and current tendencies

Epidemiological and demographic studies report the appendicitis incidence to vary according to age, gender, race, socioeconomic status, food culture, and seasonal changes (Adamidis et al., 2000; Ergul, 2007; Noudeh et al., 2007; Oguntola et al., 2010; Sulu et al., 2010). Therefore, the frequency of AA is different in each country. For example, the rate of appendicitis in Europe during the 1980s was 116 per 100.000 while this rate was 96-120 in the USA, 75 in Ontario, 200 in Hong Kong, and 32-37 in Thailand for the same years (Al-Omran et al., 2003; Chatbanchai et al., 1989; Luckmann & Davis,1991; Zoguéreh et al., 2001).

Epidemiological studies report that the incidence of AA within a single country tends to increase or decrease at different times of the year. In fact, differences have even been reported between people living in the same country when the society is formed from individuals from various geographical locations, cultures, and races. Walker et al. reported the prevalence of appendicitis as 0.5% in rural blacks, 1.2% in urban blacks, and 14% in urban whites (Walker & Segal, 1979). Walker et al. also evaluated the relationship between ethnicity and appendicitis in a study of 56 high school age (16-18 years) young people in South Africa and found that the rate of appendectomies was 0.6% in rural Blacks, 0.7% in urban Blacks, 2.9% in Indians, 1.7% in Coloureds (Eur-African-Malay), and 10.5% in Caucasians (Walker et al., 1982). This situation is similar within different ethnic communities in western societies, where the gap between gender and ethnic origins has shown similar distributions. In California, the incidence of appendicitis was 137.5 per 100.000 for Caucasian males while this incidence was 162.7 for Hispanics, 98.0 for Asian/others, and 70.7 for blacks. The same was true in female patients (Andersson, 2008) with rates per 100,000 of 98.8, 97.5, 64.6, and 49.6 for the above groups respectively. The authors reported that the difference observed between whites and blacks was associated with their consumption of different amounts of fiber.

However, the fact that studies performed in the last decade have reported a decrease in the incidence of AA in western countries (Andersson, 2008; Andersen et al., 2009; Andreu-Ballester et al., 2009; Cirocchi et al., 2008) but an increase in some African and Asian countries is interesting (Chavda et al., 2005; Lee et al., 2010). The rate of patients undergoing an appendectomy has decreased in the UK, the USA, and Europe (Williams et al., 1998). Even though there has been no change in the amount of fiber consumed in food in England and Wales during the 20st century, the mortality rate from appendicitis, which was 40 to 70 per millon in the first decade, dropped to 5 per million in the last decade (Barker, 1985). A study on Danish children has found a decreased appendicitis incidence in children from every age group (Andersen et al.,2009). The effect of better socioeconomic conditions created as a result of improving water supplies and hygienic conditions, has been found to be the reason for this decrease in Western societies. A recent study from Spain found a decrease in appendicitis in the last 10 years (Andreu-Ballester et al.,2009). A study from Greece evaluating the last 30 years found the age-standardized appendicitis rate to fall 75% from 652/100.000 to 164/100.000 (Papadopoulos et al.,2008). Both countries eat a Mediterranean diet rich in fiber but the decrease in Spain may be due to improved hygienic conditions with socioeconomic development. It is believed that the spread of the western-type diet in African and Asian societies today is responsible for the increase in the number of AA cases observed. However, we found in a previous study that short-term dietary changes had no effect on an increase in AA incidence (Papadopoulos et al., 2008). Studies conducted on the effects of fasting seem to support this conclusion. More than one billion Muslims consider the month of 'Ramadan' to be sacred and abstain from food or drink from sunrise to sunset for one month. During this month, devotees avoid performing any daily habitual action, such as the consumption of any food, drinks, drug therapy, smoking, or having sexual intercourse for a total of 12-19 hours each day. Since the body is used to receiving two meals a day, these changes in diet and the number of meals consumed each day change the metabolism (Sulu et al., 2010). This behavior has provided an ideal model for many researchers to investigate the effect that long-term hunger has on the human body. We have also used this opportunity to investigate the effect of changes in hunger and dietary habits on the development of AA in a study conducted throughout the month of Ramadan. We compared the frequency of AA before and after Ramadan in a 4-year study that included 4288 AA cases in two different cities. Of the 992 patients investigated, 37.1% developed AA in the period before Ramadan, 32.1% during the month of Ramadan, and 30.8% were diagnosed after the month of Ramadan. There was no significant difference between the values of these three periods. Based on these results, it is possible to infer that there is no short-term increase in the frequency of AA in societies starting to follow a western-type diet nor is there expected to be an increase in cases where migrants have moved to a new geographical location.

One further subject of discussion is whether environmental conditions have an influence on the frequency of the development of AA. It has been reported that seasonal changes, in particular, and moisture in the air (humidity) do have an effect (Al-Omran et al., 2003; Gallerani et al., 2006; Lee et al., 2010; Noudeh et al., 2007; Oguntola et al., 2010; Trepanowski & Bloomer, 2010). An increase in the frequency of cases in the AA summer months has been reported in many studies. However, studies have shown that this increase is observed in regions situated in low altitudes and close to the seaside **(Table 1)**.

Altitude (meters)		Appendicitis	Perforated
Ferrara	9	Summer	
Jersey City	25	Summer	
Ontario	86	Summer	
Beer Sheva	260	Autumn-Summer	
Hail	988	Spring-Summer	
Shahr-e-Rey	1050	Summer	
Kirman	1749	Winter	Summer-Autumn
İstanbul	100	Spring-Summer	Summer-Autumn
Kars	1750	Winter	

Table 1. The seasonal tendency of total and perforated appendicitis according to the altitude of different regions

In a study conducted in two Turkish cities with different climatic characteristics and altitudes, we found that the number of patients with acute appendicitis increases at low altitude in Istanbul during spring and summer ($p<0.05$). At high altitude in Kars, this increase is seen during winter ($p>0.05$). **(Table 2).**

Hospital	Season				Age Groups					
	1*	2*	3*	4*	0-9	10-19	20-29	30-39	40-49	≥50
KSH	503	476	458	434	300	814	349	204	113	91
HNTEH	712	846	762	686	22	664	1133	606	289	292

KSH : Kars State Hospital, HNTEH: Haydarpasa Numune Teaching and Research Hospital 1*: Winter, 2*: Spring, 3*: Summer, 4*: Autumn

Table 2. A comparison of the seasonal and age distribution of patients with appendicitis in Kars and Istanbul (2004-2007)

A further study reported that AA was seen more frequently in the winter months in Kerman, an Iranian city with an altitude similar to that of Kars (Nabipour & Mohammad, 2005; Sulu et al., 2010). In other words, an increase in altitude resulted in more appendicitis cases being seen during the winter months. The reason for this trend is unclear, but it has been reported that several factors may play a part: 1) the varying effects of bacterial or viral pathogens that cause infections at different temperatures, 2) the effect of allergens occurring in summer and warmer months, 3) changes in the form of nutrition, and 4) the effect of migration for touristic purposes during the summer. Another controversial environmental factor is daytime humidity. In a study by Brummer, a significant relationship was observed between humidity and AA, and it was reported, in their study on the physiology of hunger, that a decrease in body fluid loss, fecal stasis, and fecal dehydration prepared the ground for inflammation (Brumer, 1970). In contrast, van Nieuwenhoven et al. reported that changes in intestinal system functions such as intestinal permeability and orocaecal transit time were not the reason for dehydration occurring (van Nieuwenhoven et al., 2000). We also determined, during a 4-year (2004-2007) study using meteorological data in our region, that such data as moisture and amount of rain did not have an effect on the frequency of AA **(Table 3)**.

	Appendicitis	Perforated	z value	p value
Humidity (%)				
Winter	76.7±7.95 (54.0 - 94.0)	76.7±8.01 (60.7 - 94.0)	-0.054	0.957
Spring	68.2±10.24 (30.0 - 93.3)	67.7±10.77 (40.0 - 89.3)	-0.047	0.963
Summer	63.9±8.75 (35.0 - 87.8)	64.7±10.33 (36.0 - 87.8)	-1.191	0.234
Autumn	71.9±9.60 (47.3 - 94.0)	71.7±9.91 (48.7 - 93.3)	-0.148	0.882
General	70.4±10.32 (30.0 - 94.0)	69.6±10.75 (36.0 - 94.0)	-0.548	0.584
Temperature (°C)				
Winter	-5.8±6.41 (-21.1 - 8.5)	-6.5±7.19 (-19.7 - 7.2)	-0.751	0.453
Spring	10.7±5.14 (-4.6 - 19.7)	9.6±5.63 (-2.8 - 18.5)	-1.209	0.227
Summer	17.2±3.34 (8.7 - 28.6)	16.6±3.38 (6.2 - 23.3)	-1.031	0.302
Autumn	0.2±7.90 (-21.2 - 14.4)	0.8±9.48 (-21.2 - 14.4)	-0.912	0.362
General	5.3±10.81 (-21.2 - 28.6)	6.2±10.77 (-21.2 - 23.3)	-1.193	0.233

Table 3. Seasons, Humidity, and Temperature Distribution Levels by Group

Other factors said to influence AA development include vascular disorders, non-specific viral infections, depression and emotional problems due to a stressful lifestyle, being the child of a mother who smoked while pregnant, air pollution, and anemic diseases these have not, however, been widely accepted (Ahmed et al., 2005; Butland & Strachan, 1999; Ewald et al., 2001; Kaplan et al., 2009; Walker & Segal, 1995). As with the development of many diseases, the effect of genetics on the development of AA is unknown. In a survey of 282 patients, it was discovered that 21% of patients undergoing appendectomies had first-degree relatives (siblings, parents, and children), 12% had second-degree relatives (grandparents, grandchildren, uncles, aunts, nieces, and nephews), and 7% had third-degree relatives with a history of appendicitis (Basta et al., 1990). However, more research to reveal the transitional property of genetics in many bowel diseases is clearly needed.

5. Conclusion

As I have discussed briefly above, the development of AA is multifactorial. Many of these reasons are not clear and require further discussion **(Figure 2)**.

The most accepted are diet and hygiene. Appendicitis is considered a preventable disease due to the effect of factors such as diet and hygiene on its development. The morbidities that can result from this disease, as well as mortality rate, may therefore be reduced by improving the socioeconomic status of poorer communities, as well as by the members of these communities modifying their dietary habits. The cost per patient for the surgical treatment of appendicitis in the United States ranges from $ 11,577 to $ 13,965 (Long et al., 2001). Therefore, a reduction in appendicitis will benefit not only public health but will also make a substantial contribution to the economy.

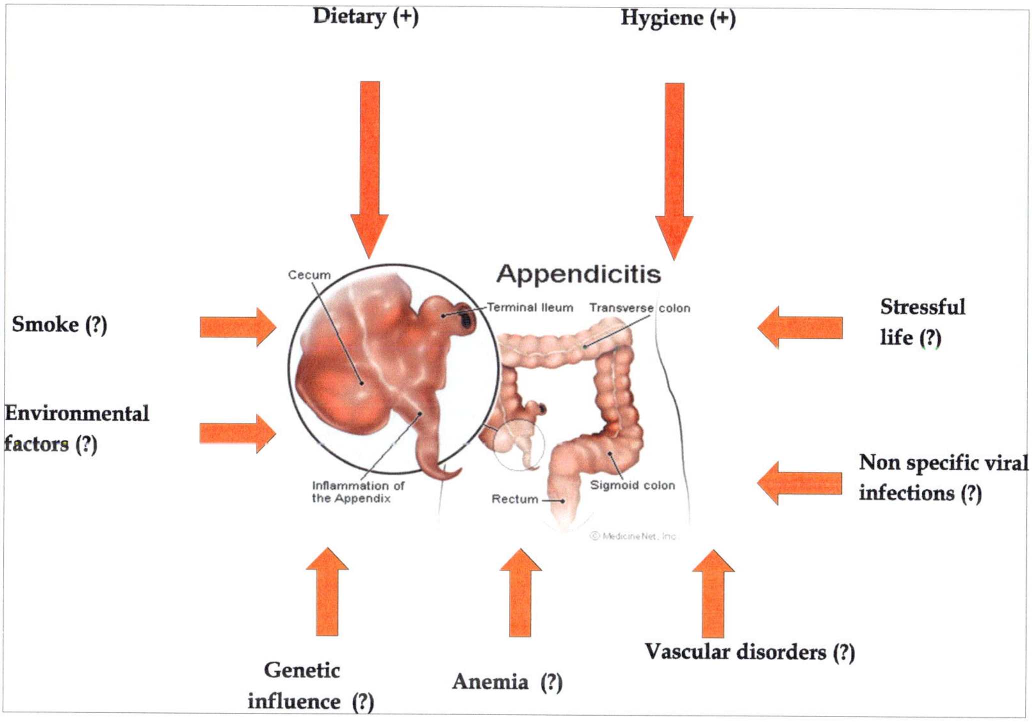

Fig. 2. Factors affecting the formation of appendicitis

6. References

Adamidis, D., Roma-Giannikou, E., Karamolegou, K., Tselalidou, E., & Constantopoulos, A. (2000). Fiber intake and childhood appendicitis. *Int J Food Sci Nutr*, Vol.51, No.3, pp.153-157, ISSN: 0963-7486

Addiss, DG., Shaffer, N., Fowler, BS., & Tauxe, RV. (1990). The epidemiology of appendicitis and appendectomy in the United States. *Am J Epidemiol*, Vol.132, No.5, pp.910-925, ISSN: 0002-9262

Ahmed, S., Shahid, RK., & Russo, LA. (2005). Unusual causes of abdominal pain: sickle cell anemia. *Best Pract Res Clin Gastroenterol*, Vol.19, No.2, pp.297-310, ISSN: 1521-691

Ajao, OG. (1979). Appendicitis in a tropical African population. *J Natl Med Assoc*, Vol.71, No.10, pp.997-999, ISSN: 0027-9684.

Al-Omran, M., Mamdani, M., & McLeod, RS. (2003). Epidemiologic features of acute appendicitis in Ontario, Canada. *Can J Surg*, Vol.46, No.4, pp.263-268, ISSN: 0008-428X

Andersson, RE. (2008). Changing trends in surgery for acute appendicitis (Br J Surg 2008; 95: 363-368). *Br J Surg*. Vol.95, No.9,pp.1187-1188, ISSN: 0007-1323

Andersen, SB., Paerregaard, A., & Larsen, K. (2009). Changes in the epidemiology of acute appendicitis and appendectomy in Danish children 1996-2004. *Eur J Pediatr Surg,* Vol.19, No.5,pp.286-289, ISSN: 0939-7248

Andreu-Ballester, JC., González-Sánchez, A., Ballester, F., Almela-Quilis, A., Cano-Cano, MJ., Millan-Scheiding, M., & del Castillo, JR. (2009). Epidemiology of appendectomy and appendicitis in the Valencian community (Spain), 1998-2007. *Dig Surg,* Vol.26, No.5, pp.406-412, ISSN: 0253-4886.

Arnbjörnsson, E. (1983). Acute appendicitis risk in various phases of the menstrual cycle. *Acta Chir Scand,* Vol.149, No.6,pp.603-605, ISSN: 0001-5482

Barker, DJ. (1985). Acute appendicitis and dietary fibre: an alternative hypothesis. *Br Med J (Clin Res Ed),* Vol. 290, No.6475,pp.1125-1127, ISSN: 0267-0623

Barker, D.J, Morris, JA., Simmonds, SJ., & Oliver, RH. (1988). Appendicitis epidemic following introduction of piped water to Anglesey. *J Epidemiol Community Health,* Vol.42, No.2,pp.144-148, ISSN: 0143-005X

Basta, M., Morton, NE., Mulvihill, JJ., Radovanović, Z., Radojicić, C., & Marinković, D. (1990). Inheritance of acute appendicitis: familial aggregation and evidence of polygenic transmission. *Am J Hum Genet, Vol.*46, No.2, pp.377-382, ISSN: 0002-9297

Brumer, M. (1970). Appendicitis. Seasonal incidence and postoperative wound infection. *Br J Surg,* Vol.57, No.2, pp.93-99, ISSN: 0007-1323

Butland, BK., & Strachan, DP. (1999). Smoking and acute appendicitis. *Lancet, Vol.*353, No.9165,pp.1712, ISSN: 0140-6736

Chatbanchai, W., Hedley, AJ., Ebrahim, SB., Areemit, S., Hoskyns, EW., & de Dombal, FT. (1989). Acute abdominal pain and appendicitis in north east Thailand. *Paediatr Perinat Epidemiol,* Vol.3, No.4, pp.448-459, ISSN: 0269-5022

Chavda, SK., Hassan, S., & Magoha, GA. (2005). Appendicitis at Kenyatta National Hospital, Nairobi. *East Afr Med J,* Vol.82, No.10, pp.526-530, ISSN: 0012-835X

Cirocchi, R., Morelli, U., La Mura, F., Cattorini, L., Napolitano, V., Galanov, I., Covarelli, P., Giustozzi, G., & Sciannameo, F. (2008). Acute appendicitis: a descending trend? *Minerva Chir,* Vol.63, No.2, pp.109-113. ISSN: 0026-4733

Deng, Y., Chang, DC., Zhang, Y., Webb, J., Gabre-Kidan, A., & Abdullah, F. (2010). Seasonal and day of the week variations of perforated appendicitis in US children. *Pediatr Surg Int,* Vol.26, No.7, pp.691-696, ISSN: 0179-0358

Ergul, E. (2007). Heredity and familial tendency of acute appendicitis. *Scand J Surg,* Vol.96, No.4,pp.290-292, ISSN: 1457-4969

Ewald, H., Mortensen, PB., & Mors, O. (2001). Decreased risk of acute appendicitis in patients with schizophrenia or manic-depressive psychosis. *Schizophr Res,* Vol.49, No.3, pp.287-293, ISSN: 0920-9964

Freud, E., Pilpel, D., & Mares, AJ. (1988). Acute appendicitis in childhood in the Negev region: some epidemiological observations over an 11-year period (1973-1983). *J Pediatr Gastroenterol Nutr,* Vol.7, No.5,pp.680-684. ISSN: 0277-2116

Gallerani, M., Boari, B., Anania, G., Cavallesco, G., & Manfredini, R. (2006). Seasonal variation in onset of acute appendicitis. *Clin Ter.* Vol.157, No.2, pp.123-127. ISSN: 0009-9074

Jones, BA., Demetriades, D., Segal, I., & Burkitt, DP. (1985). The prevalence of appendiceal fecaliths in patients with and without appendicitis. A comparative study from Canada and South Africa. *Ann Surg.* Vol.202, No.1, pp.80-82. ISSN: 0003-4932

Kaplan, GG., Dixon, E., Panaccione, R., Fong, A., Chen, L., Szyszkowicz, M., Wheeler, A., MacLean, A., Buie, WD., Leung, T., Heitman, SJ., & Villeneuve, PJ. (2009). Effect of ambient air pollution on the incidence of appendicitis. *CMAJ, Vol.*181, No.9, pp.591-597, ISSN: 0008-4409

Lee, JH., Park, YS., & Choi, JS. (2010). The epidemiology of appendicitis and appendectomy in South Korea: national registry data. *J Epidemiol,* Vol.20, No.2,pp.97-105, ISSN: 0917-5040

Long, KH., Bannon, MP., Zietlow, SP., Helgeson, ER., Harmsen, WS., Smith, CD., Ilstrup, DM., Baerga-Varela, Y., & Sarr, MG. (2001). Laparoscopic Appendectomy Interest Group. A prospective randomized comparison of laparoscopic appendectomy with open appendectomy: Clinical and economic analyses. *Surgery,* Vol.129, No.4, pp.390-400. ISSN: 0263-9319

Luckmann, R., & Davis, P. (1991). The epidemiology of acute appendicitis in California: racial, gender, and seasonal variation. *Epidemiology,* Vol.2, No.5, pp.323-330, ISSN: 1044-3983

Morris, J., Barker, D.J, & Nelson, M. (1987). Diet, infection, and acute appendicitis in Britain and Ireland. *J Epidemiol Community Health,* Vol.41, No.1, pp.44-49, ISSN: 0143-005X

Nabipour, F., & Mohammad, BD. (2005). Histopathological features of acute appendicitis in Kerman-Iran from 1997 to 2003. *American J. Environmental Sci,* Vol.1, No.2, pp.130-132, ISSN: 1553-345X

Noudeh, YJ., Sadigh, N,. & Ahmadnia, AY. (2007).Epidemiologic features, seasonal variations and false positive rate of acute appendicitis in Shahr-e-Rey, Tehran. *Int J Surg, Vol.*5, No,2,pp.95-98, ISSN: 1743-9191

Oguntola, AS., Adeoti, ML., & Oyemolade, TA. (2010). Appendicitis: Trends in incidence, age, sex, and seasonal variations in South-Western Nigeria. *Ann Afr Med,* Vol. 9, No.4,pp.213-217, ISSN: 1596-3519

Papadopoulos, AA., Polymeros, D., Kateri, M., Tzathas, C., Koutras, M., & Ladas, SD. (2008). Dramatic decline of acute appendicitis in Greece over 30 years: index of improvement of socioeconomic conditions or diagnostic aids? *Dig Dis,* Vol.26, No.1, pp.80-84. Epub 2008 Feb 15. ISSN: 0257-2753

Simpson, J., Samaraweera, AP., Sara, RK., & Lobo, DN. (2008). Acute appendicitis--a benign disease? *Ann R Coll Surg Engl,* Vol.90, No.4, pp.313-316, ISSN: 0035-8843

Sulu, B., Gunerhan, Y., Ozturk, B., & Arslan, H. (2010). Is long-term hunger (Ramadan model) a risk factor for acute appendicitis? *Saudi Med J,* Vol.31, No.1, pp.59-63, ISSN: 0379-5284

Sulu, B., Günerhan, Y., Palanci, Y., Işler, B., & Cağlayan, K. (2010). Epidemiological and demographic features of appendicitis and influences of several environmental factors. *Ulus Travma Acil Cerrahi Derg, Vol.*16, No.1, pp.38-42, ISSN: 1306-696X

Terada, T. (2009). Schistosomal appendicitis: incidence in Japan and a case report. *World J Gastroenterol,* Vol.15, No.13, pp.1648-1649, ISSN: 1007-9327

Trepanowski, JF., & Bloomer, RJ. (2010). The impact of religious fasting on human health. *Nutr J,* Vol.9, No.57, ISSN: 1475-2891

van Nieuwenhoven, MA., Vriens, BE., Brummer, RJ., & Brouns, F. (2000). Effect of dehydration on gastrointestinal function at rest and during exercise in humans. *Eur J Appl Physiol,* Vol.83, No.6, pp.578-584, ISSN: 1439-6319

Walker, AR., & Segal, I. (1979). Is appendicitis increasing in South African blacks? *S Afr Med J*, Vol.56, No.13, pp.503-504, ISSN: 0256-9574

Walker, AR., Walker, BF., Duvenhage, A., Jones, J., Ncongwane, J., & Segal, I. (1982). Appendicectomy prevalences in South African adolescents. *Digestion*, Vol.23, No.4, pp.274-278, ISSN: 0012-2823

Walker, AR., & Segal, I. (1995). Appendicitis: an African perspective. *J R Soc Med*, Vol. 88, No.11, pp.616-619, ISSN: 0141-0768

Williams, NM., Jackson, D., Everson, NW., & Johnstone, JM. (1998). Is the incidence of acute appendicitis really falling? *Ann R Coll Surg Engl*, Vol.80, No.2, pp.122-124, ISSN: 0035-8843

Zoguéreh, DD., Lemaître, X., Ikoli, JF., Delmont, J., Chamlian, A., Mandaba, JL., & Nali, NM. (2001). [Acute appendicitis at the National University Hospital in Bangui, Central African Republic: epidemiologic, clinical, paraclinical and therapeutic aspects]. *Sante*, Vol.11, No.2,pp.117-125, ISSN: 1157-5999

10

Current Evidence and Recommendations for Laparoscopic Appendectomy

Hurng-Sheng Wu[1,3,4,5,6], James Wall[2],
Hung-Wen Lai[1] and Jacques Marescaux[2]
[1]*Asia Institute Tele-Surgery*
[2]*European Institute Tele-Surgery*
[3]*Show-Chwan Memorial Hospital, Chang-Hua*
[4]*Chang-Bin Show Chwan Memorial Hospital, Chang-Hua*
[5]*Tri-service General Hospital, Taipei*
[6]*National Defense Medical Center, Taipei*
R.O.C.

1. Introduction

Acute appendicitis is the most common etiology of the acute abdomen, generally requiring urgent surgical intervention. The lifetime incidence of acute appendicitis is approximate 7%. In 1886, Fitz described the natural course of appendicitis. He began advocating early appendectomy to prevent perforation with subsequent complications of sepsis, shock and potential mortality. In 1894 McBurney introduced the right lower quadrant incision to approach the appendix. The open appendectomy (OA) through a McBurney incision came into favour more than a century ago. It is a simple, safe, quick, and effective operation that can be performed by a general surgeon with the basic surgical instruments.

2. Laparoscopic appendectomy

During the past two decades, general surgery has seen a major shift from open to minimally invasive surgery. This has been driven by the development of laparoscopic technology that enables surgeons to perform increasingly complex tasks through small incisions. Laparoscopic appendectomy (LA) was one of the first reported laparoscopic cases in general surgery by de Kok in 1977[1]. Despite an early start, it did not enjoy the same popularity as other general surgery procedures such as laparoscopic cholecystectomy.

There are over 2000 articles on LA and over 60 randomized clinical trials comparing OA to LA. In the 2004 Cochrane review of OA versus LA several key differences were noted[2]. Wound infections were less likely after LA than after OA; however the incidence of intraabdominal abscesses was higher after LA. The duration of surgery was on average 10 minutes longer for laparoscopic procedures. Pain on day 1 after surgery was modestly reduced after LA on a 100 point visual analog scale and hospital stay was shortened by 1.1 days after LA. Return to normal activity, work, and sport occurred earlier after laparoscopic procedures than after open procedures. While the operation costs of laparoscopic procedures were significantly higher, the costs outside hospital were reduced. The conclusion of the review was that young female, obese, and employed patients seem to benefit from the laparoscopic procedure more than other groups. The European Association of Endoscopic Surgeons (EAES) has recently released guidelines on appendectomy that clearly favor the laparoscopic approach[3]. The justification includes the benefits of decreased wound infection and faster return to activity. EAES additionally highlights that the highest level of evidence for benefit of LA over OA is in women of childbearing age and obese patients.

We performed a retrospective analysis of 1366 patients with acute appendicitis at Changhua and Chang-Bing Show-Chwan Memorial Hospitals from January 1, 2004 to December 31, 2009[4]. Compared with OA, LA was associated with a lower complication rate (9.5% versus 5.8%; P=0.013), a lower wound infection rate (8.6% versus 4.2%; P=0.001), and a shorter hospital stay (4.60±3.64 versus 4.06±1.84 days; P=0.001), but a higher mean cost (32,670±28,568 versus 37,567±12,064 New Taiwan dollars). In the subgroup analysis, the patients with complicated appendicitis, female patients, and pediatric and elderly patients benefited from a reduced hospital stay.

A global trend toward an increased use of laparoscopic appendectomy has been observed. Hove et al. reported an increase in the United States from 19.1% in 1997 to 37.9% in 2003 based on the Nationwide Inpatient Sample[5]. Sporn et al. reported a further increase to 58% in 2005 based in the same sampling technique[6]. In our institution the rate has increased rapidly, from 8.1% in 2004 to 90.3% in 2009[4]. The reasons for such a rapid increase are not entirely clear in light of the modest benefits of LA over OA at significantly increased cost. The increased adoption of LA is undoubtedly multifactorial and includes motivations of the surgeon, patient and medical device industry that go beyond the measurable outcome benefits. From the surgeons' perspective, laparoscopy offers greater flexibility for both diagnosis and intervention in the event of finding unexpected pathology when operating on suspected appendicitis. In addition, the current generation of surgeons is significantly more familiar and comfortable with laparoscopy. Satisfaction with improved cosmetic results and a perception of decreased surgical trauma is driving patient demand for less invasive surgical approaches. Finally, the medical device industry profits from the increased use of laparoscopic technologies and has gone to great lengths to promote minimally invasive approaches.

Findings	**Statistical Significance**
Lower wound infection rate for LA	0.43 odds ratio (0.34 - 0.54 95% CI)
Higher intra-abdominal abscess rate	2.48 odds ratio (1.45 - 4.21 95% CI)
12 minute longer operating time for LA	12 min (7-16 95% CI)
Decreased post-operative pain after LA on a 100 point visual analog scale	2.48 odds ratio (1.45 - 4.21 95% CI)
Decreased hospital stay by 1.1 day after LA	1.1 day (0.6 - 1.5 95%CI)
Reduced risk of negative appendectomy with diagnostic laparoscopy in women of child bearing age	0.20 odds ratio (0.11 - 0.34)
Reduced risk of negative appendectomy with diagnostic laparoscopy in the general adult population	0.37 odd ratio (0.13 - 1.01)

Table 1. Summary of findings from the 2004 Cochrane review of LA vs OA.

3. Minimally invasive training

Appropriate laparoscopic training is important in assuring good surgical outcomes. Iatrogenic bowel perforations and vascular injuries from both trocar placement and out of field instruments have been reported in LA[7,8]. These injuries should be avoidable with appropriate training and experience. With the growing popularity of minimally invasive surgery, there is an increasing need to training surgeons to become proficient in minimally invasive techniques. In Asia, the Asia Institute Tele-Surgery (AITS) laparoscopic training center has played a major role in increasing surgeons' preference for laparoscopic appendectomy.

4. Complex appendicitis

Complex appendicitis includes the presence of an intraabdominal abscess or a phlegmon. The risk of surgical complications is increased in these situations. Conservative treatment with antibiotics followed by interval appendectomy has been proposed since the 1920s in patients who do not have generalized peritonitis[9]. This approach has been reported to carry significantly fewer complications, wound infections, abdominal/pelvic abscesses, ileus/bowel obstructions, and reoperations while not increasing hospitalization or length of antibiotic use[10]. Interval appendectomy after successful conservative treatment of an appendiceal mass remains controversial. The rate of recurrent appendicitis in patients has been reported as high as 10-20% and interval appendectomy was generally recommended in all but the highest risk patients [11]. More recent studies show that the failure rate of conservative treatment ranges from 5-15% and those patients will require surgical intervention within the first few moths[12]. However, recurrent appendicitis beyond one year of successful conservative management is low at 2% and interval appendectomy in those patients may not be justified[13]. We believe there is still a role for interval appendectomy with benefits for a substantial group of patients, but it is not routinely necessary. If it is to be performed a laparoscopic approach is appropriate.

5. Technique for laparoscopic appendectomy

5.1 Patient positioning and room setup

The patient is positioned as for an open appendectomy in the supine position with the legs together, right arm angled on a board, and left arm tucked alongside the body (Image 1). This position allows the surgeon and their assistant to work on the left side of the patient. A single monitor is placed over the right side of the patient. In order to facilitate maximal exposure of the appendix after trocar placement, the operating table is placed in a Trendelenburg position and tilted to the left.

5.2 Instrumentation

We use the following instrumentation at our institution for standard laparoscopic appendectomy.

1. 0° laparoscope
2. Fine dissection scissors
3. Peanut swab
4. Fenestrated grasping forceps
5. Bipolar cauterizing grasper

6. Clip applicator
7. Electrocautery hook
8. Suction-irrigation device
9. 2 endoloops
10. Extraction bag.

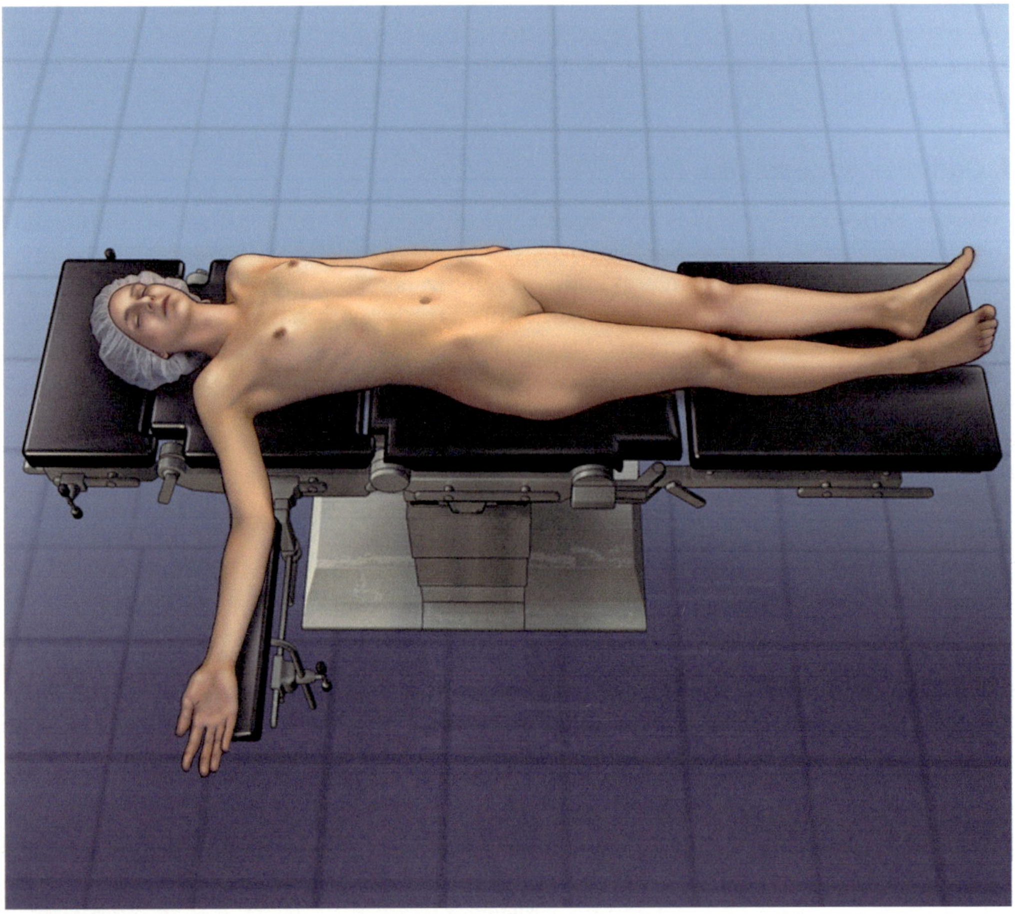

Image 1. Patient positioning for laparoscopic appendectomy. The left arm is tucked by the side and the right arm is angled on a board.

5.3 Trocar placement

Three trocars placed in triangular formation are generally needed: one optical trocar and two operating trocars. The optical trocar is generally a 10/11mm trocar placed in the peri-umbilical position. Smaller 3-5mm optics can be used, particularily in children. Two operating trocars are placed ideally at a minimum of 8 to 10cm from one another. One operating trocar (5 or 10/11mm) is placed in the midline suprapubic position and another operating trocar (5 or 10/11mm) is placed in left iliac fossa position (Image 2). Some authors place the second operating trocar in the right iliac fossa, however we find that this places a working instrument too close to the field of interest. Another notable variation is placement of the two working ports adjacent to one another in the suprapubic position. This reduces the benefits of the triangulation of the working instruments described above, but leaves scars generally hidden below the waistline. Another option is to use two 5mm operating ports placed similarly. As with any laparoscopic case, as difficulty arise with retraction and visualization, additional ports can be added.

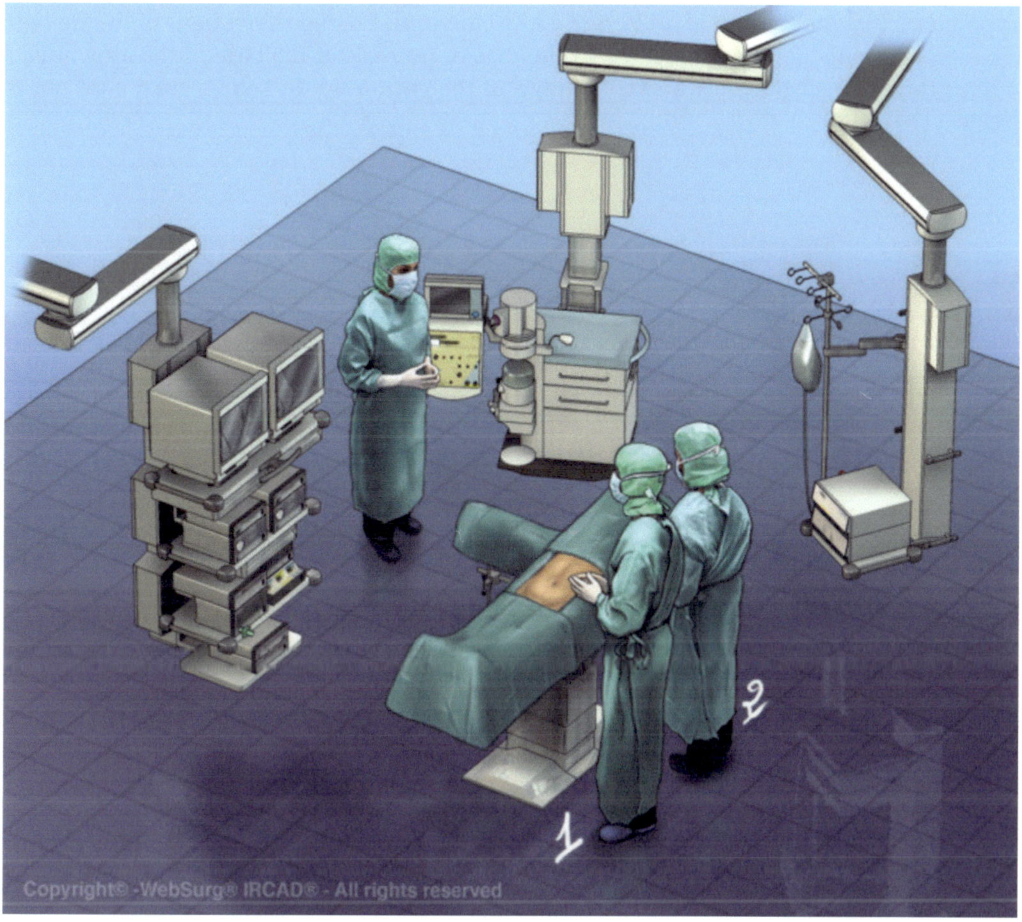

Image 2. Operating room setup for laparoscopic appendectomy. The surgeon and assistant are positioned on the left side of the patient with a monitor on the right side of the patient.

5.4 Dissection

The procedure begins with an exploration to confirm the diagnosis of acute appendicitis. Laparoscopy is clearly superior to the surgeons' finger through a McBurney's point incision in the diagnosis of alternative abdominal pathologies.

If acute appendicitis is confirmed, any adhesions between the appendix and the peritoneal wall are divided to expose the appendix from its tip to its base. The appendix is frequently located laterally or posterior to the cecum. Next the mesoappendix is controlled using either bipolar forceps or a harmonic scalpel for coagulation of the appendicial artery. Finally the ligation of the appendix and control of the appendiceal stump are performed. Double ligation of the base of the appendix is performed with a Surgitie™ Loop (Covidien) or an ENDOLOOP® Ligature (Ethicon) and the appendix is amputated with scissors. The appendix can be extracted through a port site directly or placed into a specimen bag to prevent contamination. The specimen is extracted through the largest port site, which is typically the 10/11mm periumbilical trocar. Alternative approaches include the use of an Endo GIA™ Universal Stapler (Covidien) to divide both the mesoappendix and the appendix. In the case of necrosis of the base of the appendix, a stapler can be used to resect a small wedge of the cecum while taking great care not to create a stenosis.

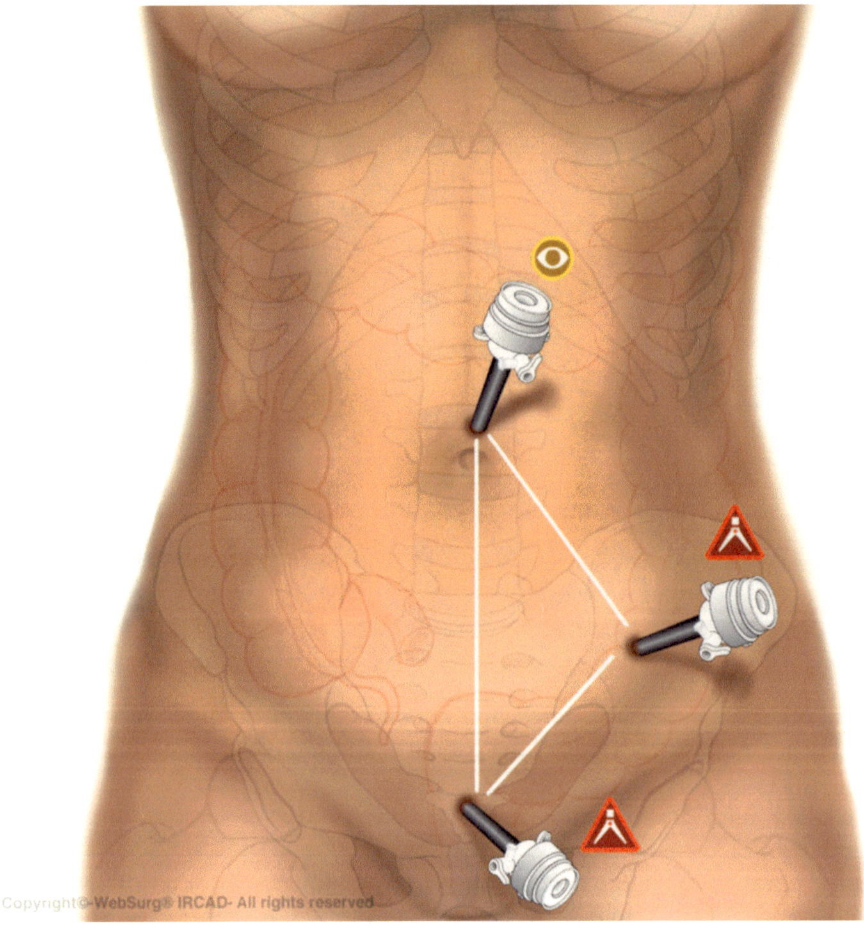

Image 3. Preferred trocar placement for laparoscopic appendectomy. An optical trocar in the umbilicus and working trocars in the suprapubic and left lower quadrant.

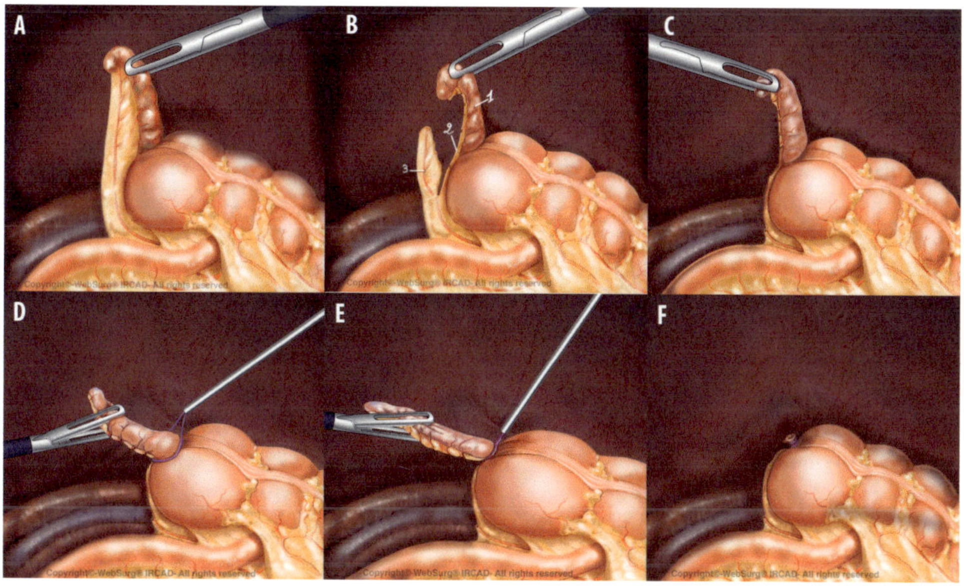

Image 4. Basic technique of laparoscopic appendectomy. (A) exposure of the appendix and meso appendix (B) division of the mesoappendix and appendicial artery (C) isolation of the appendicial base (D) placement of endoloop at the base of the appendix (E) ligation of the base of the appendix (F) completed appendectomy.

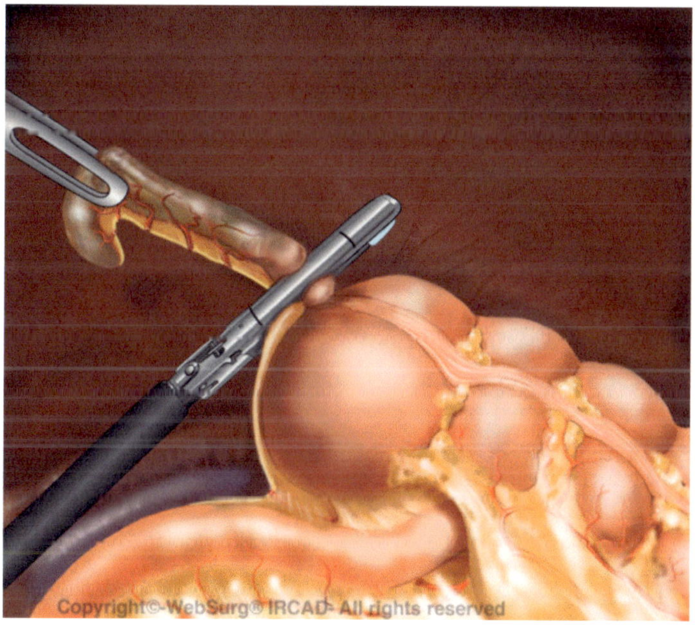

Image 5. Alternative approach to division of the appendix using an EndoGIA stapler. This approach is useful for a necrotic appendicial base that may require a small wedge resection of the cecum taking care not to create a stenosis.

6. Emerging technologies

6.1 Single Incision Laparoscopic Surgery (SILS)

Minimally invasive surgery has seen the emergence of two new techniques that attempt to further minimize surgical trauma for the benefit of the patient. Single Incision Laparoscopic Surgery (SILS) attempts to limit abdominal wall trauma by performing procedures through a single incision that can accommodate multiple working instruments. SILS procedures are technically demanding due to multiple factors including 1) internal and external conflicts between operating instruments and the optical system, 2) lack of triangulation for working instruments, 3) in-line view, and 4) limited ability to retract and expose. Early reports used more endoscopic techniques[14], but a recent emergence of single port operating systems have begun to address the challenges of SILS with such innovations as angulated instruments. Appendectomy may be ideally suited for SILS as the procedure rarely requires significant retraction, the dissection is not complex and the operative field is limited to the right lower quadrant. Initial reports have shown the feasibility of SILS[15,16], and trials are ongoing to compare the benefits with traditional LA. While awaiting the results of definitive trials, SILS appears to be a reasonable approach in highly skilled hands.

6.2 Natural Orifice Transluminal Endoscopic Surgery (NOTES)

Natural Orifice Transluminal Endoscopic Surgery goes a step beyond SILS in minimizing abdominal wall trauma by avoiding any abdominal incisions. The concept of NOTES is to introduce a flexible operative platform through natural orifices including the mouth, vagina or anus. A vicerotomy is made in the wall of the stomach, vagina, or rectum respectively to gain access into the peritoneal cavity. The procedure is then performed and any specimen extracted through the natural orifice, leaving behind no abdominal scar. Both transvaginal and transgastric NOTES appendectomy have been performed in humans[17,18], but major concerns exist around the need to create a vicerotomy in an otherwise healthy organ and then securely close the defect. NOTES appendectomy can currently only be considered appropriate for experienced surgeon in the setting of approved clinical trials.

7. Conclusion

The management of appendicitis is at the core of general surgery practice. The development of minimally invasive surgery has offered the surgeon a wider range of options in the treatment of this age-old disease. Laparoscopy is a robust and safe platform that allows the surgeon more flexibility in exploring the abdomen than the traditional McBurney's incision. Overall benefits of LA are modest but measurable and multiple factors have combined to significantly increase the choice of LA over OA in recent years. Appropriate training is necessary for all new technologies and techniques in the OR. Emerging technologies are on the horizon that may further minimize surgical trauma for the benefit of patients.

8. References

[1] de Kok HJ. A new technique for resecting the non-inflamed not-adhesive appendix through a mini-laparotomy with the aid of the laparoscope. *Arch Chir Neerl.* 1977;29(3):195-198.

[2] Sauerland S, Lefering R, Neugebauer EA. Laparoscopic versus open surgery for suspected appendicitis. *Cochrane Database Syst Rev.* 2004(4):CD001546.

[3] Vettoretto N, Gobbi S, Corradi A, et al. Consensus conference on laparoscopic appendectomy: development of guidelines. *Colorectal Dis.* Jul 2011;13(7):748-754.

[4] Wu HS, Lai HW, Kuo SJ, et al. Competitive edge of laparoscopic appendectomy versus open appendectomy: a subgroup comparison analysis. *J Laparoendosc Adv Surg Tech A.* Apr 2011;21(3):197-202.

[5] Van Hove C, Hardiman K, Diggs B, Deveney C, Sheppard B. Demographic and socioeconomic trends in the use of laparoscopic appendectomy from 1997 to 2003. *Am J Surg.* May 2008;195(5):580-583; discussion 583-584.

[6] Sporn E, Petroski GF, Mancini GJ, Astudillo JA, Miedema BW, Thaler K. Laparoscopic appendectomy--is it worth the cost? Trend analysis in the US from 2000 to 2005. *J Am Coll Surg.* Feb 2009;208(2):179-185 e172.

[7] Long KH, Bannon MP, Zietlow SP, et al. A prospective randomized comparison of laparoscopic appendectomy with open appendectomy: Clinical and economic analyses. *Surgery.* Apr 2001;129(4):390-400.

[8] Guloglu R, Dilege S, Aksoy M, et al. Major retroperitoneal vascular injuries during laparoscopic cholecystectomy and appendectomy. *J Laparoendosc Adv Surg Tech A.* Apr 2004;14(2):73-76.

[9] Soresi AL. Technic of Appendectomy: Description of a Rational, Safe and Easy Technic of the Operation for Acute and Interval Appendicitis. *Ann Surg.* Mar 1920;71(3):315-346.

[10] Simillis C, Symeonides P, Shorthouse AJ, Tekkis PP. A meta-analysis comparing conservative treatment versus acute appendectomy for complicated appendicitis (abscess or phlegmon). *Surgery.* Jun 2010;147(6):818-829.

[11] Bradley EL, 3rd, Isaacs J. Appendiceal abscess revisited. *Arch Surg.* Feb 1978;113(2):130-132.

[12] Willemsen PJ, Hoorntje LE, Eddes EH, Ploeg RJ. The need for interval appendectomy after resolution of an appendiceal mass questioned. *Dig Surg.* 2002;19(3):216-220; discussion 221.

[13] Tekin A, Kurtoglu HC, Can I, Oztan S. Routine interval appendectomy is unnecessary after conservative treatment of appendiceal mass. *Colorectal Dis.* Jun 2008;10(5):465-468.

[14] Inoue H, Takeshita K, Endo M. Single-port laparoscopy assisted appendectomy under local pneumoperitoneum condition. *Surg Endosc.* Jun 1994;8(6):714-716.

[15] Lee J, Baek J, Kim W. Laparoscopic transumbilical single-port appendectomy: initial experience and comparison with three-port appendectomy. *Surg Laparosc Endosc Percutan Tech.* Apr 2010;20(2):100-103.

[16] Chow A, Purkayastha S, Paraskeva P. Appendicectomy and cholecystectomy using single-incision laparoscopic surgery (SILS): the first UK experience. *Surg Innov.* Sep 2009;16(3):211-217.

[17] Park PO, Bergstrom M. Transgastric peritoneoscopy and appendectomy: thoughts on our first experience in humans. *Endoscopy.* Jan 2010;42(1):81-84.

[18] Palanivelu C, Rajan PS, Rangarajan M, Parthasarathi R, Senthilnathan P, Prasad M. Transvaginal endoscopic appendectomy in humans: a unique approach to NOTES--world's first report. *Surg Endosc.* May 2008;22(5):1343-1347.

11

Laparoscopic Appendicectomy

Maheswaran Pitchaimuthu
SpR in General/HPB Surgery,
Department of Surgery, Queens Medical Centre,
Nottingham University Hospitals NHS Trust, Nottingham,
UK

1. Introduction

Appendicitis is the most common surgical emergency, with the greatest incidence in the 2nd decade of life. It is 40% more common in males than females [1]. The clinical presentation, investigations and management options are discussed elsewhere in this text book. The laparoscopic or keyhole approach has become widespread where facilities are available. Kurt Semm from Switzerland performed the first laparoscopic appendicectomy in 1980 [2]. However, it was not widely practiced until the success of elective laparoscopic cholecystectomy was well established. Improvements in instruments, video equipment and training have made this a routine approach for the emergency appendicectomy.

2. Advantages

There are benefits for laparoscopy when the diagnosis of appendicitis is in doubt especially in young women when other diagnoses are relatively common. There is evidence for reduced wound infection rates, less postoperative pain and earlier return to normal activities. It may also reduce postoperative adhesion formation and it provides better cosmesis.

3. Patient selection

Most patients with suspected appendicitis can undergo a laparoscopic appendicectomy. It is particularly also useful in obese patients in whom it avoids a large wound. However, laparoscopic appendicectomy is generally avoided in patients with major cardio-respiratory problems. In patients who have had previous lower abdominal surgery, it may be difficult to visualize the appendix due to adhesions. Some consider that laparoscopic appendicectomy is contraindicated in patients who are septic and have generalized peritonitis, where laparotomy may be preferable. In advanced pregnancy laparoscopic appendicectomy may be difficult due to the gravid uterus which interferes with adequate visualization and instrumentation [3]

4. Preoperative assessment and preparation

The preoperative assessment and preparation for laparoscopic appendicectomy is similar to any surgical procedure. Patients are assessed for fitness for general anesthesia and coagulation

is corrected if necessary prior to surgery. When obtaining consent, it is important to explain the procedure to the patient, especially the possibility of open conversion. Patients should also be informed about potential complications including bleeding, wound infection, intra abdominal collections, appendicular stump leak and faecal fistula.
All patients should be kept fasting at least 6 hrs prior to the procedure and should be given intravenous fluids to avoid dehydration. Antibiotics should be given preoperatively especially in those who show signs of sepsis (spiking temperature, high white cell count and CRP).

5. Procedure

5.1 Position

After general anesthesia with muscle relaxation, the patient is placed in the supine position with the left arm by the side. This is very important to allow sufficient space for the surgeon and the assistant who stand on the left side of the patient. The position of the surgeon and the assistant differs depending upon the port sites. Some surgeons prefer the lithotomy position, especially in women to allow access to the perineum, so that a cervical manipulator can be used to get a better visualization of the pelvic organs [4]. The monitor is on the right side of the patient. The bladder is catheterized to get a better view of the pelvis and to avoid bladder injury during suprapubic port insertion. The catheter can be removed at the end of the procedure.

5.2 Recommended Instruments

1. 5 -12mm trocar (camera port)
2. Two 5mm trocars or one 5mm and one 10mm trocar with reducer
3. Two atraumatic bowel grasping forceps
4. One dissecting curved forceps
5. One curved scissors
6. One hook
7. Bipolar / Monopolar diathermy
8. Endoloop x 3 (Ethicon Endoloop®Ligature PDS II/Vicryl Suture)
9. Clip applicator with clips if necessary
10. Vascular and intestine stapler if necessary
11. Retrieval bag if necessary
12. Drain if necessary

5.3 Ports

Usually 3 ports are required to perform a laparoscopic appendicectomy. The first trocar is introduced through an infra or supra umbilical incision by using either a Veress needle or through an open technique. Once the umbilical port is inserted a pneumoperitoneum is created and the intraperitoneal pressure is set at 12 mmHg with a maximum of 14mmHg being accepted in adults. In children the maximum pressure is lower at around 8 -10 mmHg [5]. A 0 or 30 degree telescope is inserted and other ports are inserted under vision. If there is fogging of the telescope lens an anti fogging solution is used. The other two port positions are placed depending upon surgeon's preference. The author's standard practice is to have a left iliac fossa and a supra pubic working port [Fig. 1], where the assistant stands on the surgeon's right.

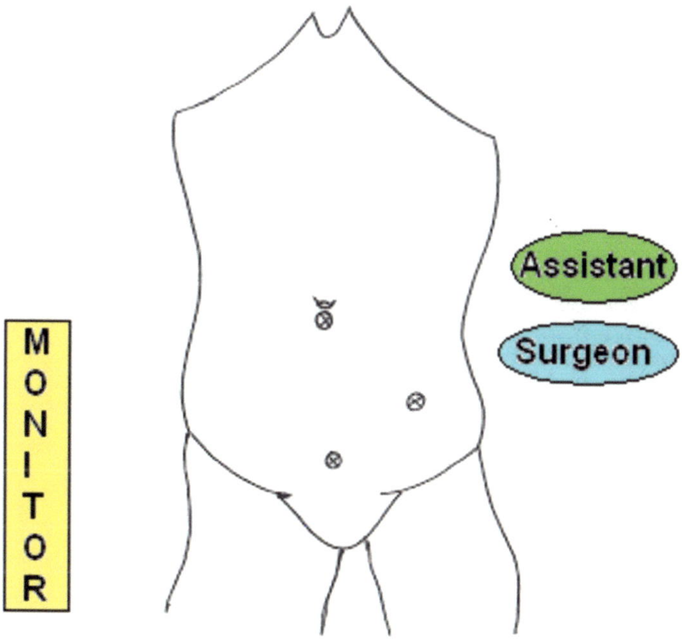

Fig. 1. Port positions for laparoscopic appendicectomy

Other port positions include,

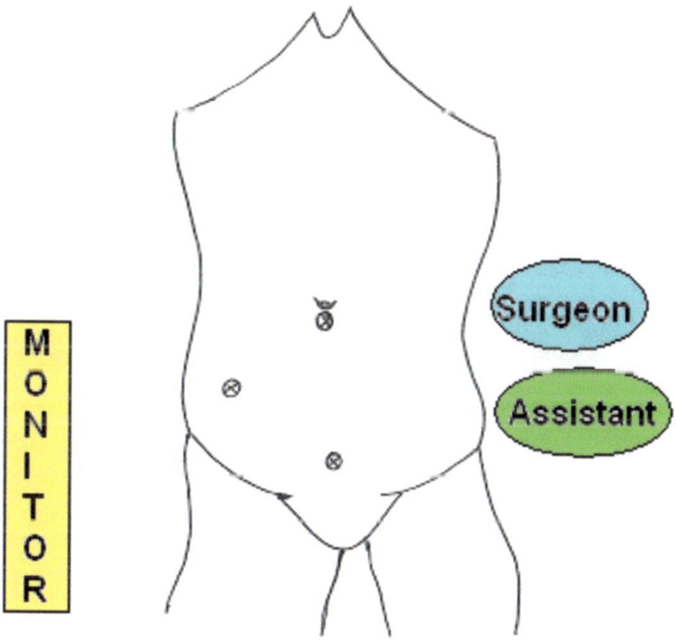

Fig. 2. a) Umbilical, suprapubic and right iliac (assistant on surgeon's left)

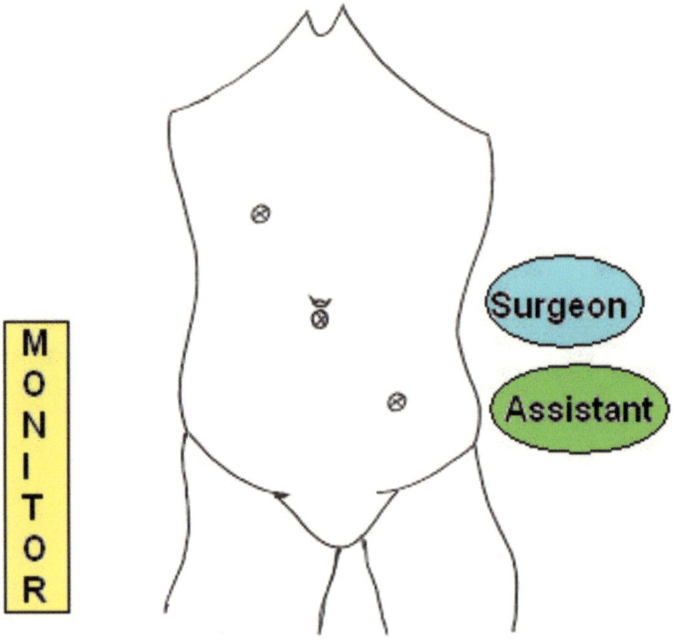

Fig. 2. b) Umbilical, left iliac and right hypochondrium (assistant on surgeon's left)

5.4 Diagnostic laparoscopy

Once the telescope is inserted, a general laparoscopy of the entire abdomen is performed to rule out any other intra abdominal pathology and to assess the degree of peritonitis from the spread of purulent peritoneal fluid. Then the patient is placed in the trendelenburg position to visualize the pelvic organs, especially in women to rule out gynecological pathology. Then the patient is tilted with the right side up to get a view of the caecum and appendix. If the appendix is inflamed the appendicectomy is performed as detailed below.

5.5 Management of the macroscopically normal appendix

If the appendix is macroscopically normal [Fig. 3], then a careful search should be made for other pathology such as caecal diverticulitis, terminal ileitis, terminal ileal Crohn's disease, Meckel's diverticulitis. In females, pelvic inflammatory disease, salphingitis, ovarian cyst rupture or torsion, tubo ovarian abscess, and endometriosis should be looked for. If any of the above pathology is encountered, then the operation should be modified according to the unexpected findings.

If every thing is normal, the author's preference is to take the normal appendix out. The reasons as follows a) 75% of patients get improvement in their pain symptoms [6] b) There may be a pathological inflammation, even if the appendix is grossly normal [7] c) adequate inspection of the appendix needs mobilization, which may cause trauma to the appendix and mesoappendix, where it is not advisable to leave the appendix d) In one study patients who only had diagnostic laparoscopy without removal of appendix, presented later with recurrent abdominal pain [8] e) Performing laparoscopic appendicectomy for a normal appendix is simple and quick [9] f) to avoid future appendicitis.

Some surgeons prefer to leave the normal appendix to avoid the complications related to the procedure.

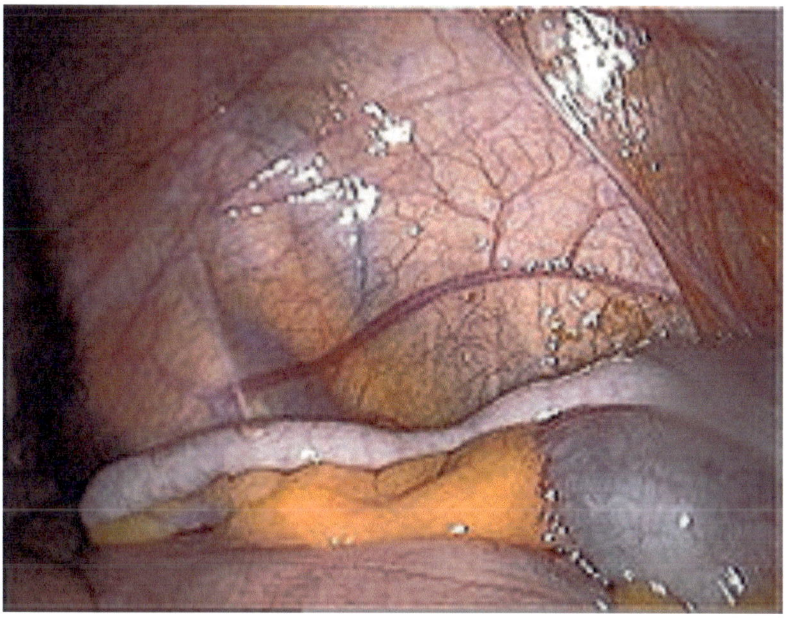

Fig. 3. Normal looking appendix on laparoscopy

5.6 Dissection of the appendix

Once the diagnosis of appendicitis is confirmed [Fig. 4], the tip of the appendix is grasped with atraumatic bowel grasping forceps inserted through the lower port and the appendix is lifted towards the anterior abdominal wall with the surgeon's left hand. Then a curved dissecting forceps is inserted through the upper port to start the dissection. If the tip is not visualized due to omental adhesions, which is usually the case, the adhesions are gently teased away from the appendix. Then a relatively healthy, non necrotic part of the appendix is grasped with left hand and the dissection continues towards the base.

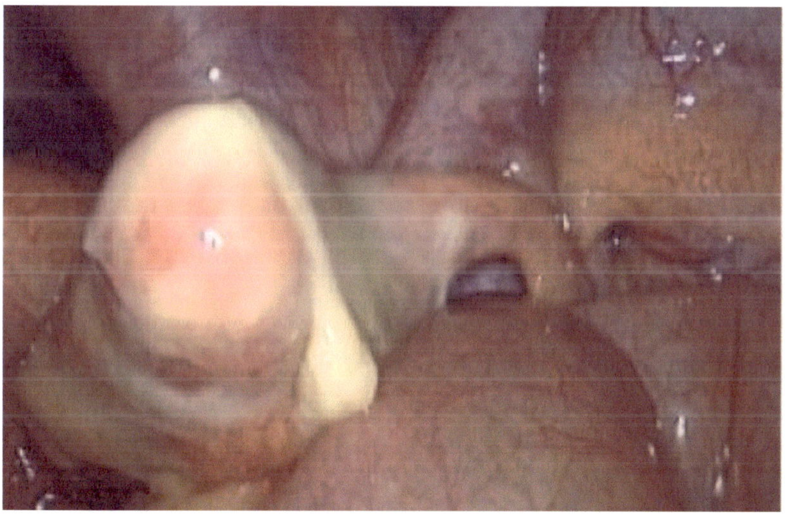

Fig. 4. Inflamed appendix on laparoscopy

If the tip is not visualized due to an unusual position [Fig. 5], then the base should be identified, which is usually 2cm lateral and inferior to ileo-caecal junction. If the base is correctly identified then there are 2 options. 1) grasp the base and dissect towards the tip without dividing it. 2) Divide the base between two ligations (intra or extra corporeal sutures), within 5mm of the attachment to the caecum and then continue the dissection of the appendix and the mesoappendix towards the tip.

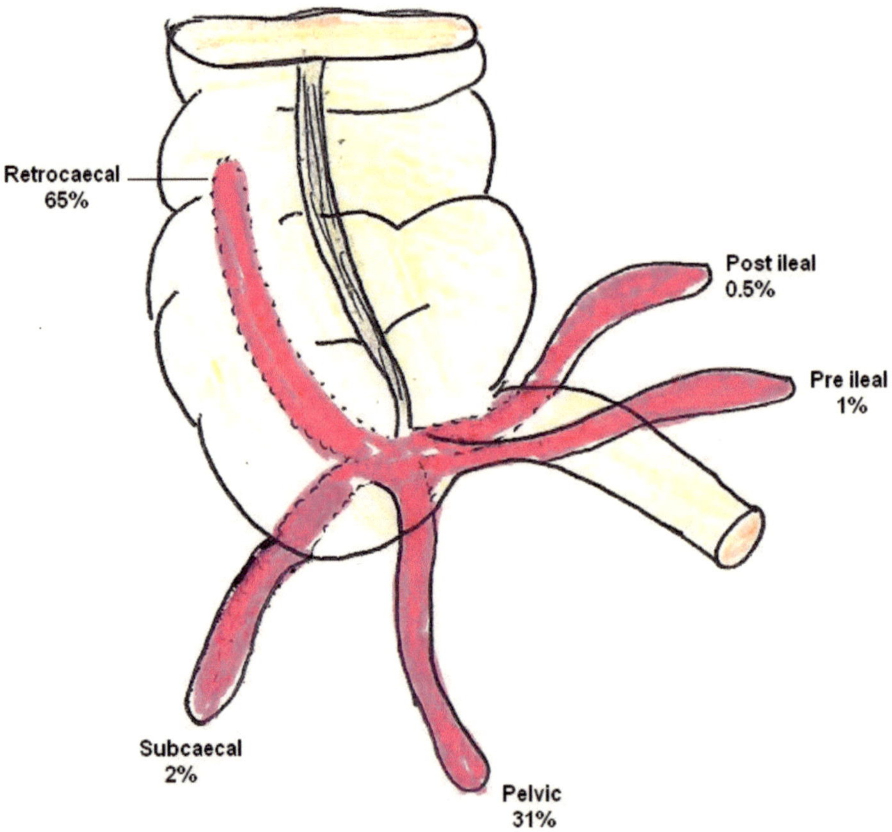

Fig. 5. Different positions of the appendix

If there is an appendicular mass or abscess, gentle dissection should be carried out to visualize the anatomical structures appropriately and there should be a low threshold to convert to an open procedure as prolong dissection carries the risk of causing more damage.

5.7 Division of the mesoappendix and appendix

The options to divide the mesoappendix and appendix are as follows:

- Diathermy dissection of the mesoappendix and ligation of the appendix
- Ligation of both appendix and mesoappendix
- Clip application for the appendicular artery and ligation of the appendix
- Stapled division of both structures

5.7.1 Diathermy dissection of the meso appendix and ligation of the appendix

Bipolar diathermy is safely used to divide the meso appendix, as it has minimal lateral spread of energy, thus avoid tissue damage. Monopolar diathermy can also be safely used with short burst of energy rather than using it for prolonged periods. The dissection is started at the middle part of free edge of meso appendix and directed towards the appendix. Once dissection is close to the appendix the dissection is carried towards the base. The reason for starting in the middle part of meso appendix is, in case the appendicular artery is injured, it can be easily grasped and dealt with. Diathermy causes thrombosis of the appendicular artery and coagulates the surrounding tissue. Once the meso appendix is completely divided then the appendix base is ligated [Fig. 6]. Some surgeons prefer to free the meso appendix from the appendix from the tip to the base using diathermy, where the meso appendix is left intact. The appendix base is ligated twice with an endoloop (Ethicon Endoloop®Ligature PDS II/Vicryl Suture) at the base and a third loop is placed about 1cm from the previous one. The appendix is divided at least 5mm from the ligation at the base side.

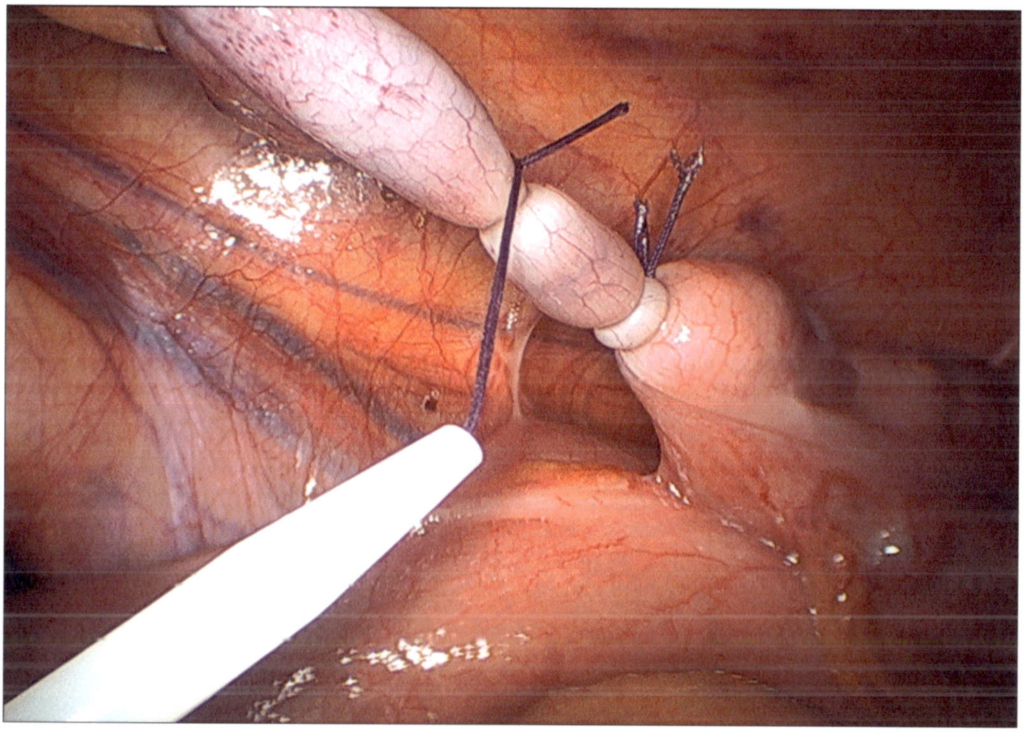

Fig. 6. Ligation of base of the appendix using an endoloop

5.7.2 Ligation of both appendix and meso appendix

Both the appendix and meso appendix can be safely ligated with either intra corporeal or extra corporeal knots. For this a window is created [Fig. 7] in the meso appendix near the base of the appendix using curved dissecting forceps. Then the suture material (2-0 Vicryl or PDS) is passed through the window and the meso appendix and appendix are ligated twice and divided between the ligatures. The other option is to ligate the mesoappendix as described and ligate the base of the appendix using endoloop

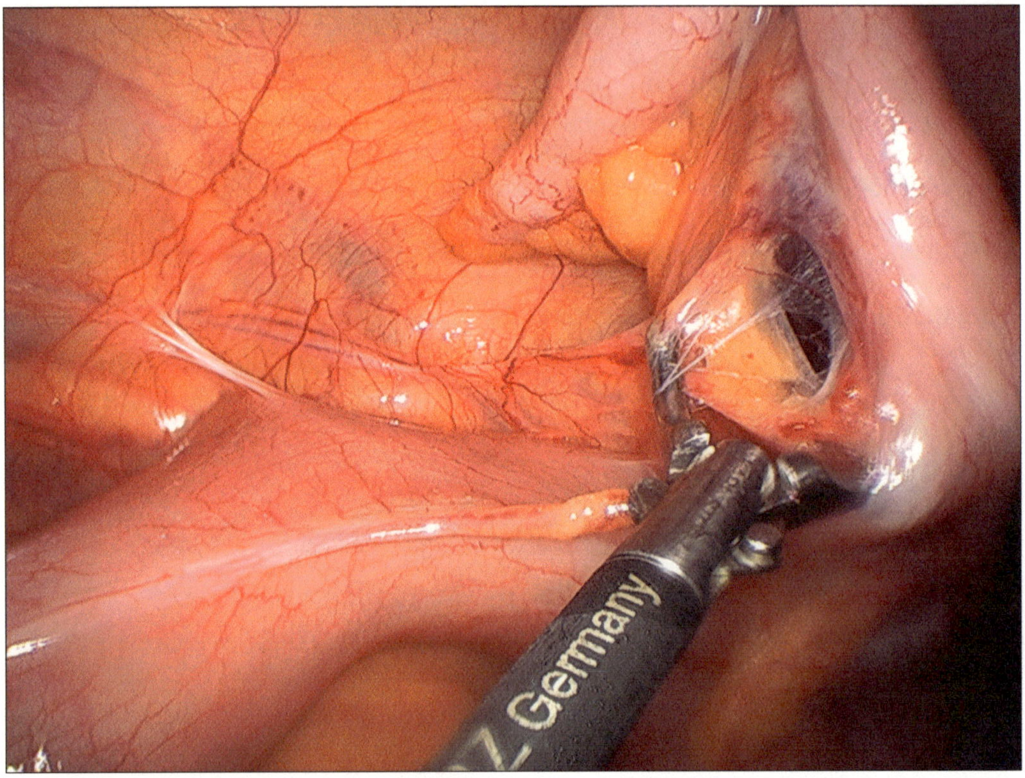

Fig. 7. Creation of window in the mesoappendix near the base

5.7.3 Clip application for appendicular artery and ligation of the appendix

This is possible where the meso appendix is not grossly inflamed and friable. The fat over the meso appendix is gently dissected and the appendicular artery is identified. Then 3 clips are applied to the artery [Fig. 8] (2 towards the base and 1 proximal to these) and the artery is divided between the clips. Then the base of the appendix is ligated as mentioned above.

5.7.4 Stapler division of appendix and meso appendix

The principal advantage of using a stapler device is the ability to divide the appendiceal mesentery and appendix in a single maneuver [Fig. 9], even in the presence of severe inflammation and thickening of meso appendix. The main disadvantage of the stapler includes the cost and the requirement for a larger trocar size. In general a minimally inflamed or an uninflammed appendix only needs ligation with an endoloop, but a stapler can greatly facilitate the surgery in the presence of severe inflammation with a thickened mesoappendix and appendix base. It is also useful, where the base of the appendix is necrotic. In these cases the stapler is applied at the healthy caecal wall.

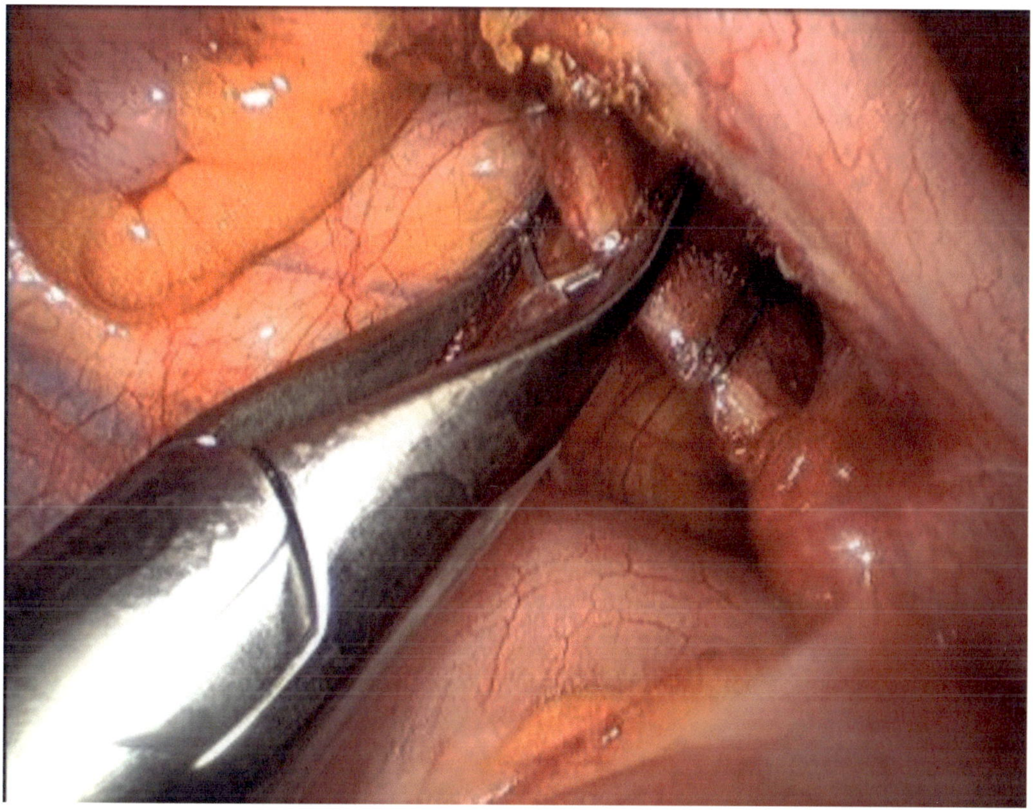

Fig. 8. Application of clip to the appendicular artery

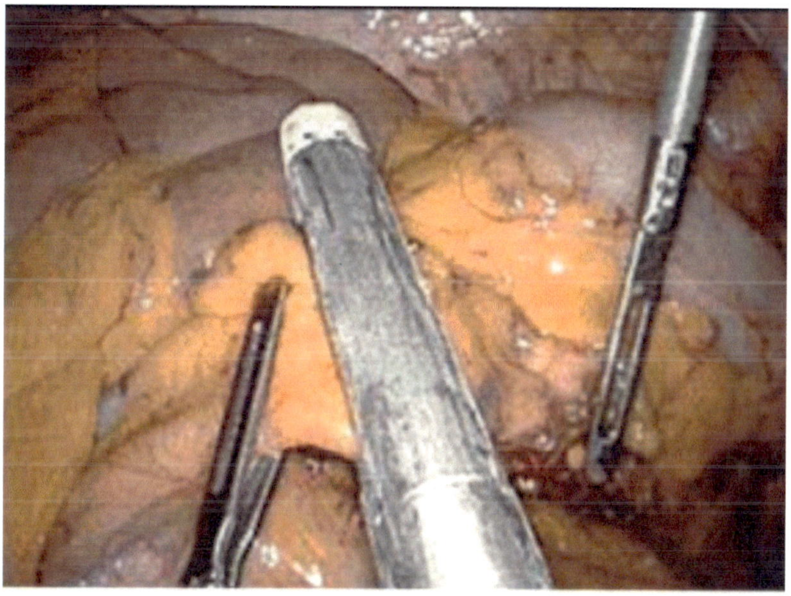

Fig. 9. Stapler division of appendix and mesoappendix

To use the stapler the surgeon will need to use a 5mm telescope, so that the stapler device can be introduced through the larger umbilical port or one of the 5mm existing working ports should be converted to a larger 12mm port. When using a single stapler to divide both appendix and meso appendix, careful inspection of the meso appendix is performed to check hemostasis. The other option is to use a vascular stapler for the meso appendix and an intestinal stapler for the base of the appendix. For this a window is created in the mesoappendix adjacent to the appendicular base and both structures are divided separately using the stapler devices. When the stapling device is used, care should be taken not to include the terminal ileum, right ureter or gonadal vessel in the jaws of the stapling device. Very rarely a harmonic scalpel (Ethicon Endo-Surgery inc.,) or the Ligasure (Ligasure TM, Covidien plc, USA) are used to divide the meso appendix.

5.8 Removal of the appendix

Once the appendix and meso appendix are divided the appendix specimen should be removed. If the appendix is thin and normal or minimally inflamed then it is removed through the umbilical port by feeding the appendix to the umbilical port when the camera is in situ. Then the whole umbilical port is removed along with the specimen.

If the appendix is thick and highly inflamed then either a 5mm telescope is used in the lateral port or one of the 5mm ports is converted to a 10mm port to remove the appendix under vision. If the meso appendix is thick and the appendix is friable, gangrenous and filled with pus, then an endobag (Endobag® retrieval bags, Tyco Healthcare USA) [Fig. 10] or BERT (Synergy Health (UK) Limited) bag is used to remove the appendix to avoid rupture of the specimen in the peritoneal cavity. A BERT bag can be inserted (attached with Vicryl suture with long ends left outside) and removed along with the specimen through the umbilical port if a 5mm telescope is not available and to avoid conversion of a 5mm to 10mm port.

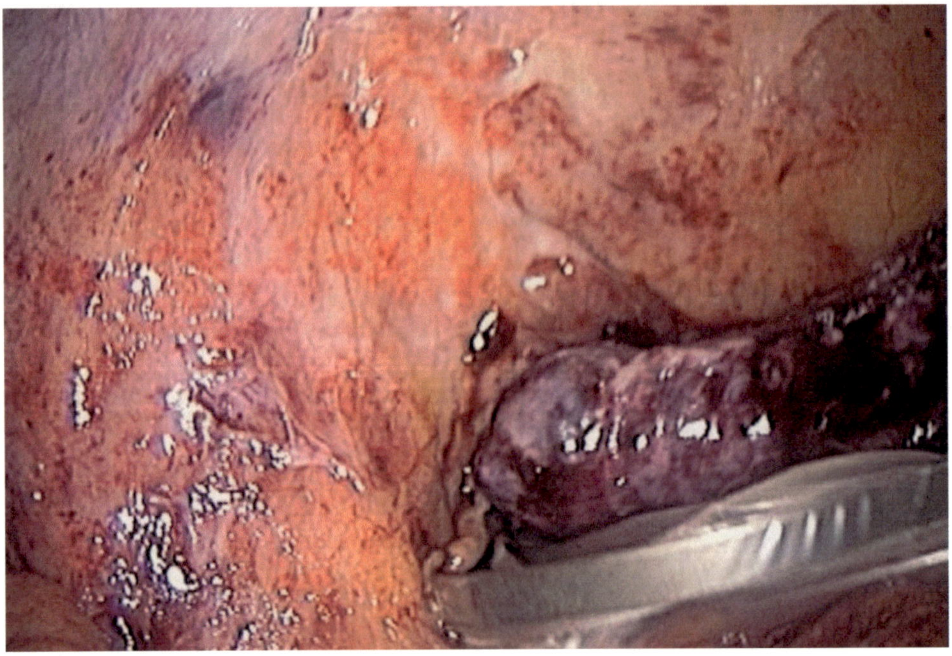

Fig. 10. Removal of appendix using endobag

Care should be taken to avoid the contact between the specimen and the anterior abdominal wall to prevent wound infection. Once the specimen is retrieved the port is reinserted and the pneumoperitoneum is created for a final check.

5.9 Wash and close

Careful inspection should be performed to check for hemostasis and any residual contamination. If there is gross contamination then a local wash should be performed with normal saline. If there is extensive contamination of the peritoneal cavity then all quadrants of the abdomen should be irrigated with copious amount of normal saline until the returned fluid is clear. Once this has been done the patient is placed in the head up position and the fluid gravitating to the pelvis is sucked out. Some surgeons place a drain if there has been gross contamination with perforation of the appendix, though there is no evidence for the benefit of drains.

Ports should be withdrawn under vision; especially the lateral port to make sure that there is no injury to the inferior epigastric artery. The umbilical port is closed with 2-0 vicryl / PDS and the skin is closed with either subcuticular suture or skin glue.

5.10 Postoperative management

Oral fluids and diet can be started when the patient tolerates them. Adequate analgesia with initial parentral then oral analgesics and thrombo prophylaxis are prescribed. Antibiotics are continued for a few days if there is gross contamination, perforation or gangrenous appendicitis. The drain can be removed, if placed, when the out put is minimal and clear. With early mobilization patients are usually discharged before the 2nd post operative day.

6. Difficult dissection

6.1 Retrocaecal appendix

The retrocaecal appendix comprises about 65% of the normal appendix positions. Performing an appendicectomy for retrocaecal appendicitis may be challenging. In this situation, the caecum and the ascending colon are mobilized, similar to the dissection for a right hemicolectomy. By this maneuver the appendix can be visualized, which then should be gently dissected off from the caecum. Care should be taken to avoid injury to the adjacent retroperitoneal structures i.e right ureter or gonadal vessels. Once the entire appendix is mobilized then the appendicectomy is completed as above. If the surgeon is not experienced in mobilization of the colon or the dissection is found to be difficult, then there should be no hesitation to convert to an open procedure.

6.2 Subhepatic appendix

Sometimes the appendix tip may be in the subhepatic space. If the appendix is mildly inflamed, it may be easy to mobilize it. But in case of gross inflammation, the appendix may be completely stuck in the paracolic position. In these cases it is ideal to find the base by identifying the ileo caecal junction. Then the base can be divided between ligatures and proceed with dissection of the appendix and meso appendix towards the tip. It is also acceptable to proceed without dividing the base. When the dissection reaches the tip, care should be taken to avoid injury to the gall bladder or liver.

6.3 Gangrenous base

Some times the inflammation extends up to the base and the base is found to be necrotic. All precautions should be taken to avoid accidental avulsion of the appendix. The appendix should be removed along with a healthy cap of caecum, by using endo staplers as mentioned earlier. If the stapler is not available then the appendix is removed and intracorporeal suturing with the healthy caecal wall should be applied. If that is not possible then the procedure should be converted to an open operation.

6.4 Appendicular mass

An appendicular mass is formed by adhesions between the appendix, small bowel, caecum and the omentum. In this situation all the adhesions are gently teased away to find the appendix. If it is difficult then the procedure is converted. In elderly patients caecal malignancy should be considered when dealing with a mass in the right iliac fossa.

6.5 Perforated appendix

While most patients are found to have a perforated appendix only after laparoscopic or open exploration, some have preoperative evidence with generalized peritonitis, SIRS or radiological findings [10]. When there is obvious evidence of appendicular perforation, some surgeons prefer to proceed directly to an open procedure, as there is some evidence of an increased risk of a pelvic abscess following a laparoscopic approach [11]. Further, in contrast to patients with simple appendicitis, the recovery period is similar with the open or the laparoscopic method in patients with perforation and generalized peritonitis, because the recovery depends on resolution of the intra abdominal pathology rather than the abdominal incision [12]. However, when perforated appendix is identified unexpectedly during a laparoscopic approach, it is acceptable to proceed with appendicectomy laparoscopically, if it is safe and feasible.

7. Special situations (children, pregnancy, previous surgeries)

7.1 Children

Laparoscopic appendicectomy is considered to be safe in children, provided the operator has ample experience in performing the procedure. The procedure is similar to that of adults. But the instruments required for paediatric patients differ according to their age. Usually 3mm - 5mm scopes are used. The size of the additional trocars varies between 3 - 5mm. Even though there is little published data regarding safe intra abdominal pressures lower pressures are used and are age related [5]. The result of one of the meta analyses suggests that laparoscopic appendicectomy in children reduces the complications in comparison with the open procedure [13]

7.2 Pregnancy

Appendicectomy is the most common non obstetric operation performed during pregnancy [14, 15] with a reported incidence of 0.05% - 0.1% [16]. Twenty-five per cent of all pregnant women who have acute appendicitis will progress to perforation [17]. A 66% perforation incidence has been reported where surgery is delayed by more than 24 hours compared with 0% incidence when surgical management is initiated prior to 24 hours after presentation [18]

Laparoscopic appendicectomy has potential advantages with a small incision, less postoperative pain and early return to normal activity [19 - 23]

Laparoscopy can result in less manipulation of the uterus while obtaining optimum exposure of the surgical field and can reduce delays in diagnosis and treatment. Laparoscopy also affords an easier visualization and treatment of the ectopically located appendix and helps in detecting other unexpected sources of pain [23, 24]

A recent review of laparoscopic appendicectomy in pregnancy reported a significantly higher fetal loss rate compared with open appendicectomy and has raised some concerns [25]. Fetal loss is due to spontaneous abortion in the first trimester and premature labour in 3rd trimester [26]. The areas of concern were the effect of the pneumoperitoneum and increased intra abdominal pressure on uterine blood flow, fetal distress due to maternal hypotension, fetal respiratory acidosis and trocar injury to the pregnant uterus [27].

Laparoscopic appendicectomy can be performed safely with the following measures. It is vital to get involvement of the obstetricians during the peri operative period. Place the patient slightly left lateral to avoid compression of the IVC by the uterus. Anti embolic devices should be used to prevent venous thrombosis. End tidal $CO2$ should be monitored continuously. Recent evidence suggests that it is essential to have uterine and fetal monitoring before and after operation, as continuous monitoring may be difficult. The open technique (Hassan method) should be used for induction of the pneumoperitoneum, especially after the 1st trimester, to avoid a Veress needle injury to the uterus [28]. Other port positions depend upon the position of the appendix. Intra abdominal pressure should be maintained between 10 -12mmHg. Operative time should be reduced as low as possible, ideally less than 60 minutes. Prophylactic tocolytic agents are not used routinely unless there are uterine contractions and a risk of premature birth [20, 29, 30]

7.3 Previous abdominal surgery

Previous lower abdominal surgery was a relative contraindication for laparoscopic appendicectomy. However, various techniques have been used to perform appendicectomy laparoscopically. Using Optiview (Ethicon Endo-Surgery, Cincinnati, OH) or Visiport (Autosuture, USA) helps to place the camera port and the secondary ports under vision. If the adhesions are found to be flimsy they can be released with blunt and sharp dissection. If the appendix is visualized, then the procedure can be done as described earlier. But if the adhesions are found to be dense and the appendix is not visualized, then it is safer to convert the procedure to an open technique.

8. Complications

8.1 Bleeding

Aggressive or careless dissection of the mesoappendix can cause significant bleeding. If the appendix is highly inflamed and forms an early mass then dissection of the omentum, small bowel and caecum can also cause bleeding. Early control of the meso appendix and gentle dissection prevent this complication. Once bleeding is noted, it is controlled with an adequate view, gentle suction and simple pressure. Additional trocar may be necessary to solve this issue. Once the bleeding vessel is identified it is better to control it with a clip or endoloop, than continuous diathermy, which may potentially cause lateral damage.

Bleeding and haematoma can also arise from the port site, due to accidental injury to an anterior abdominal wall muscle/vessel, especially the inferior epigastric artery. This can be avoided by placing the incision away from the vascular structures by creating trans-illumination of the abdominal wall with the telescope. If there is a significant bleeding, it should be controlled with a suture at the port site.

8.2 Wound infection

One of the principal advantages of laparoscopy is the reduced rate of wound complications [31]. But still patients can get infections at the port sites. This may be due to delivery of the highly inflamed, gangrenous or perforated appendix through the port. This can be avoided by using a retrieval bag. If the patient develops a wound infection, it should be dealt with similar to any surgery.

8.3 Intra abdominal collection/ abscess

This is related to the degree of contamination caused by the inflamed appendix. This may also be due to the pneumoperitoneum, increased operative time and a prolonged dependant position [32]. A Cochrane review of 34 trials in 2003 showed an increased rate of intra abdominal abscess (pooled odds ratio 2.77, 95% CI 1.61 - 4.77) [33]. But later on it was proved that the pooled data was highly influenced by one large study and more perforated and gangrenous appendix were included in the laparoscopic group [11].

Patients who develop intra abdominal collections show signs of sepsis, including fever, abdominal pain and rising inflammatory markers. A CT scan is the investigation of choice to identify intra abdominal collections. Patients are treated with antibiotics and percutaneous radiological drainage if possible. If these measures fail then they should be dealt with surgically with either a re-look laparoscopy with liberal wash or a formal laparotomy.

8.4 Leakage of appendicial pus and faecoliths

Leakage of pus happens when the appendix is distended with pus and about to perforate. This can be prevented by gentle dissection and by using a retrieval bag for specimen removal. If there is accidental perforation of the appendix and leakage of pus or a faecolith, thorough irrigation should be performed and any visible faecolith should be removed immediately to prevent intra abdominal abscess formation.

8.5 Appendix stump leak

Leakage from the appendix stump occurs when an endoloop is applied to the gangrenous base. As there is no viable tissue the loop can cut through and cause leakage of caecal contents. This can be prevented by dividing the appendix with a healthy cuff of caecum by using a stapler device.

9. Open conversion

Open conversion should not be considered as a failure of laparoscopic appendicectomy. The common reasons for open conversion include, unable to find the appendix or mobilize the appendix, appendicular mass which is difficult to dissect, necrotic or perforated appendix, suspicion of a caecal malignancy where a right hemicolectomy is needed. The choice of incision depends on surgeon's preference and the findings on laparoscopy

10. Comparison with the open procedure

There is no evidence in the published literature that laparoscopic appendicectomy is less safe than open appendicectomy [34]. Whether the laparoscopic appendicectomy is better than open procedure depends on the outcomes measured, such as resource utilization, diagnostic accuracy, duration of surgery and stay, postoperative recovery and complications. Many randomized trials compared one or more of the above outcome measures. A Cochrane review in 2003 showed no difference in overall healthcare resource consumption between these groups [33].

A Cochrane review in 2011 found a significant difference favouring laparoscopy in diagnostic accuracy (7 RCTs, 561 participants; OR 4.1, 95% CI 2.50 - 6.71). Although the operative time is significantly less in the open appendicectomy group (by 14.55 mins, 95% CI 3.62 - 25.48, 5 RCTs, 355 participants), there was no difference in the overall length of hospital stay (6 RCTs, 455 participants; WMD -0.07, 95%CI -0.63 - 0.49).

The rate of removal of normal appendix was reduced with the laparoscopic approach compared to open appendicectomy (7 RCTs, OR 0.13, 95% CI 0.07 - 0.24). Laparoscopic appendicectomy was superior in regards to measures of postoperative recovery, such as pain reduction on a 10cm visual analogue scale (by 0.8cm, 95% CI 1.3 - 0.3), wound infection (pooled odds ratio 0.47, 95% CI 0.36 - 0.62) and reduced time to return to normal activity (by 5.09 days, 95% CI 5.56 - 4.61) [35]. Overall it appears that laparoscopic appendicectomy has obvious benefits in view of diagnostic accuracy and post operative outcome, with no overall increase in health care cost.

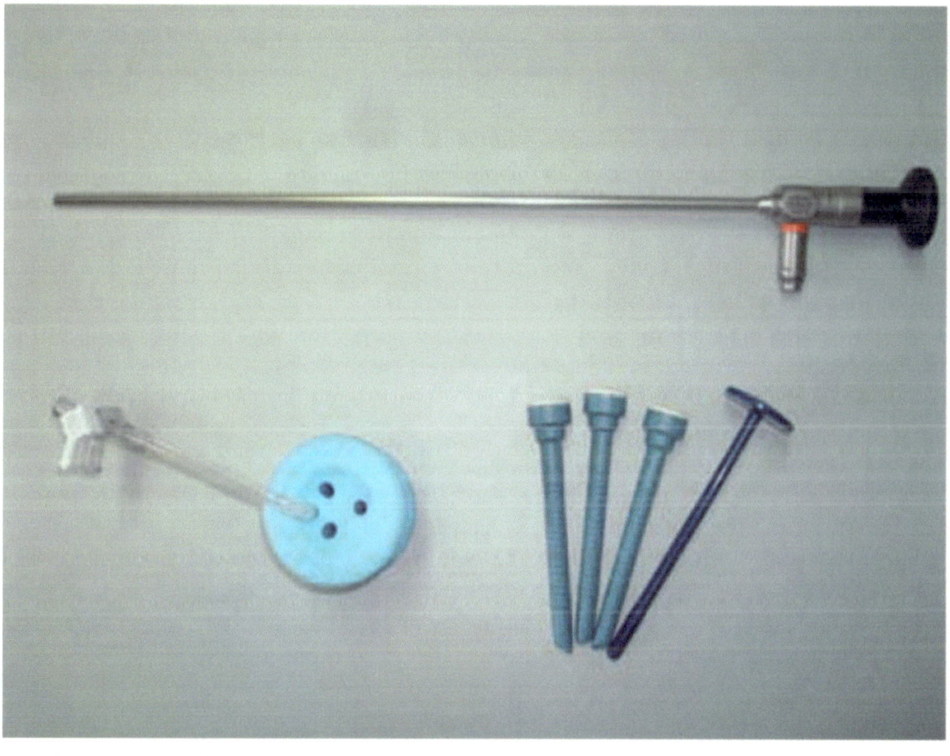

Fig. 11. SILS ports and 5mm 30 degree scope

11. SILS appendicectomy

SILS (Single Incision Laparoscopic Surgery) appendicectomy involves appendicectomy through a single incision through the umbilicus. Esposito C reported single trocar appendicectomy in 1998 [36], where the appendix was tied off laparoscopically and the appendicectomy was performed extracorporeally. Now the complete procedure is performed with a single umbilical incision with multiple ports [Fig. 11]. It improves the cosmetic outcome and minimizes the pain as it is not penetrating the muscle. It also avoids injury to the inferior epigastric vessels [37]. However, it needs great technical ability.

12. Conclusion

Laparoscopic appendicectomy is well tolerated by patients with reduced postoperative wound complications, improved cosmetic appearance and earlier return to normal activity. It is a preferred method in obese patients and young women, especially when the diagnosis is uncertain.

13. References

[1] Addiss DG et al. (1990). The epidemiology of appendicitis and appendectomy in the United States. *Am J Epidemio* 132:910-25

[2] Semm K. (1983). Endoscopic appendicectomy. *Endoscopy* 15:59-64

[3] Barnes SL et al. (2004). Laparoscopic appendectomy after 30 weeks pregnancy: report of two cases and description of technique. Am Surg. 70:733–736.

[4] Keith N Apelgren. (2006). Laparoscopic Appendicectomy.. *The SAGES manual. Fundamentals of Laparoscopy, Thoracoscopy and GI Endoscopy.* Carol E.H. Scott-Conner :350 -56. Springer, ISBN : 13: 978-0387-23267-6, USA

[5] Jean-Louis Dulucq. (2003). *Tips and Techniques in laparoscopic surgery.* 103 -118. Springer, ISBN 3-540-20902-6, Berlin Heidelberg New York

[6] Roumen R. M. et al. (2008). Randomized clinical trial evaluating elective laparoscopic appendicectomy for chronic right lower-quadrant pain. Br J Surg; 95: 169-174

[7] Grunewald B, Keating J. (1993). Should the 'normal' appendix be removed at operation for appendicitis? *J R Coll Surg Edin;* 38:158 – 60.

[8] Van den Broek WT et al. (2001). A normal appendix found during laparoscopic appendectomy should not be removed. *Br J Surg;* 88:251-4.

[9] Greason KL, Rappold JF, Liberman MA. (1998). Incidental laparoscopic appendicectomy for acute right lower quadrant abdominal pain. Its time has come. *Surg Endosc;* 12:223 -25.

[10] Horrow MM, White DS, Horrow JC. (2003) Differentiation of perforated from nonperforated appendicitis on CT. *Radiology;* 227:45-51.

[11] Pedersen AG, Petersen OB, Wara P, et al. (2001) Randomised controlled trial of laparoscopic versus open appendicectomy. *Br J Surg;* 88:200 – 5.

[12] Piskun G, Kozik D, Rajpal S, Shaftan G, Fogler R (2001). Comparison of laparoscopic, open and converted appendectomy for perforated appendicitis. *Surg Endosc;* 15:660-2.

[13] Omer Aziz, Thanos Athanasiou et al. (2006) Laparoscopic Versus Open Appendicectomy in Children – A meta analysis. *Ann Surg ;* 243: 17-27

[14] Kammerer WS. Nonobstetric surgery during pregnancy. (1979) *Med Clin North Am.;* 63:1157–1164

[15] Kort B, Katz VL, Watson WJ. (1993). The effect of nonobstetric operation during pregnancy. *Surg Gynecol Obstet.;* 177:371–376.

[16] Curet MJ. Special problems in laparoscopic surgery. (2000) Previous abdominal surgery, obesity and pregnancy. *Surg Clin North Am.* ;80:1093–1110.

[17] Cappell MS, Friedel D. Abdominal pain during pregnancy. (2003) *Gastroenterol Clin North Am.;* 32:1–58.

[18] Tamir IL, Bongard FS, Klein SR (1990). Acute appendicitis in the pregnant patient. *Am J Surg.;* 160:571–575.

[19] Affleck DG, Handrahan DL, Egger MJ, Price PR (1999). The laparoscopic management of appendicitis and cholelithiasis during pregnancy. *Am J Surg.;* 178:523–529.

[20] Moreno-Sanz C et al. (2007) Laparoscopic appendectomy during pregnancy: between personal experiences and scientific evidence. *J Am Coll Surg.;* 205(1):37–42.

[21] Rollins MD, Chan KJ, Price RR. (2004) Laparoscopy for appendicitis and cholelithiasis during pregnancy: a new standard of care. *Surg Endosc.;* 18:237–241.

[22] Halkic N et al. (2006) Laparoscopic management of appendicitis and symptomatic cholelithiasis during pregnancy. *Langenbecks Arch Surg.;* 391:467–471.

[23] Lyass S et al. (2001) Is laparoscopic appendicectomy safe in pregnant women? *Surg Endosc.;* 15:377–379.

[24] de Perrot MD et al. (2000) Laparoscopic appendicectomy during pregnancy. *Surg Laparosc Endosc Percutan Tech.;* 10(6):368–371.

[25] McGory ML et al. (2007) Negative appendectomy in pregnant women is associated with a substantial risk of fetal loss. *J Am Coll Surg.;* 205:534–540.

[26] Al-Fozan H, Tulandi T. (2001). Safety and risks of laparoscopy in pregnancy. *Curr Opin Obstet Gynecol ;* 14:375-9

[27] Amos JD, Schorr SJ, Norman PF, et al. (1996) Laparoscopic surgery during pregnancy. *Am J Surg;* 171:435 – 7.

[28] Friedman JD, Ramsey PS, Ramin KD, Berry C. (2003). Pneumoamnion and pregnancy loss after second-trimester laparoscopic surgery. *Obstet Gynecol ;* 99:512-3

[29] Walsh CA, Tang T, Walsh SR. (2008). Laparoscopic versus open appendectomy in pregnancy: a systematic review. *Int J Surg.* 6:339–344 Epub 2008 Feb1.

[30] Jackson H, Granger S, Price R, et al. (2008). Diagnosis and laparoscopic treatment of surgical diseases during pregnancy: an evidence based review. *Surg Endosc.;* 22:1917–1927.

[31] Holzman MD et al. (1997). Laparoscopic ventral and incisional hernioplasty. Surg Encosc; 11:32-5.

[32] Balague Ponz C, Trias M. (2001). Laparoscopic surgery and surgical infection. *J Chemother* ;13 Spec No 1:17-22

[33] Sauerland S, Lefering R, Neugebauer EAM (2003). Laparoscopic versus open surgery for suspected appendicitis (Cochrane Review) In: *The Cochrane Library,* Issue 1. Oxford: update Software, 2003.

[34] Edmund AM Neugebaue et al. (2006). *EAES guidelines for Endoscopic Surgery.* ISBN-10 3-540-32783-5, Springer Berlin Heidelberg New York

[35] Gaitan HG, Reveiz L, Farquhar C (2011). Laparoscopy for the management of acute lower abdominal pain in women of childbearing age (Cochrane review). *The Cochrane Library,* Issue 1.

[36] Esposito C. One trocar appendicectomy in pediatric surgery (1998). *Surg Endosc.;* 12:177-78

[37] Maria DF et al. (2011) Single incision transumbilical laparoscopic appendicectomy: initial experience. *CIR ESP.;* 89(1):37-41

12

An Animal Model of Sepsis in Appendicitis: Assessment of the Microcirculation

Eduardo Ryoiti Tatebe, Priscila Aikawa, José Jukemura,
Paulina Sannomiya and Naomi Kondo Nakagawa
University of São Paulo School of Medicine
Brazil

1. Introduction

Acute appendicitis is one of the most common causes of inflammation in the abdomen. Appendicitis, characterized by inflammation of the appendix, is an urgent clinical illness with significant morbidity, which increases with diagnostic delay. Perforation and peritonitis are associated with increased morbidity and mortality, especially in the very young, the elderly and immune-suppressed patients.

The diagnosis is based on the patient's history by the classic signs and symptoms of appendicitis (abdominal pain in the right iliac fossa, fever, anorexia, nausea, and vomiting) and physical examination. Children and the elderly have fewer signs and symptoms, or cannot adequate describe them. In pregnant women, particularly during the second and third trimester, the diagnosis of acute appendicitis is often delayed because of the nonspecific clinical abdominal presentation. In these conditions, diagnosis often requires imaging methods (ultrasound and/or CT scanning), and the incidence of complications is more frequent. Most patients usually recover well after surgical treatment, but complications can occur if treatment is delayed or if perforation that results in peritonitis or sepsis is present.

Sepsis and septic shock are clinical syndromes that result from complex interactions between the host and infectious agents. These events are characterized by hemodynamic derangements, widespread microcirculatory disturbances and cellular alterations leading to heterogeneous flow distribution, capillary obstruction and, therefore, to an uncoupling between cellular oxygen need and oxygen supply (De Backer et al., 2002; Hinshaw, 1996; Sakr et al., 2004). Despite improvements in treatments for sepsis, there are still gaps in our knowledge of the physiopathology and therapeutic interventions.

1.1 Cecal Ligation and Puncture as an experimental model of appendicitis

Among several experimental animal models, perforated appendicitis by cecal ligation and puncture (CLP), particularly in rodents, has been used to investigate the pathophysiology and assess the effectiveness of therapies in sepsis and septic shock. The CLP model begins with bowel exposure, followed by cecal ligation distal to the ileocecal valve. Thereafter, the cecum is perforated by a needle and the contents squeezed into the peritoneal cavity. The number of punctures, the diameter of the hole and the total amount of squeezed bowel content can introduce several variations of the model that will directly induce lethal or non-lethal sepsis. Sepsis in the CLP model is caused by contamination of the peritoneal cavity with a mixed flora of microorganisms and by the ischemic/necrotic tissue complications. Without the appropriate clinical (fluid resuscitation and antibiotics) and surgical treatment (necrotic tissue resection and peritoneal lavage), a rapid onset of septic shock can be observed.

1.1.1 Advantages of the CLP model

In this work, we will focus on the experimental model of CLP in rodents that is a simple and reproducible model widely used in research. The CLP model allows for control of the setting and reduction of some of the variables. We have focused on the mechanisms responsible for the altered immunological, cardiovascular, respiratory and metabolic changes as a model for acute perforated appendicitis in humans.

The CLP model can also be used to evaluate cardiac output/total and regional blood flow (Angle et al., 1998; Jarrar et al., 2000; Yang et al., 2002), metabolism (Lang et al., 1990; Wang et al., 1999), immune function (Ayala & Chaudry, 1996; Kato et al., 2004; Schneider et al., 2000), apoptosis (Reddy et al., 2001; Ayala &Chaudry, 1996; Chung et al., 2003; Coopersmith et al, 2002), cytokines (Schneider et al., 2000; Vianna et al., 2004), resuscitation (Esmon, 2004; Marx et al., 2004; Yang et al., 2002), antibiotics (Doerschug et al., 2004; Vianna et al., 2004), and microbial components (Ayala & Chaudry, 1996; Esmon, 2004; Mollitt, 2002; Yang et al., 2001).

1.1.2 Limitations of the CLP model

The CLP model in small mammals, particularly rodents, has some limitations on the translation to humans. One difference that is common between rodents and humans is that the mice or rats can tolerate quite well the cecal ligation alone without puncture. These animals can block the necrotic tissue and survive. Humans, in turn, are not able to overcome by theirselves. Another aspect is related to the size of the animal. Several technical and physiological difficulties may appear. Among them, the inability to obtain large quantities of blood and other fluids for tests over long periods of observation (Hubbard et al., 2005), and the technology to obtain accurate physiological measurements in these small animals.

1.2 Other models of acute appendicitis

Rabbits and pigs have also been used as experimental models of acute appendicitis. However, due to anatomical differences, the use of pigs is very limited. Pig does not have an appendix and the occlusion is performed in the uterine horn to study surgical procedures, such as an endoscopic transgastric appendectomy (Sumiyama et al., 2006) . In rabbits, investigators use the vascular partial or total clamping method to obtain necrotic tissue mimicking the acute appendicitis (Nunes & Silva, 2005).

2. Intravital microscopy in the assessment of microcirculation

A well-established technique applied in many experimental models of sepsis is the intravital microscopy (Figure 1). This technique allows the *in vivo* and *in situ* observation of the microvascular bed of different tissues, such as the mesentery, ileum, liver, and skeletal muscle of rats, mice, rabbits and felines. Suitable tissues are selected if they can be easily exteriorized and transilluminated, as illustrated in Figure 2. It is important to minimize the preparative surgery and to maintain the physiological conditions: temperature, extracellular fluid composition, pH, and gas tensions. The introduction of close circuit television has facilitated quantification of many of the variables, such as leukocyte-endothelial interactions, through the possibility to store images on videotape for detailed off-line analysis. More recently, analyses have been performed online by using image-computer software (Nakagawa et al, 2006).

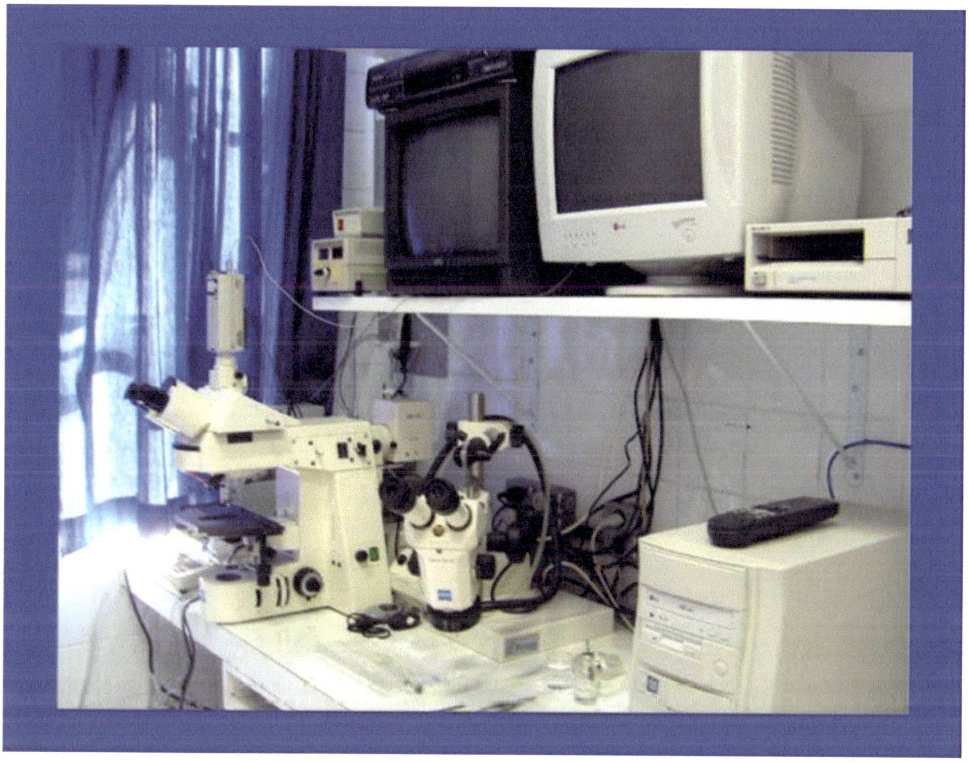

Fig. 1. Equipment for Intravital Microscopy.

Intravital microscopy has been applied to evaluate different pathophysiological aspects of the microcirculation during several challenges. In addition, intravital microscopy has also been used to test novel prophylactic and therapeutic approaches that aim to prevent or attenuate manifestations of sepsis-associated microvascular disorders and cellular dysfunctions. In the mesentery, microcirculatory observations have focused on capillary obstruction, capillary or arteriolar density, microvessel reactivity and leukocyte-endothelial interactions in post-capillary venules (Harris, 2006; Kim & Harris, 2006; Nakagawa et al., 2006, 2007; Schimidt et al., 1997; Smalley et al., 2000; Walther et al., 2004; Woodman et al., 2000). A representative photomicrograph of rat mesenteric microcirculation is shown in Figure 3. In other organs, such as lungs and heart, increased leukocyte-endothelial interactions have been observed mostly induced by physical trapping in pre-capillary microvessels and capillaries (Kubo et al., 1999; Waisman et al., 2006). In liver, blood flow/perfusion regulation is at the arteriolar and sinusoidal level (Baveja et al., 2002; Kamoun et al., 2005).

Microcirculatory dysfunctions, as seen in humans (De Backer & Dubois, 2001; De Backer et al., 2002; Groner et al., 1999; Trzeciak et al., 2007), have been shown to occur in most experimental models of sepsis (Baveja et al., 2002; Kamoun et al., 2005; Kim & Harris, 2006; Kubo et al., 1999; Nakagawa et al., 2006, 2007; Nakajima et al., 2001; Schimidt et al., 1997; Smalley et al., 2000; Waisman et al., 2006; Walther et al., 2004; Woodman et al., 2000). Endotoxin infusion is a widely used experimental model (Kim & Harris, 2006; Schimidt et al., 1997; Smalley et al., 2000; Nakajima et al., 2001). Increased leukocyte-endothelial interactions and protein leakage in mesenteric microvessels have been shown to occur after acute endotoxemia in rats (Schimidt et al., 1997; Woodman et al., 2000) and cats (Walther et al., 2004). However, there are two major concerns regarding this experimental model: 1) clinical sepsis typically evolves over many days, in contrast to studies on the early effects (1 to 6 hours) of endotoxin administration, and 2) rats are generally more resistant to the effects of endotoxin.

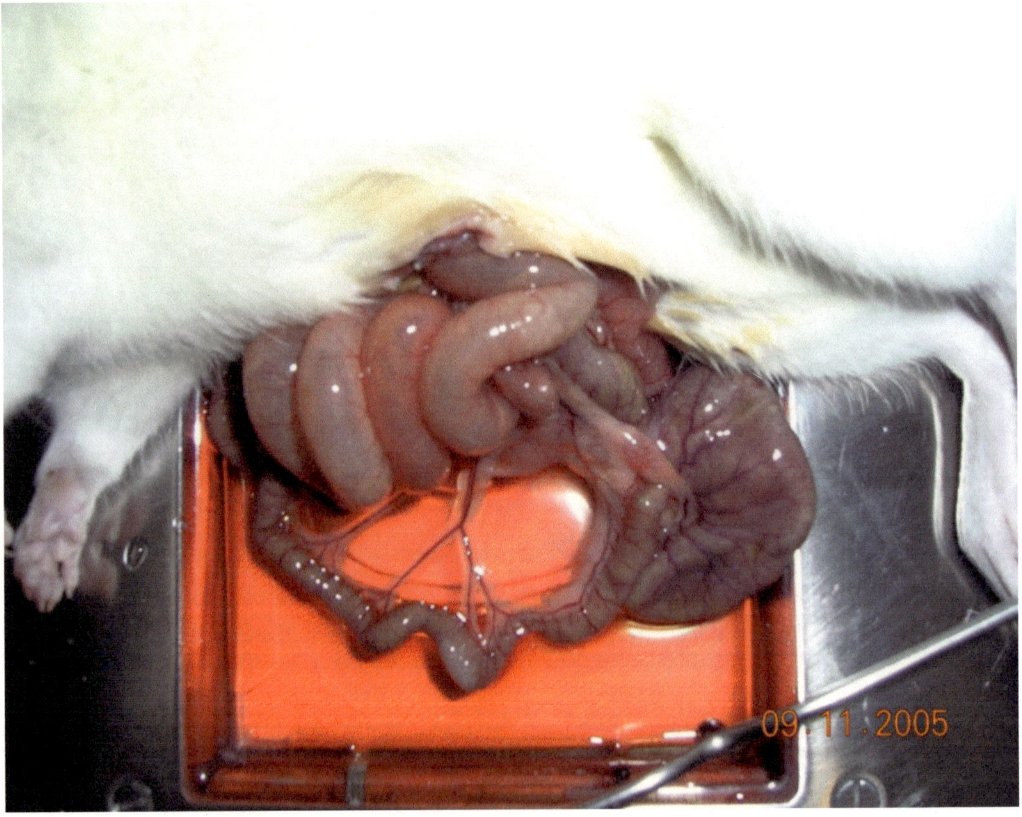

Fig. 2. Positioning of the mesentery in the platform for intravital microscopy.

Therefore, many microvascular changes seen in animal models of endotoxemia may not occur in humans (Chaudry, 1999). On the other hand, laparotomy complicated by sepsis is a common clinical presentation of sepsis. This rationale was used in selecting CLP as a model of polymicrobial and normotensive sepsis (Chaudry, 1999; Chaudry et al., 1979; Farquhar et al., 1996; Hersch et al., 1998; Madorin et al., 1999; Nakagawa et al., 2006, 2007).

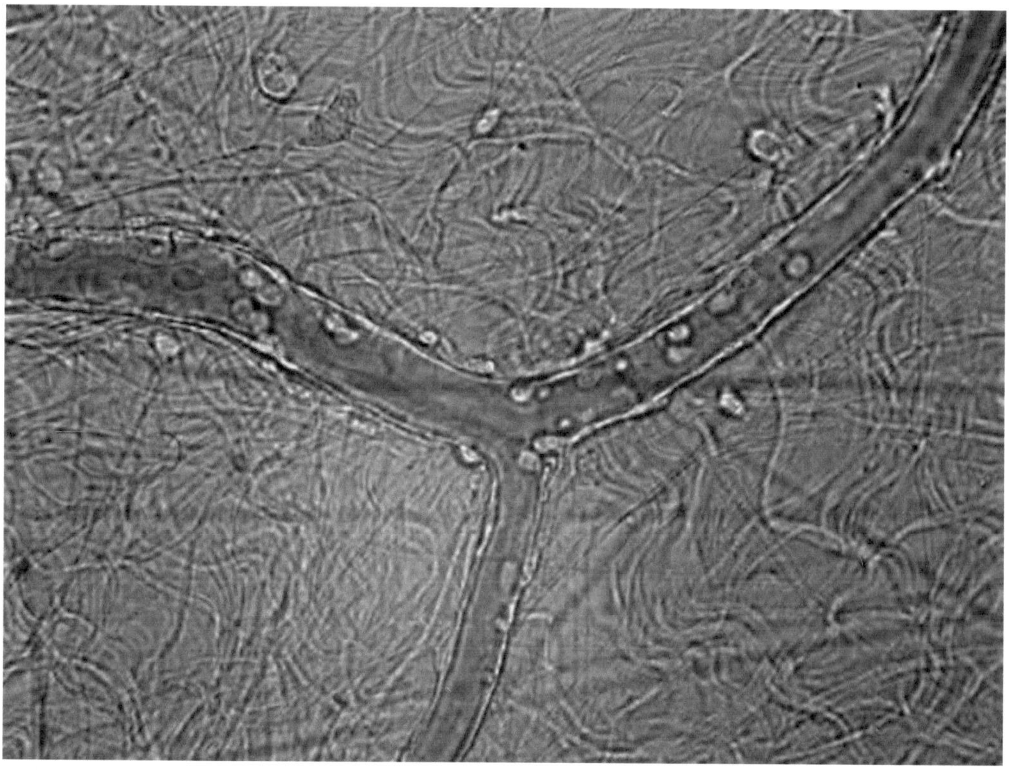

Fig. 3. Photomicrograph of rat mesenteric microcirculation by intravital microscopy showing leukocyte-endothelial interactions under inflammation (425x)

In the CLP model (Figure 4), many microvascular derangements occur such as increased total blood flow to the ileum with preferential redistribution toward the muscularis and away from the mucosa (Farquhar et al., 1996; Hersch et al., 1998; Madorin et al., 1999; Nakajima et al., 2001). The abnormal microvascular blood flow may result in tissue hypoxia and increased permeability (Farquhar et al., 1996). CLP induces an inflammatory response characterized by an increased number of white blood cells, increased leukocyte-endothelial interactions in mesenteric microvessels and lung neutrophil infiltration (Nakagawa et al., 2006).

3. CLP in a double-injury model

In attempting to understand the pathophysiology of septic shock, several investigators have performed double-injury models to study the microcirculation by intravital microscopy in different tissues. Hoffman et al. (1999) observed increased leukocyte adhesion and reduced capillary perfusion in skin microvessels of hamsters submitted to persistent endotoxemia (72 hours) induced by a double-LPS exposure. Swartz et al. (2000) performed CLP followed by the local application of *E. coli* on cremaster muscle. Despite an intra-abdominal infection, there was no increase in leukocyte adhesion in the cremaster muscle. In contrast, Pascual et al. (2003) observed increased leukocyte adhesion to microvessels of cremaster muscle after hemorrhagic shock/reperfusion followed by intratracheal injection of LPS in mice. Smalley et al. (2000) reported no changes in leukocyte adhesion in the mesentery in an acute model (4 hours) of CLP. However, a topical application of highly diluted fecal matter increased leukocyte adhesion in the mesenteric microcirculation, which was mediated by platelet activation factor. More recently, Nakagawa et al. (2006) observed leukocyte-endothelium interactions in the mesenteric microcirculation after hemorrhagic shock/reperfusion followed by an intra-abdominal sepsis (CLP). Twenty-four hours after the double-injury, rats exhibited an increased number of rolling, adherent and migrated leukocytes accompanied by an increased expression of P-selectin and intercellular adhesion molecule (ICAM)-1 at the mesentery and by leukocyte infiltration and ICAM-1 up-regulation at the lungs.

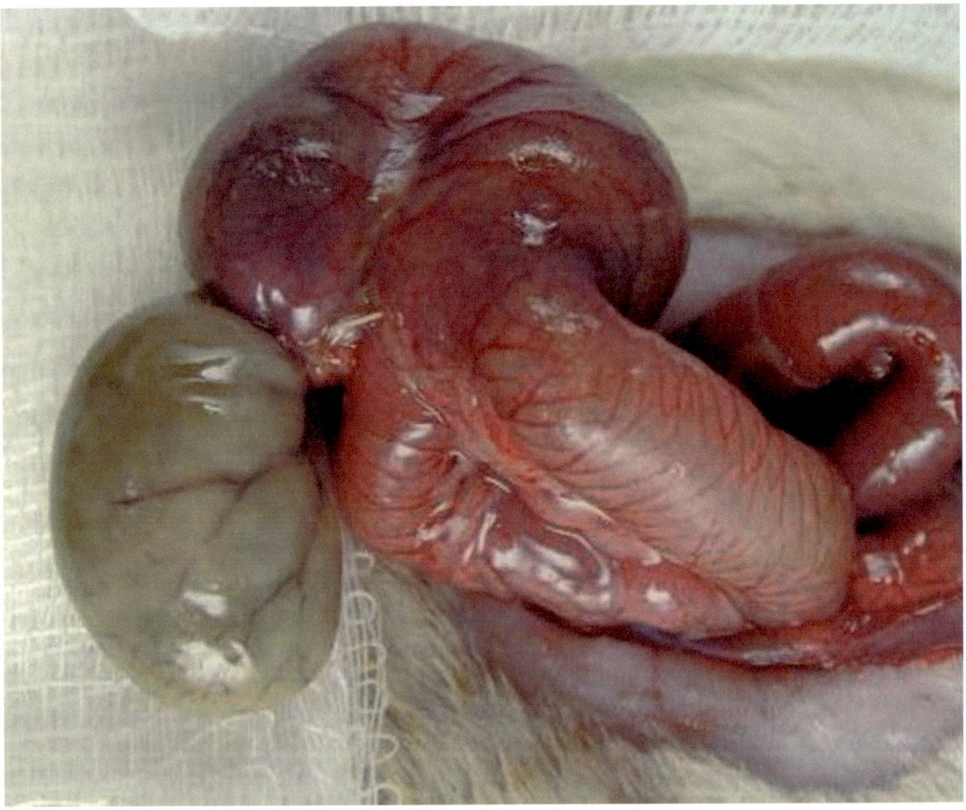

Fig. 4. Twenty-four hours after cecal ligation and puncture model. Note the impressive intestinal edema around the necrotic tissue.

4. Surgical control of the septic focus

In the model of single-injury (CLP) the surgical removal of the septic focus followed by peritoneal lavage partially controls the inflammatory reaction in these animals. By intravital microscopy, leukocyte-endothelial interactions at the mesentery were normalized by the surgical control. These results support surgical source control as a therapy contributing to resolving the immune dysfunction observed in this specific septic challenge (Nakagawa et al., 2007).

5. Conclusion

Cecal ligation and puncture in rodents is a useful experimental model that mimics appendicitis with pathophysiological alterations enrolled in this process. Surgical removal of the septic focus improves clinical condition and normalizes physiological aspects that are clearly observed in this model. In addition, the study of the microcirculation by intravital microscopy represents a unique research tool to analyse complex biological interactions and disease-related mechanisms.

6. References

Angle, N.; Hoyt, D.B.; Coimbra, R.; Liu, F.; Herdon-Remelius, C.; Loomis, W. & Junger, W.G. (1998). Hypertonic saline resuscitation diminishes lung injury by suppressing neutrophil activation after hemorrhagic shock. Shock, Vol. 9, No. 3, (March 1998), pp. 164-170, ISSN 1073-2322

Ayala, A.; Chaudry, I.H. (1996). Immune dysfunction in murine polymicrobial sepsis: mediators, macrophages, lymphocytes and apoptosis. *Shock*, Vol. 6, No. 4, (October 1996), pp. S27-S38, ISSN 1073-2322

Baveja, R.; Kresge N.; Ashburn, J.H.; Keller, S.; Yokoyama, Y.; Sonin, N.; Zhang, J.X.; Huynh, T. & Clemens, M.G. .(2002). Potentiated hepatic microcirculatory response to endothelin-1 during polymicrobial sepsis. *Shock*, Vol.18, No. 5, (November 2002), pp. 415-422, ISSN 1073-2322

Chaudry, I.H.; Wichterman, K.A. & Baue, A.E. (1979). Effect of sepsis on tissue adenine nucleotide levels. *Surgery*, Vol. 85, No. 2 (February 1979), pp. 205-211, ISSN 0039-6060

Chaudry, I.H. (1999). Sepsis: lessons learned in the last century and future directions. *Archives of Surgery*, Vol. 134, No. 9, (September 1999), pp. 922-929, ISSN 0004-0010

Coopersmith, C.M.; Chang, K.C.; Swanson, P.E.; Tinsley, K.W.; Stromberg, P.E.; Buchman, T.G.; Karl, I.E. & Hotchkiss, R.S. (2002). Overexpression of Bcl-2 in the intestinal epithelium improves survival in septic mice. Critical Care Medicine, Vol. 30, No. 1, (January 2002), pp. 195-201, ISSN 0090-3493

De Backer, D. & Dubois, M.J. (2001). Assessment of the microcirculatory flow in patients in the intensive care unit. *Current Opinion in Critical Care*, Vol. 7, No. 3, (June 2001), pp. 200-203, ISSN 1070-5295

De Backer, D.; Creteur, J.; Preiser, J.C.; Dubois, M.J. & Vincent, J.L. (2002). Microvascular blood flow is altered in patients with sepsis. *American Journal of Respiratory and Critical Care Medicine*, Vol. 166, No. 1, (July 2002), pp. 98-104, ISSN 1535-4970

Doerschug, K.C.; Powers, L. S.; Monick, M.M.; Thorne, P.S. & Hunninghake, G.W. (2004). Antibiotics delay but do not prevent bacteremia and lung injury in murine sepsis. *Critical Care Medicine*, Vol. 32, No. 2, (February 2004), pp. 489-494, ISSN 0090-3493

Esmon, C.T. (2004). Why do animal models (sometimes) fail to mimic human sepsis? *Critical Care Medicine*, Vol. 32, No. 5, (May 2004), pp.S202-S208, ISSN 0090-3493

Farquhar, I.; Martin, C.M.; Lam, C.; Potter, R.; Ellis, C.G. & Sibbald, W.J. (1996). Decreased capillary density in vivo in bowel mucosa of rats with normotensive sepsis. *Journal of Surgical Research*, Vol. 61, No. 1, (February 1996), pp. 190-196, ISSN 0022-4804

Groner, W.; Winkelman, J.W.; Harris, A.G.; Ince, C.; Bouma, G.J.; Messmer, K. & Nadeau, R.G. (1999). Orthogonal polarization spectral imaging: a new method for study of the microcirculation. *Nature Medicine,* Vol. 5, No. 10, (October 1999), pp. 1209-1213, ISSN 1078-8956

Hersch, M.; Madorin, W.S.; Sibbald, W.J. & Martin, C.M. (1998). Selective gut mirocirculatory control (SGMC) in septic rats: a novel approach with a locally applied vasoactive drug. *Shock,* Vol. 10, No. 4, (October 1998), pp. 292-297, ISSN 1073-2322

Hinshaw, L.B. (1996). Sepsis/septic shock: participation of the microcirculation: an abbreviated review. *Critical Care Medicine,* Vol. 24, No.6, (June 1996), pp. 1072-1078. ISSN 0090-3493

Hoffman, J.N.; Vollmar, B.; Inthorn, D.; Schildberg, F.W. & Menger, M.D. (1999). A chronic model for intravital microscopic study of microcirculatory disorders and leukocyte/endothelial cell interactions during normotensive endotoxemia. *Shock,* Vol. 12, No.5, (November 1999), pp. 355-364, ISSN 1073-2322

Hubbard, W.J.; Choudhry, M.; Schwacha, M.G.; Kerby, J.D.; Rue III, L.W.; Bland, K.I. & Chaudry, I.H. (2005). Cecal Ligation and Puncture. Shock, Vol. 24, No. 1, (December 2005), pp. 52-57, ISSN 1073-2322

Jarrar, D.; Wang, P.; Song, G.Y.; Cioffi, W.G.; Bland, K.I. & Chaudry, I.H. (2000). Inhibition of Tyrosine Kinase Signaling After Trauma-Hemorrhage: A Novel Approach for Improving Organ Function and Decreasing Susceptibility to Subsequent Sepsis. Annals of Surgery, Vol. 231, No. 3, (March 2000), pp. 399-407, ISSN 0003-4932

Kamoun, W.S.; Shin, M.C.; Keller, S.; Karaa, A.; Huynh, T. & Clemens, M.G. (2005). Induction of biphasic changes in perfusion heterogeneity of rat liver after sequential stress in vivo. *Shock,* Vol. 24, No. 4, (October 2005), pp. 324-331, ISSN 1073-2322

Kato, T.; Hussein, M.H.; Sugiura, T.; Suzuki, S.; Fukuda, S.; Tanaka, T.; Kato, I. & Togari, H. (2004). Development and characterization of a novel porcine model of neonatal sepsis. *Shock;* Vol. 21, No. 4, (April 2004), pp. 329-335, ISSN 1073-2322

Kim, M.H. & Harris, N.R. (2006). Leukocyte adherence inhibits adenosine-dependent venular control of arteriolar diameter and nitric oxide. *American Journal of Physiology-Heart and Circulatory Physiology,* Vol. 291, No. 2, (August 2006), pp. H724-731, ISSN 0363-6135

Kubo, H.; Doyle, N.A.; Graham, L.; Bragwan, S.D.; Quinlan, W.M. & Doerschuk, C.M. (1999). L- and P-selectin and CD11/CD18 in intracapillary neutrophil sequestration in rabbit lungs. *Am J Respir Crit Care Med* 1999;159:267-274.

Lang, C.H.; Dobrescu, C. & Mészáros, K. (1990). Insulin-mediated glucose uptake by individual tissues during sepsis. Metabolism, Vol. 39, No.10, (October 1990), pp. 1096-1107, ISSN 0026-0495

Madorin, W.S.; Martin, C.M. & Sibbald, W.J. (1999). Dopexamine attenuates flow motion in ileal mucosal arterioles in normotensive sepsis. *Critical Care Medicine,* Vol. 27, No. 2 (February 1999), pp. 394-400, ISSN 0090-3493

Marx, G.; Pedder, S.; Smith, L.; Swaraj, S.; Grime, S.; Stockdale, H. & Leuwer, M. (2004). Resuscitation from septic shock with capillary leakage: hydroxyethyl starch (130 Kd), but not Ringer's solution maintains plasma volume and systemic oxygenation. *Shock,* Vol. 21, No. 4, (April 2004), pp. 336-341, ISSN 1073-2322

Mollitt, D.L. (2002). Infection control: avoiding the inevitable. *Surgical Clinics of North America,* Vol. 82, No. 2, (April 2002), pp 365-378, ISSN 0039-6109

Nakagawa, N.K.; Nogueira, R.F.; Correia, C.J.; Shiwa, S.R.; Costa Cruz, J.W.M.; Poli de Figueiredo, L.F.; Rocha e Silva, M. & Sannomiya, P. (2006). Leukocyte-endothelium interactions after hemorrhagic shock/reperfusion and cecal ligation/puncture: an intravital microscopic study in rat mesentery. *Shock,* Vol. 26, No. 2, (August 2006), pp. 180-186, ISSN 1073-2322

Nakagawa, N.K.; Jukemura, J.; Aikawa, P.; Nogueira, R.A.; Poli de Figueiredo, L.F. & Sannomiya, P. (2007). In vivo observation of mesenteric leukocyte-endothelial interactions after cecal ligation/puncture and surgical source control. *Clinics,* Vol. 62, No. 3, (May-June 2007), pp. 321-326, ISSN 1807-5932

Nakajima, Y.; Baudry, N.; Duranteau, J. & Vicaut, E. (2001). Microcirculation in intestinal villi. *American Journal of Respiratory and Critical Care Medicine,* Vol. 164, No. 8, (October 2001), pp. 1526-1530, ISSN 1535-4970

Nunes, F.C. & Silva, A.L.(2005). Acute ischaemic Appendicitis in rabbits: new model with histopathological study. *Acta Cirurgica Brasileira,* Vol. 20, No. 5, (September-October 2005), pp. 399-404, ISSN 1678-2674

Pascual, J.L.; Khwaja, K.A.; Ferri, L.E.; Giannias, B.; Evans, D.C.; Razek, T.; Michel, R.P. & Christou, N.V. (2003). Hypertonic saline resuscitation attenuates neutrophil lung sequestration and transmigration by diminishing leukocyte-endothelial interactions in a two hit model of hemorrhagic shock and infection. *Journal of Trauma* Vol. 54, No. 1, (January 2003), pp. 121-132, ISSN 0022-5282

Sakr, Y.; Dubois, M.J.; De Backer, D.; Creteur, J. & Vincent, J.L. (2004). Persistent microcirculatory alterations are associated with organ failure and death in patients with septic shock. *Critical Care Medicine,* Vol. 32, No. 9, (September 2004), pp. 1825-1831, ISSN 0090-3493

Schmidt, H.; Schmidt, W.; Muller, T.; Bohrer, H.; Gebhard, M.M. & Martin, E. (1997). N-acetylcysteine attenuates endotoxin-induced leukocyte-endothelial cell adhesion and macromolecular leakage in vivo. *Critical Care Medicine, Vol. 25, No. 5, (May* 1997), pp. 858-863, ISSN 0090-3493

Schneider, C.P.; Nickel, E.A., Samy, A.T.S.; Schwacha, M.G.; Cioffi, W.G.; Bland, K.I.; Chaudry, I.H.(2000). The aromatae inhibitor, 4-hydroxyandrostenedione, restore immune responses following trauma-hemorrhages in males and decreases mortality from subsequent sepsis. *Shock*; Vol. 14, No. 3, (September 2000), pp. 347-353, ISSN 1073-2322

Smalley, D.M.; Childs, E.W. & Cheung, L.Y. (2000). The local effect of PAF on leukocyte adherence to small bowel mesenteric venules following intra-abdominal contamination. *Inflammation,* Vol. 24, No. 5, (October 2000), pp. 399-410, ISSN 0360-3997

Sumiyama, K.; Gostout, C.J.; Rajan, E.; Bakken, T.A.; Deters, J.L.; Knipschield, M.A.; Hawes, R.H.; Kalloo, A.N.; Pasricha, P.J.; Chung, S.; Kansevoy, S.V. & Cotton, P.B. (2006). Pilot Study of the porcine uterine horn as an in vivo appendicitis model for development of endoscopic transgastric appendectomy. Gastrointestinal Endoscopy, Vol. 64, No. 5, (November 2006), pp. 808-812, ISSN 0016-5107

Swartz, D.E.; Seely, A.J.E.; Ferri, L.; Giannias, B. & Christou, N.V. (2000). Decreased systemic polymorphonuclear neutrophil (PMN) rolling without increased PMN adhesion in peritonitis at remote sites. *Archives of Surgery,* Vol. 135, No. 8, (August 2000), pp. 959-966, ISSN 0004-0010

Trzeciak, S.; Dellinger, R.P.; Parrillo, J.E.; Guglielmi, M.; Bajaj, J.; Abate, N.L.; Arnold, R.C.; Colilla, S.; Zanotti, S.; & Hollenberg, S.M. (2007). Early microcirculatory perfusion derangements in patients with severe sepsis and septic shock: relationship to hemodynamics, oxygen transport, and survival. *Annals of Emergency Medicine*, Vol.49, No. 1 (January 2007), pp. 88-98, ISSN 0196-0644

Vianna, Rosa C.S.; Gomes, R.N.; Bozza, F.A.; Amancio, R.T.; Bozza, P.T.; David, C.M.N. & Castro-Faria-Neto, H.C. (2004). Antibiotic Treatment in a Murine Model of Sepsis: Impact on Cytokines and Endotoxin Release. *Shock*, Vol. 21, No. 2, (February 2004), pp. 115-120, ISSN 1073-2322

Waisman, D.; Abramovich, A.; Brod, V.; Lavon, O.; Nurkin, S.; Popovski, F.; Rotschild, A. & Bitterman, H. (2006). Subpleural microvascular flow velocities and shear rates in normal and septic mechanically ventilated rats. *Shock*, Vol. 26, No. 1, (July 2006), pp. 87-94, ISSN 1073-2322

Walther, A.; Czabanka, M.; Gebhard, M.M. & Martin, E. (2004). Glycoprotein IIB/IIIA-inhibition and microcirculatory alterations during experimental endotoxemia - an intravital microscopic study in the rat. *Microcirculation*, Vol. 11, No. 1, (January-February 2004), pp. 79-88, ISSN 1073-9688

Wang, P.; Ba, Z.F.; Cioffi, W.G.; Bland, K.I. & Chaudry, I.H.(1999). Salutary effects of ATP-MgCl2 on the depressed endothelium-dependent relaxation during hyperdynamic sepsis. *ritical Care Medicine*, Vol. 27, No. 5,(May 1999), pp. 959-964, ISSN 0090-3493

Woodman, R.C.; Teoh, D.; Payne, D. & Kubes, P. (2000). Thrombin and leukocyte recruitment in endotoxemia. *American Journal of Physiology-Heart and Circulatory Physiology*, Vol. 279, No. 3, (September 2000), pp. H1338-1345, ISSN 0363-6135

Yang, S.; Zhou, M.; Chaudry, I.H. & Wang, P. (2001). The role of lipopolysaccharide in stimulating adrenomedullin production during polymicrobial sepsis. *Biochimica et Biophysica Acta-Molecular Basis of Disease*, Vol. 1537, No. 2, (September 2001), pp 167-174, ISSN 0925-4439

Yang, S.; Zhou, M.; Chaudry, I.H. & Wang, P. (2002). Novel Approach to prevent the transition from the hyperdynamic phase to the hypodynamic phase of sepsis: role of adrenomedullin and adrenomedullin-binding protein-1. *Annals of Surgery*, Vol. 236, No 5, (November 2002), pp. 625-633, ISSN 0003-4932

13

Parasitic Appendicitis

Omer Engin[1], Bulent Calik[2] and Sebnem Calik[3]
[1]*Tepecik Training and Research Hospital,*
[2]*Buca Large State Hospital,*
[3]*Urla State Hospital*
Turkey

1. Introduction

The etiologic factors and the incidence of appendicitis differ from country to country.(Francis et al, 1992; Jones et al, 1985) In this chapter, we discuss parasitic appendicitis. Enterobious vermicularis and Tenia sp are frequently found in the appendectomy specimens in Izmir, Turkey. Other parasites include: Trichuris trichiura, Schistosoma haematobium, Schistosoma mansoni, Ascaris lumbricoides, Entamoeba histolytica which are reported in different city and countries. (Okolie et al, 2008; Pasupati et al, 2008; Terada et al, 2009) .
It is important to understand about parasitic appendicitis for both local populations at risk and for travelers.
This chapter asks if the incidence of parasitic appendicitis be reduced with preventive medicine?
Whenever parasites are found at an appendicectomy antiparasitic treatments are necessary and the rest of the immediate family should be treated. Education about hand washing, hygiene, cooking and animal management may be required.

2. Histology

Appendix wall has four layers from out to in that serosa, muscular layer, submucosa and mucosa respectively. Muscular layer contains circular and longitudinal muscles. Appendix has intestinal structure but there is not villus in the mucosa. Lamina propria and submucosal layers have got large amounts of lymphoid tissue. (Erbengi, 1985; lab.anhb.uwa.edu.au, 2011; Skandalakis et al, 2004)

3. Clinical features

The clinical features of appendicitis in the context of parasitic infections are varied.

Etiology of parasitic appendicitis:

Appendicitis is more common in males than females (1.4:1) and can be seen at any age but it is more commonly seen in older children and in young adults. Obstruction of the appendiceal lumen can occur with parasites and their eggs. If the lumen is obstructed, continued secretion and proliferation of bacteria or the parasites may cause an increase in the intraluminal pressure. Increased pressure impairs the circulation of the appendix wall and mucosal damage may cause bacterial invasion, inflammation, sepsis and finally necrosis and perforation. If the lumen is obstructed, pain can be partially or exclusively reported at the umbilicus, and can be difficult to localize. (Bilgin, 2004; Engin O et al, 2010,2011; Lally et al, 2004; Smink et al, 2007; Turhan et al, 2009)

Taenia

Taenia saginata, is a parasite of both cattle and humans, causing taeniasis in humans and is frequently seen in Turkey, Africa, Southeast Asia, other parts of Eastern Europe and in Latin America where cattle are managed by infected humans who have poor hygiene. Preventative measures include better education, proper disposal of faeces and rigorous meat inspection programs and the thorough cooking of beef. The organisms are killed if meat is heated to 75^0C for 5 minutes or until no longer pink or cooled to -10^0C for 5 days.
T. saginata can grow to over 10 m in length. The worm is divided into an anterior scolex, a short neck and a long body called the strobila. The worm has four strong suckers to anchor it in the intestine where it can live for over 20 years passing out gravid segments containing eggs. These segments dry up and release eggs which can infect cattle. Inside the bovine duodenum the eggs hatch and gain entry to the circulation and then the connective tissues over muscle where they develop into infective cysticercoid cysticerci.
The most commonly infected muscles are the masticatory muscles, heart, tongue, thorax and diaphragm. If meat containing adult Ciysticerci bovis are eaten undercooked or raw, scolexs adhere to the human small intestine and the rings begin to develop. After 10 weeks, adult rings are passes from the anus.
The life cycle of T. saginata is human-cow-human. Oral intake may follow from the unclean hands of workers handling infected meats in slaughterhouses. It is impotant to note that an infected person may have no clinical symptoms.
The diagnosis is made on seeing the falling rings. If eggs are seen in the stool, it can not be easily determined to which tenia the eggs belong.
Treatment for tenia infection is the drug praziquantel which opens calcium channels causing paralysis of the worm, aiding expulsion of the parasite through peristalsis. Albendazole is also effective.
Taenia solium lives in the human small intestine and their cysticercus cellulosa live in the pig which is the intermediate host. The life cycle is human-pig-human. Infection occurs in humans eating undercooked pork. The diagnosis is made on find rings or scolex of T.solium. For prevention the contact of human stool with pigs should be avoided and undercooked pork should not be eaten.(Cetin et al, 1983; Gonzales et al, 2002; Sartorelli et al, 2005; Unat et al, 1982)

Appendicitis and tapeworms

Though infected individuals may be asymptomatic tape worms can cause non-specific symptoms such as abdominal pain, diarrhea and a decreased appetite with nausea. There may be abdominal swelling and on investigation a leucocytosis. Confusion with appendicitis is easily understood. However, distinguishing features may include an increased appetite and eosinophila which are seen with tape worms and not with appendicitis. Protoglottids of the adult tapeworms may be found in the lumen of the appendix but if they casue the appendicitis or not is unclear.

Enterobius vermicularis

Enterobius vermicularis or Occiyur vermicularis, is a small white nematod. The length of the male parasite is 3-6mm, and the width is 0.1-0.25mm. The dimensions in the female parasite are 8-13mm and 0.3-1.3mm respectively. The host of the parasite is the human. The female parasite leaves the bowel and goes out from anus where it spawns on the perianal region at night and then dies. Male enterobious may be rarely found in the perianal area. Perianal pruritus may occur when the parasite is there. The parasitic embryo becomes an adult in 6-7 hours in the presence of the appropriate heat and humidity. The adult egg is infectious for humans and when the adult egg enters the human gastrointestinal tract, it changes into the to adult parasite. After 15-43 days from oral intake the adult eggs are changed into the spawning adult parasites. The life cycle of the parasite is thus human-human-human. The parasite generally stays in the caecum taking nourishment from the bowel wall where it takes blood, epithelial cells and organic mater

Clinical symptoms caused by the parasite include perianal pruritus, macroscopic and microscopic blood in the stool, appetite disorders, abdominal pain, diarrhoea, weight loss, nasal itching, teeth grinding, dizziness, a singing in the ears and on investigation anemia, and eosinophilia.

Female parasite may go out from the anus and come in to the vagina or urethra and so cause urogenital symptoms. The diagnosis is made on finding the parasite and its eggs on the perianal area, in stool, or under the nails of patient's.

The parasite may infect humans in different ways. The eggs may be taken in through the digestive system. Eggs found in powders may go into foods or be inhaled and after that swallowed. The patient may contaminate others. If contaminated underwear and bed linen are shaken, infection can be transmitted to others. Sometimes, hatched parasites from the matured eggs in the perianal region may enter the bowel retrogradely.

For prevent of infection the vectors must be treated and beds should not be shared and nails should be cut short. Hands must be washed well before cooking and eating. Children must not scratch their perianal regions and rooms should be well ventilated. (Cetin et al, 1983; Chang et al, 2009; Fukushima et al, 2010; Ok et al, 1999; Unat, 1982)

Enterobius vermicularis has been reported in 1.4% of 1549 appendicectomies in the USA (Arcaet al 2004) and is not much higher in many other series.

Trichuriasis

Trichuriasis is a world wide parasite from infected vegetables, fruits, drinking water and dirty fingers. The eggs hatch in the small intestine and the larvae become adults on their way to the caecum and large bowel. Adult worms are 3-4 cm in length and they feeds on food residue and blood. Female parasite spawns in the bowel and the eggs go out with the stool. Embryo grows in appropriate conditions. From egg to spawning adult parasite takes 12-14 weeks from orally intake (Ok et al, 2009; Unat, 1982; Vavricka et al, 2009) The worms can be asymptomatic but can be visible in the stools and they can cause rectal prolapse and appendicitis. Diagnosis is on seeing the eggs or worms in the stools and treatment is with Flubendazole.

Schistosoma haematobium and S. mansoni

S.hematobium and S.mansoni are the most commonly seen Scistosomia types in humans. The male's length is 10-15mm and female's length is 20mm. They live in the venous system and feed on blood and the final host is the human. After the male and female parasite mate the eggs pass through the urinary bladder and bowel. The parasite is expelled from in the urine or stools and on contact with fresh water they hatch. and infect the intermediate host which is a mollusc. Bulinus truncatus, Bulinus africanus, Bulinus globus are the important intermediate host molluscs. Hundreds of larvae (cercariae) ar released back into the water

after 5-6 weeks from the onset of invasion of the molluscs. The cercariae enter the human through softened skin and migrate to the lungs and the liver. The life cycle of the parasite is human-molluscs (e.g. Bulinus truncatus)-human. To prevent the spread of Scistosomiasis human's urine and stool should be treated before entering rivers. In endemic region, gloves and boots are important because transmission occurs in water. (Cetin et al, 1983; Djuikwo-Teukeng et al, 2011; Keiser et al, 2010; Kosinski et al, 2011)
After appendicectomy eggs have been found in the lumen of the appendix together with transmural inflammation granulomatous reactions and purulent exudates. Sometimes the fibrosis that follows a schistosomal infection causes a luminal obstruction and later secondary bacterial appendicitis.

Ascaris lumbricoides: A round worm

The male parasite's length is 15-20 cm and in female parasites the length is 20-30 cm. The life cycle is human-human-human and infection follows with the oral in take of eggs containing live larvae. Larvaes exit from the egg in the bowel lumen and enter the venous system through bowel wall. They then go to liver, lung, trachea, pharynx, esophagus, stomach, and small bowel. They become adults in 2-3 months. Different clinical symptoms may be found during the 2-3 month period. Clinical symptoms include pain located in the right upper quadrant, nasal itching and intestinal obstruction and discomfort in the chest with a cough producing sputum which may contain parasites. Investigations may show an eosinophilia and icterus due to bile duct obstruction,. The diagnosis is made on finding the parasites and eggs in the stool. Eggs are not found in the stool if there are only male parasites or no adult female parasites in the bowel. The eggs are taken in orally with foods and drinks contaminated with human stool. (Bailey et al, 2010; Cetin et al, 1983; Gupta et al, 2009 ;Unat, 1982)
Treatment is with albendazole or mebendazole. Appendicitis due to ascriasis has been made on Ultrasound and CT scanning showing long filling defects in the right iliac fossa.

Entamoeba histolytica

The main host of the parasite is the human were it stays in the lumen or wall of the large bowel. The parasite may stay in the appendix, small intestine, liver, lung, brain or testis. Spread is via fecal-oral contamination of food and drinks. Clinical symptoms include abdominal pain, diarrhoea and bloody stools. (Ali et al, 2008; Biller et al, 2009; Tan et al, 2010)

Cryptosporidium parvum

This is an intestinal parasite. It is mainly affects the ileum of humans.(Borowsi et al, 2010) Clinical symptoms are diarrhea, nausea, vomiting, fever and abdominal pain. Oocysts are found in the stools of infected humans. The diagnosis is made on finding cysts in the stools or on showing torfozoits in intestinal biopsy specimens. The diagnosis of pulmonary and tracheal cryptosporisidiasis is made by biopsy and staining. The disease is transmitted by the fecal-oral route. (Hannahs et al, 2011; www.fda.gov/Food/FoodSafety/, accessed:16 April 2011))

Microsporidia

This is a mandatory intracellular parasite. It causes a small intestinal infection. Other than this, the parasite may cause biliary tractus, oculary, pulmonary and renal infections. Granulomatous lesions may occur. The most common species of parasite infections are Enterocytozoon bieneusi and Encephalitozoon intestinalis. Enteritis, cholangitis. The diagnosis is made by microscopic examination of biopsy specimens, stools, urine, bile, or from bronco-alveolar-nasal lavage fluid. Transmission of the disease is: fecal-oral, oral-oral, aerosol inhalation, or eating contaminated foods. (Sancak et al, 2005; Turk et al, 2009)

Blastocystis hominis

B. hominis infection is seen all over the World especially in tropical and subtropical areas. Orally ingested cysts cause an intestinal infection leading to diarrhea, abdominal pain, abdominal distention, weight loss, rectal hemorrhage and pruritus. (Dogruman et al, 2007; Ertug et al, 2009)

Isospora belli

This parasite lives in epithelial cells of the small intestine. The disease is transmitted by contaminated foods and drinks. The symptoms include anorexia, abdominal pain, nausea, diarrhea and fever. The diagnosis is made by identification of oocysts in the host feces. (Nagamani et al, 2008; Walther et al, 2009)

4. Discussion

Though parasites may be found in appendicectomy specimens it does not follow that they always cause the appendicitis. It is well know that an appendicolith may be asymptomatic so to may be parasitic infections in the appendix..(Huwart et al, 2006)
Turan at al. reported a retrospective study that consisted of 56 patients who underwent surgery for gynecologic pathologies. Incidental appendectomy materials were examined microscopically. The appendices were abnormal in 31 cases (55.36%), as follows: acute appendicitis in 3 cases, lymphoid hyperplasia in 21 cases, fibrotic obliteration in 6 cases, and endometriotic implants in one case. Thus lymphoid hyperplasia does not equate to acute appendicitis. (Turan et al, 1994). Likewise some minor degree of lymphoid hyperplasia may follow parasitic infection and not always cause symptoms.
Nonetheless obstruction of the appendicular lumen may start acute appendicitis. Pieper at al.'s experimental model in which the rabbit's appendix was obstructed with a balloon showed a role for obstruction in the pathogenesis of acute appendicitis. (Pieper et al, 1982)
Parasitic appendicitis is reported all over the World but, it is more frequently seen in some areas than another.
Izmir is the third biggest city in Turkey with a population of 3.6million. Two retrospective clinical studies were made in Izmir. The first study was made by Dicle et al between 1990-1996. The second study was made by Engin et al between 2002-2009. The two investigations were made in different two hospitals close to each other in the city center. The numbers of patients attending the emergency departments were similar in the two hospitals.
Dicle et al investigated retrospectively 2473 cases operated between 1990-1996 years and found 45 (1.8%) cases of parasitic appendicitis. The female/male ratio was 30/15. There were 5 Tenia, 34 E.vermicularis, and 6 undetermined parasites in 45 cases. Investigators reported histopathologic changes from mucosal hemorrhage to ulceration in some of the excised appendices: mucosal hemorrhage in 12 cases, eosinophilia in 18 cases, neutrophil infiltration in 6 cases.(Dicle et al, 1997)
Engin et al investigated parasitic appendicitis operated between 2000-2009 years in Izmir, Turkey. In this study, there were 1969 cases of acute appendicitis and 9 parasitic cases (0.45%). These parasites were E.vermicularis and Tenia. Tenia in 2 cases and E.vermicularis in 7 cases. The female/male ratio was 8/1. Fecaliths with parasites were found in two cases and parasites alone in 7 cases.

If Dicle and Engin et al's studies are compared, parasitic appendicitis fell from 1.8% to 0.45%. During this time the literacy ratio rose form 87.13% in 1990 to 95,3% in 2009. (http://ekutup.dpt.gov.tr/bolgesel/gosterge ; http://www.yeniasir.com.tr)
Let us consider another geographic region. The literacy ratio is lower in Adana than some cities in Turkey and parasitic appendicitis is high in Adana. It has been argued that if the literacy ratio is increased to 88% or higher then the parasitic appendicitis ratio may decreased. (Engin et al, 2010)
However, it should be noted that the incidence of parasitic appendicitis was in the early study similar to that found in the USA and the most recent study has one of the lowest incidences reported anywhere in the world.
Hazir et al had made a study in Ankara, Turkey. In this investigation, Screening for E.vermicularis was explored in different districts of Ankara. The following were determined: the student's age, sex, and socioeconomic status of their families, and knowledge about E.vermicularis infection. Significant gender-related differences were not found. Infections declined with increased educational level of the family. The mothers are usually the primary carers of children in Turkey, and for this reason, the mother's educational level affects her child's. In this study, 86.4% of Mothers of children with parasitosis had been graduated from primary school, and only 4,5% of the mothers had graduated from university. This shows that a mother's educational level affects her child's health.(Hazir et al, 2009)

5. Antiparasitic therapy should be given after finding parasitic appendicitis

Antiparasitic therapy must be given to confirmed cases of parasitic infection. Close friends and family members may be examined for parasitic infection and carrier state. Additionally education about hygiene and sanitation must be given.
Community health programs and individual training are important to prevent parasitic infections. People working in the food industry must be appropriately educated and trained. Wastewater treatment plants should be sufficient for the population.
If parasitic infestations are prevented, the rate of appendicitis caused by parasites will also decrease.(Kazemzadeh et al, 2008; Okolie et al, 2008)

6. References

Ali IK, Mohammadi SS, Akhter J, Roy S, Gorrini C, Calderaro A, Parker SK, Haque R, Petri WA, Clark CG. (2008). Tissue invasion by Entamoeba histolytica: Evidence of genetic selectionand/or DNA reorganization events in organ tropism. PLoS Negl Trop Dis, Vol. 2, No. 4, (Apr 2008), pp.(e219)

Arca MJ, Gates RL, Groner JI, Hammond S, Caniano DA. Clinical manifestations of appendiceal pinworms in children: an institutional experience and a review of the literature. Pediatric Surgery International 2004;20(5):372-5.

Bailey JK, Warner P. (2010). Respiratory arrest from Ascaris lumbricoides. Pediatrics, Vol. 126, No. 3, (Sep 2010), pp.(e712-715)

BBB - Cryptosporidium parvum. Bad Bug Book: Foodborne Pathogenic Microorganisms and Natural Toxins Handbook Cryptosporidium parvum http://www.fda.gov/Food/FoodSafety/FoodborneIllness/FoodborneIllnessFoodbornePathogensNaturalToxins/BadBugBook/ucm070753.htm (accessed:16 April 2011)

Bilgin N. (2004). Akut Apandisit, In: Temel Cerrahi, Sayek İ. editor, pp. (1191-1197), Güneş Kitabevi, Ankara

Biller L, Schmidt H, Krause E, Gelhaus C, Matthiesen J, Handal G, Lotter H, Janssen O, Tannich E, Bruchhaus I. (2009). Comparison of two genetically related Entamoeba histolytica cell lines derived from the same isolate with different pathogenic properties. Proteomics, Vol. 9, No. 17, (Sep 2009), pp.(4107-4120)

Binnebosel M, Stumpf M, Mahnken AH, Gassler N, Schumelick V, Truonq S. (2009). Acute appendicitis. Modern diagnostics—surgical ultrasound. Chirurg, Vol. 80, No. 7, (Jul 2009), pp.(579-587)

Borowsi H, Thompson RCA, Armstrong T, Clode PL. (2010). Morphological characterization of Cryptosporidium parvum life-cycle stages in an in vitro model system. Parasitology, Vol. 137, No. 1, (Jan 2010), pp.(13-26)

Cetin ET, Ang O, Toreci K. (1983). Tıbbi parazitoloji, I.U.İstanbul Tıp Fakultesi Yayinlari, Rektörlük No:3073,Fak no:146, Istanbul

Chang TK, Liao CW, Huang YC, Chang CC, Chou CM, Tsay HC, Huang A, Guu SF, Kao TC, Fan CK. (2009). Prevalence of Enterobius vermicularis infection among preschool children in Kindergartens of Taipei City, Taiwan in 2008. Korean J Parasitol, Vol. 47, No. 2, (Jun 2009), pp.(185-187)

Ching TK, Jeng DT, Hung CL, Nien LW, Shin LS, Chun CL, Fu YH. (2002). Right perinephric abcess: a rare presentation of ruptured retrocecal appendicitis. Pediatr Nephrol, Vol. 17, No. 3, (Mar 2002), pp.(177-80)

Cohen-Kerem R, Railton C, Oren D, Lishner M, Koren G. (2005). Pregnancy outcome following non-obstetric surgical intervention. The American Journal of Surgery, Vol. 190, No. 3, (Sep 2005), pp. (467-473)

Dogruman F, Hokelek . (2007). Is Blastocystis hominis an opportunist agent? Türkiye Parazitoloji Dergisi, Vol. 31, No. 1, (Jan 2007),pp.(28-36)

Dicle N, Sayin AY, Eliyatkin N, Selek E, Postaci H. (1997). Parasitic appendicitis. SSK Izmir Eğitim Hastanesi TipDergisi (Medical Journal of Izmir Hospital), Vol. 3 No. 4, (Oct 1997), pp. (105-108)

Djuikwo-Teukeng FF, Njiokou F, Nkengazong L, De Meeus T, Ekobo AS, Dreyfuss G. (2011). Strong genetic structure in Cameroonian populations of Bulinus truncates (Gastropoda: Planorbidae), intermediate host of Schistosoma haematobium. Infection, Genetics and Evolution, Vol. 11, No. 1, (Jan 2011), pp.(17-22)

Engin O, Calik S,Calik B, Yildirim M, Coskun G.(2010). Parasitic appendicitis from past to present in Turkey. Iranian J Parasitol, Vol. 5, No.3, (Jul 2010), pp. (57-63)

Erbengi T. (1985). Histoloji 2, Beta Basim Yayim Dagitim AS, Yayin no:46,Tip Dizisi No:11 , Istanbul

Engin O, Calik B, Yildirim M, Coskun A, Coskun GA.(2011). Gynecologic pathologies in our appendectomy series and literature review.J Korean Surg Society, Vol. 80, No. 4, (Apr 2011), pp. (267-271)

Engin O, Yildirim M, Yakan S, Coskun G.(2011). Can fruit seeds and undigested plant residuals cause acute appendicitis. Asian Pacific Journal of Tropical Biomedicine, Vol. 1, No. 2, (Apr 2011), pp. (99-101)

Ertug S, Dost T, Ertabaklar H, Gultekin B.(2009). The effect of trimethoprim-sulfamethoxazole in Blastocystis hominis infection. Türkiye Parazitoloji Dergisi, Vol. 33, No. 4 (Oct 2009), pp.(270 - 272)

Flum DR, Morris A, Koepsell T, Dellinger EP. (2001). Has misdiagnosed of appendicitis decreased over time? JAMA, Vol. 286, No. 14, (Oct 2001), pp. (1748-1753)

Francis IM, Hira PR, Matusik J, Farid L, Tungekar FM. (1992). Parasite infestation of the vermiform appendix: The experience in Kuwait. Medical Principles and Practice, Vol. 3, No. 1, (Jan 1992/1993), pp. (31-39)

Fukushima S, Marui E, Hamada A. (2010). The prevalence of Enterobius vermicularis among Japanese expatriates living in developing countries. Kansenshoqaku Zasshi, Vol. 84, No. 1,(Jan 2010), pp. (19-23)

Gayer G, Zissin R, Apter S, Shemesh E, Heldenberg E. (1999). Acute diverticulitis of the small bowel: CT findings. Abdom Imaging, Vol.24, No. 5,(Oct 1999), pp. (452-455)

Gonzales LM, Montero E, Puente S, Lopez-Velez R, Hernandez M, Sciutto E, Harrison LJS, Michael R, Parkhouse E, Garate T. (2002). PCR tools for the defferential diagnosis of Taenia saginata and Taenia solium taeniasis/cysticercosis from different geographical locations. Parasitology, Vol. 42, No. 4, (Apr 2002), pp. (243-249)

Gupta P, Sundaram V, Abraham G, Shanta GPS, Mathew M. (2009). Obstructive uropathy from Ascaris lumbricoides. Kidney International, Vol. 75, No. 11, (Jun 2009), pp. (1242)

Hannahs G, Cryptosporidium parvum: an emerging pathogen. http://biology.kenyon.edu/slonc/bio38/hannahs/crypto.htm (accessed:16-April 2011)

Hardin M. (1999). Acute appendicitis: Review and update. Am Fam Physician, Vol. 60, No. 7, (Nov 1999), pp. (2027-2034)

Hazir C, Gundesli H, Ozkirim A, Keskin N. (2009). Distribution of Enterobius vermicularis Among the Schoolchildren of Two Primary Schools with Different Social-Economic Status in the Ankara Province. Türkiye Parazitoloji Dergisi, Vol. 33, No. 1, (Jan 2009), pp. (54 - 58)

http://ekutup.dpt.gov.tr/bolgesel/gosterge/1997-04/24.pdf

http://www.lab.anhb.uwa.edu.au/mb140/CorePages/GIT/git.htm (accessed: 08 Apr 2011)

http://www.yeniasir.com.tr/HayatinIcinden/2010/04/19/izmir_okuryazar_oraninda_ortalamanin_ustunde(accessed 08 Apr 2011)

Huwart L, El Khoury M, Lesavre A, Phan C, Rangheard AS, Bessoud B, Menu Y. (2006). Is appendicolith a reliable sign for acute appendicitis at MDCT? J.Radiol, Vol. 87, No. 4, (Apr 2006), pp. (383-387)

Jones BA, Demetriades D, Segal I, Burkitt DP. (1985). The prevalence of appendiceal fecaliths in patients with and without appendicitis. A comparative study from Canada and South Africa. Ann Surg, Vol. 202, No. 1, (Jul 1985), pp.(80-82)

Kazemzadeh H, Afshar-Moghadam N, Meamar AR, Rahimi HR, Kia EB. (2008) Enterobious vermicularis and the Appendix: Report of Five Cases. Iranian J Parasitol, Vol 3, no. 3, (Jul 2008), pp. (54-55)

Keiser J, N'Guessan NA, Adoubryn KD, Silue KD, Vounatsou P, Hatz C, Utzinger J, N'Goran EK. (2010). Efficacy and safety of mefloquine, artesunate, mefloquine-artesunate, and praziquantel against Schistosoma haematobium:Randomized, exploratory open-label trial. Clinical Infectious Disease, Vol. 50, No. 9, (May 2010), pp. (1205-1213)

Kosinski KC, Bosompem KM, Stadecker MJ, Wagner AD, Plummer J, Durant JL, Gute DM. (2011). Diagnostic accuracy of urine filtration and dipstick tests for Schistosoma haematobium infection in a lightly infected population of Ghanaian achoolchildren. Acta Tropica, Vol. 118, No. 2, (Feb 2011) pp. (123-127)

Lally KP, Cox CS, Andrassy RJ. (2004). Appendix, In: Sabiston Textbook of Surgery 17th Edition, Townsend CM, Beauchamp RD, Evers BM, Mattox KL. editors. Pp. (1381-1397) ,Saunders, ISBN:0-7216-0409-9 , Philadelphia

Liu K, Ahancie S, Pisaneschi M, Lin I, Walter R. (2007). Can acute appendicitis be treated by antibiotics alone? The American Surgeon, Vol. 73, No. 11, (Nov 2007), pp. (1161-1165)

Nagamani K, Rao PPR, Mathur G, Krishna GTP, Rajalingam AP, Saxena NK. (2008). Prevalance of Cryptosporidium, Cyclospora cayetanensis and Isospora belli infection among diarrheal patients in South India. Tropical Medicine and Health, vol. 36, No. 3, (Aug 2008), pp. (131-136)

Ok KS, Kim YS, Song JH, Lee JH, Ryu SH, Lee JH, Moon JS, Whang DH, Lee HK. (2009). Trichuris trichiura infection diagnosed by colonoscopy:case reports and review of literature. Korean J Parasitol, Vol 47, No. 3, (Sep 2009), pp. (275-280)

Ok UZ, Ertan P, Limoncu E, Ece A, Özbakkaloğlu B. (1999). Relationship between pinworm and urinary tract infections in young girls. APMIS, Vol. 107, No. 1-6, (May 1999), pp. (474-476)

Okolie BI, Okonko IO, Ogun AA, Adedeji AO, Donbraye E, Nkang AO, Ihekanwa CI, Onwuchekwa EC. (2008). Incidence and Detection of Parasite Ova in Appendix from Patients with Appendicitis in South-eastern, Nigeria. World Journal of Agricultural Sciences, Vol. 4, No. S, (2008), pp. (795-802)

Paajanen H, Tainio H, Laato M. (1996). A chance of misdiagnosed between acute appendicitis and renal colic. Scandinavian Journal of Urology and Nephrology, Vol. 30, No. 5, (Oct 1996), pp. (363-366)

Pasupati MT, Yothasamutr K, Wah MJ, Sherif SET, Palayan K. (2008). A study of parasitic infections in the luminal contents and tissue sections of appendix specimens. Tropical Biomedicine, Vol. 25, No. 2, (Aug 2008), pp. (166–172)

Pedrosa I, Lafornara M, Pandharipande PR, Goldsmith JD, Rofsky NM. (2009). Pregnant patients suspected of having acute appendicitis: effect of MR imaging on negative laparotomy rate and appendiceal perforation rate. Radiology, Vol. 250, No. 3, (Mar 2009), pp. (749-757)

Pieper R, Kager L, Tidefeldt U. (1982). Obstruction of appendix vermiformis causing acute appendicitis. An experimental study in the rabbits. Acta Chir Scan, Vol. 148, No. 1, (Jan 1982), pp. (63-72)

Ripolles T, Martinez-Perez MJ, Morote V, Solaz J. (1998). Diseases that simulate acute appendicitis. The British Journal of Radiology, Vol. 71, No. 842, (Feb 1998), pp. (94-98)

Sancak B, Akyon Y. (2005). Microsporidia: General Characteristics, infections and laboratory diagnosis. Microbiyol Bult, Vol 39, No. 4 (Oct 2005), pp. (513-522)

Sartorelli AC, da Silva MG, Rodrigues MAM, da Silva RJ. (2005). Appendiceal taeniasis presenting like acute appendicitis. Parasitology Research, Vol. 97, No. 2, (2005), pp.(171-172)

Skandalakis LJ, Colborn GL, Weidman TA, Skandalakis JE, Skandalakis PN. (2004). Appendix, In: Skandalakis's Surgical Anatomy: The Embryologic and Anatomic Basis of Modern Surgery, Skandalakis JE, Editor in Chief, pp. (843-860) , PMP Ltd, ISBN:960-399-119-8, Athens

Smink DS, Soybel DI. (2007). Appendix and Appendectomy, In : Maingot's Abdominal Operations. 11th edition, Zinner MJ, Ashley SW. editors. Pp.(589-611), The McGraw-Hill Co, ISBN:978-0-07-144176-6, NewYork

Snell RS. Ceviren: Arinci K. (1993) Uygulamalı Anatomi, Turkiye Klinikleri Yayinevi, Turkiye Klinikleri yayin serisi No: 35,Istanbul

Stahfield K, Hower J, Homitsky S, Madden J. (2007). Is acute appendicitis a surgical emergency? The American Surgeon, Vol. 73, No. 6 (Jun 2007), pp. (626-630)

Tan ZN, Wong WK, Nik Zairi Z, Abdullah B, Rahmah N, Zeehaida M, Rumaizi S, Lalitha P, Tan GC, Olivos-Garcia A, Lim BH. (2010). Identification of Entemoeba histolytica trophozoites in fresh stool sample: comparison of three staining techniques and study on the viability period of the trophozoites. Tropical Biomedicine, Vol. 27, No. 1, (Jan 2010), pp. (79-88)

Terada T. (2009). Schistosomal appendicitis: Incidence in Japan and a case report. World J Gastroenterol, Vol. 15, No. 13, (Apr 2009), pp. (1648-1649)

Terasawa T, Blackmore CC, Bent S, Kohlwas JR. (2004). Systematic Review: computed tomography and ultrasonography to detect acute appendicitis in adults and adolescents. Annals of Internal Medicine, Vol. 141, No. 7, (Oct 2004), pp. (537-546)

Turan YH, Kalyoncu S, Boran N, Gungor M, Demirel LC, Ortac F. (1994). Concurrent appendectomy in gynecologic surgery. T Klin Jînekol Obst, Vol. 4 No. 3 (Jul 1994), pp. (190-192)

Turhan AN, Kapan S. (2009). Akut apandisit. In: Acil Cerrahi, Ertekin C, Guloğlu R, Taviloglu K. editors. Pp.(301-317) , Nobel Tıp Kitabevleri, ISBN: 978-9944-5104-2-4, Istanbul

Turk S, Gogruman-Al F. (2009). Microsporidia : General Characteristics and Laboratory Diagnosis. Turkish Journal of Infection, Vol. 23, No. 2 (Apr 2009), pp. (89-95)

Unat EK. (1982). Tıp Parazitolojisi 3.baskı, Cerrahpasa Tip Fakultesi Yayinlari , Rektörlük No. 3044, Dekanlık No. 113, Istanbul

Vavricka SR, Manz M, Burri E. (2009). Trichuris trichiura(Whipworm). Clinical Gastroenterology and Hepatology, Vol. 7, No. 10,(2009), pp.(A16)

Walther Z, Topazian MD. (2009) Isospora cholangiopathy: case study with histologic characterization and molecular confirmation. Human Pathology, Vol. 40, No. 9, (Sep 2009), pp. (1342-1346)

Wang WJ, Zhang SQ, Zhu M, Jin LP, Song JF. (2010). Evaluation of high and low frequency ultrasound in the diagnosis of acute appendicitis. Journal of Medical Imaging, Vol. 20, No. 11. (2010), pp. (1682-1684)

Williamson WA, Bush RD, Williams LF. (1981). Retrocecal appendicitis The American Journal of Surgery, Vol. 141, No. 4,(1981), pp. (507-509)

Zeren Z.(Kısa) (1972). Sistematik Insan Anatomisi. Ekim yayinlari, Istanbul.